Biochemistry of macrophages

Biochemistry of macrophages

Ciba Foundation Symposium 118

1986

Pitman
London

ISBN 0 272 79822 3

Published in January 1986 by Pitman Publishing Ltd., 128 Long Acre, London WC2E 9AN, UK. Distributed in North America by CIBA Pharmaceutical Company (Medical Education Division), Post Office Box 18060, Newark, NJ 07101, USA

Suggested series entry for library catalogues:
Ciba Foundation symposia

Ciba Foundation symposium 118
x + 256 pages, 33 figures, 28 tables

British Library cataloguing in publication data
Biochemistry of macrophages: [Symposium on
   biochemistry of macrophages held at the Ciba
   Foundation, 16–18 April 1985].—(Ciba Foundation symposium; 118)
   1. Macrophages   2. Biological chemistry
   I. Evered, David   II. Nugent, Jonathan
   III. O'Connor, Maeve   IV. Series
   599.08′76042   QR185.8.M3

Printed in Great Britain at The Bath Press, Avon

Contents

Participants

A. Aderem   Laboratory of Cellular Physiology and Immunology, The Rockefeller University, 1230 York Avenue, New York, NY 10021-6399, USA

P. Bellavite   Institute of General Pathology, University of Verona Faculty of Medicine and Surgery, Strada Le Grazie, 37134 Verona, Italy

Z. A. Cohn (*Chairman*)   Laboratory of Cellular Physiology and Immunology, The Rockefeller University, 1230 York Avenue, New York, NY 10021-6399, USA

F. S. Cole   Department of Pediatrics, Harvard Medical School, Division of Cell Biology, Children's Hospital, 300 Longwood Avenue, Boston, MA 02115, USA

P. R. Crocker   Sir William Dunn School of Pathology, University of Oxford, South Parks Road, Oxford OX1 3RE, UK

R. T. Dean   Cell Biology Research Group, Brunel University, Uxbridge, Middlesex UB8 3PH, UK

R. A. B. Ezekowitz   Division of Hematology and Oncology, Harvard Department of Pediatrics, 320 Longwood Avenue, Boston, MA 02115, USA

P. Goossens (*Ciba Foundation Bursar*), Unité d'Immunophysiologie Cellulaire, Institut Pasteur, 28 rue du Dr Roux, 75724 Paris Cédex 15, France

S. Gordon   Sir William Dunn School of Pathology, University of Oxford, South Parks Road, Oxford OX1 3RE, UK

Sir James Gowans   Medical Research Council, 20 Park Crescent, London, W1N 4AL, UK

J. H. Hartwig   Hematology/Oncology Unit, Harvard Medical School, Cox Building, 6th Floor, Massachusetts General Hospital, Boston, MA 02114, USA

N. Hogg   Macrophage Laboratory, Imperial Cancer Research Fund, PO Box 123, 44 Lincoln's Inn Fields, London WC2A 3PX, UK

J. Humphrey   Department of Medicine, Royal Postgraduate Medical School, Hammersmith Hospital, Ducane Road, London W12 0HS, UK

M. Moore   Department of Immunology, Paterson Laboratories, Christie Hospital and Holt Radium Institute, Wilmslow Road, Manchester M20 9BX, UK

C. F. Nathan   Laboratory of Cellular Physiology and Immunology, The Rockefeller University, 1230 York Avenue, New York, NY 10021-6399, USA

N. A. Nicola   Molecular Regulator Laboratory, Cancer Research Unit, Walter and Eliza Hall Institute of Medical Research, Post Office, Royal Melbourne Hospital, Parkville, Victoria 3050, Australia

D. Roos   Department of Blood Cell Chemistry, Netherlands Red Cross Blood Transfusion Service, Central Laboratory, Plesmanlaan 125, 1066 CX Amsterdam, The Netherlands

R. D. Schreiber   Research Institute of Scripps Clinic, 10666 North Torrey Pines Road, La Jolla, CA 92037, USA

S. J. Singer   Department of Biology, University of California at San Diego, La Jolla, CA 92093, USA

C. Sorg   Department of Experimental Dermatology, Westfälische Wilhelms-Universität Münster, Universitäts-Hautklinik, von-Esmarch-Str. 56, D-4400 Münster, Federal Republic of Germany

T. A. Springer   Membrane Immunochemistry Laboratory, Dana-Farber Cancer Institute, Harvard Medical School, 44 Binney Street, Boston, MA 02115, USA

E. R. Stanley   Department of Microbiology and Immunology, Albert Einstein College of Medicine of Yeshiva University, 1300 Morris Park Avenue, Bronx, NY 10461, USA

L. Tarcsay   Division of Biotechnology, PH2.534, K-681.5.42, CIBA-GEIGY AG, CH-4002 Basle, Switzerland

J. C. Unkeless Laboratory of Cellular Physiology and Immunology, The Rockefeller University, 1230 York Avenue, New York, NY 10021-6399, USA

R. van Furth Department of Internal Medicine and Infectious Diseases, Leiden State University Hospital, Rijnsburgerweg 10, 2333 AA Leiden, The Netherlands

Z. Werb Laboratory of Radiobiology and Environmental Health, LR-102, University of California, San Francisco, CA 94143, USA

K. Whaley Department of Pathology, University of Glasgow, Western Infirmary, Glasgow G11 6NT, UK

The first line of defence: chairman's introduction

ZANVIL A. COHN

The Rockefeller University, 1230 York Avenue, New York, New York 10021, USA

*1986 Biochemistry of macrophages. Pitman, London (Ciba Foundation Symposium 118)
p 1-6*

As mobile and long-lived cells the mononuclear phagocytes play central roles as effector cells in inflammatory reactions and cell-mediated immune responses. Inflammation, wound healing, host defence against microbes and tumours and tissue destruction all represent scenarios in which blood-borne elements differentiate in the tissue and influence the form and composition of their environment. This meeting will highlight some of the newly developed areas which pertain to these functions, with an emphasis on the more biochemical aspects. In this short discussion I will use my prerogative as Chairman to raise issues in which I have some interest. Perhaps some of these queries will be answered during our discussions.

Distribution and differentiation—the first line of defence

The recent availability of monoclonal antibodies which recognize surface determinants specific to mononuclear phagocytes is altering our awareness of the density and tissue distribution of these cells. Immunocytochemistry with such reagents in humans and animals illustrates the ubiquitous nature of mononuclear phagocytes in both normal tissues and pathological sites. As more quantitative analyses appear we will no doubt have to raise our estimates of total body pools and perhaps daily production rates as well. It seems clear, however, that the tissue content of mononuclear phagocytes, often associated with the vasculature, greatly exceeds the bone marrow replicative pool. There are, therefore, large numbers of resident cells—poised, if you will, for a prompt response to tissue injury and invasion. We know essentially nothing about their properties, but if they resemble the cells in serous cavities, they would then represent a responsive, activatable pool, capable of initiating many

1

aspects of inflammation. In a real sense they are a first line of defence, followed by secondary waves of granulocytes, lymphocytes and monocytes from the circulation. Other questions concerning their lifespan, turnover, surface phenotype and synthetic potential all remain to be resolved.

The emigratory event

Interactions between the circulating monocyte and the endothelial cell of small blood vessels probably serves to control the initial adherence and intercellular emigration of the blood-borne compartment. What factors generated during a tissue insult modify this normally quiescent relationship? Is the initial stimulus of extravascular or intravascular origin? Does it modify the circulating cell tumbling in the axial stream or the stickiness of endothelium, or both? How important are the hydrodynamic changes which occur in the microvasculature and the resulting decrease in flow rate? Do chemotaxis and the usual chemotactic factors play any role in the intravascular movement of cells and do these agents direct extravascular homing?

In a more general sense, we are also quite ignorant of the factors which regulate the emigration of T cells. Do helper and suppressor or cytotoxic phenotypes have separate regulators which control the number and localization of emigrating cells? In view of the important interactions between lymphokines and macrophages it would be useful to have helper cells close to the effector macrophage. In turn it appears that the resulting process of macrophage activation is often a highly compartmentalized event rather than a process triggered by circulating factors.

Monocytes also interact with the walls of large arteries and may lead to focal, subendothelial accumulations. The so-called 'fatty streak' of humans is one such example, in which lipid-laden monocytes initiate the earliest lesions in the arterial wall. This accumulation is seen quite early and is accelerated by cholesterol loading in both humans and experimental animals. The role of specific lipoproteins in this process and in monocyte accumulation is obviously a timely and important subject for this specialized form of inflammation.

The secretory repertoire

In addition to their classical properties of endocytosis, monocytes and macrophages are now well established as important secretory cells. Macromolecular products of macrophage biosynthetic origin are released into their environment either constitutively or after selective induction. The list of products is now quite long (>50) and encompasses complement components of the classical and alternative pathways, clotting factors, neutral and acid proteinases, other hydrolases, enzyme inhibitors, bioactive metabolites of arachidonic acid, lipoproteins, toxic oxygen intermediates and growth regulatory factors and endogenous pyrogens. Some, such as lysozyme, apolipoprotein E and factor B of the alternative pathway of C′ fixation, are bulk products whereas others are probably trace constituents. When this series of molecules is considered as a group, however, one is impressed with its wide biological potential. Scenarios come to mind in which the liberation of these agents would be appropriate for the tissue remodelling that occurs in wound healing. Enzymic débridement, angiogenesis, ingestion and digestion of damaged cells and matrix, growth stimulation and collagen synthesis by fibroblasts must all occur within secretory limits to result in a beneficial exercise. Yet, with exuberant, uncontrolled responses tissue damage may ensue and contribute to the chronic degenerative diseases of humankind.

Regulation of the secretory event is in part the result of the engagement of surface receptors. Some, such as the Fc receptor, trigger widespread secretory cascades whereas the complement receptors appear to be devoid of this activity. Mere clustering of the Fc receptor on the cell surface with multivalent ligands is sufficient to initiate release of arachidonate from membrane phospholipids and its subsequent metabolism. Neither internalization of the plasma membrane nor its pinching off to form vesicles nor fusion with lysosomes is necessary to achieve a secretory cycle. We need to know much more about the physiological triggers and the longevity of secretion to explain the heterogeneous secretory phenotypes in tissue populations.

Transmembrane signals

The existence of a series of well-defined secretory products has furthered studies on the signals linking surface receptors with internal, contractile networks and metabolic pathways. Our own studies have focused on the Fc receptor, which in the liganded state behaves as an ion channel. Monovalent cations, largely Na^+ from the environment, enter the cell in short pulses, a process associated with cellular depolarization and an increased concentration of cytosolic Ca^{2+} from intracellular sources. Perhaps in the course of this meeting some of the biochemical and molecular events associated with these phenomena will be elucidated. Clearly these events modulate not only the movement of membranes but also the export of macromolecules. In addition, specific ligand–receptor complexing leads to the simultaneous stimulation of a number of diverse and seemingly unrelated pathways which are often the expression of the activated state. An example is the ability of the

Fc receptor to trigger both an oxidative burst and arachidonic acid release and metabolism.

Other membrane-associated molecules may also play a role in this sequence. Clathrin, which is present on the cytosolic face of the plasma membrane of macrophages, is associated with the formation of coated endocytic vesicles and may even be involved in its generation. Within a short time after vesicle formation clathrin is dissociated from the vesicle and we suspect it cycles back to the surface membrane. Perhaps it is associated with the cytosolic face of important macrophage receptors as well, serving as an evanescent bridge to other elements. In any event, this general area seems worthy of more intense study and should lead to better methods for modulating both endocytic and secretory events.

To kill or not to kill

A central event in the life history of many mononuclear phagocytes is their stimulation into the cytocidal mode. In one instance resting, mature macrophages respond to the soluble products of T helper cells and are induced to form toxic oxygen intermediates and perhaps other cytocidal agents after an appreciable lag time ($\pm$ two days). All evidence points to interferon-γ as the active component of crude lymphokine preparations in both mouse and human. Yet a variety of other more rapid changes are occurring in IFN-γ targets, including the expression of genes and their products. Since IFN-γ influences many other cells, including those of the vasculature, gut and connective tissue, it is possible that these effects play significant but unknown roles in the cell-mediated immune response. Understanding the primary or secondary effects of interferon on the multicomponent oxidase system of the macrophage will be a central biochemical problem for an understanding of activation.

A second scenario is illustrated by the circulating monocyte. Here we have a cell which already is making considerable amounts of superoxide anions and hydrogen peroxide. Whether this is in response to lymphokines or to its state of differentiation is unclear; however, it can still respond to IFN-γ by increasing its production of H_2O_2 and maintaining it for longer periods *in vitro* and perhaps in the tissues. The monocyte contains an additional component in its azurophil granules—myeloperoxidase—which in the presence of halide ions and H_2O_2 forms a formidable intracellular microbicidal system, as described by Klebanoff. This enzyme is, however, lost shortly after the monocyte enters the tissues and is never re-expressed.

Age and activatability

Not all macrophage populations are capable of producing toxic oxygen inter-mediates or of being activated by IFN-γ. Two recent examples from our labora-tory will illustrate this statement. First, the murine Kupffer cell cannot produce appreciable amounts of O_2^-, H_2O_2 or mount a respiratory burst. In keeping with this finding, it is a permissive host for a number of obligate intracellular parasites and plays little role in the containment of a *Listeria monocytogenes* infection *in vivo*. Other macrophage attributes such as endocytosis and the secretion of other polypeptides and enzymes are within the usual limits. In addition, the Kupffer cell fails to respond to IFN-γ with the formation of oxygen intermediates but does react by increasing its surface expression of Ia antigen. Is this a general property of macrophages in parenchymatous organs or is it specific for the Kupffer cell? At present we cannot answer this question definitively and other sinusoidal populations in the spleen are being examined.

There is, however, a precedent for the loss in the production of oxygen radicals after prolonged *in vitro* cultivation. Monocytes, for example, demon-strate progressive reductions in their ability to form H_2O_2 and to respond to lymphokines. Such an event *in vivo* might lead to defective populations that are unable to protect the host against intracellular pathogens. The ques-tion to be answered revolves about the influence of population longevity or more selective effects of the microenvironment.

Similar end-results occur in pathological processes but with dissimilar under-lying mechanisms. In lepromatous leprosy T cells often fail to respond to *Mycobacterium leprae* antigens with the formation of lymphokines such as IFN-γ and interleukin-2. Supernatant fluids obtained from these cells fail to activate normal or lepromatous monocytes. We believe that this result, when coupled with the relative deficiency of helper T cells in the dermis, can explain the uncontrolled growth of the organism in skin macrophages. Another situa-tion occurs with the products of tumour cells which selectively reduce the capacity of macrophages to form hydrogen peroxide whereas many other sec-retory products are unaffected.

Recombinant products and delivery systems—compartmentalization of the cellular immune response

The stimulation of helper T cells, lymphokine formation and the resulting activation of effector macrophages is probably a local rather than a systemic response. It is nevertheless true that agents such as *Corynebacterium parvum* given by the parenteral route would stimulate cells in multiple loci. Whether soluble T cell factors of tissue origin would enter the circulation and work at distant sites is more conjectural. This is of more than academic interest in view of the availability of cloned products of human and animal origin such as IFN-γ. What effects these agents will have via the parenteral or local routes on macrophage activation and inflammation in general is under study. Similarly, the efficacy of these agents in promoting enhanced host resistance to intracellular parasites and tumour cell targets is under study in both humans and animals. This exciting area of the 'new immunotherapy' is in its infancy and we have much to learn about the methods for its delivery and maintenance, and about possible toxic effects. Perhaps in this meeting new information will emerge on the subject.

This will be my third Ciba Foundation Symposium and I look forward to an exciting interchange of ideas. This is a gracious and effective method to review a field in the company of colleagues and friends.

Acknowledgements

Supported by grant AI-07012 from the National Institutes of Health.

Specificity of action of colony-stimulating factors in the differentiation of granulocytes and macrophages

NICOS A. NICOLA and DONALD METCALF

Walter and Eliza Hall Institute of Medical Research, Post Office, Royal Melbourne Hospital, Parkville, Victoria 3050, Australia

Abstract. Four colony-stimulating factors (CSFs) (M-CSF, GM-CSF, Multi-CSF and G-CSF) can each stimulate the production of macrophages from progenitor cells in murine bone marrow or fetal liver. However, they differ in their relative selectivity for macrophage progenitor cells and in their dose-response characteristics for stimulating macrophage progenitors relative to other progenitors. It is unresolved whether distinct subsets of progenitor cells exist with a unique responsiveness to one or other CSF or whether the macrophages produced by different CSFs are all functionally equivalent. However, it is shown here that various CSFs can generate from blast progenitor cells an intermediate macrophage progenitor cell whose growth is specifically inhibited by a substance in lectin-stimulated spleen cell-conditioned media. It is also shown that, for at least one myelomonocytic leukaemic cell line, differentiation to macrophages and granulocytes can be induced most effectively by G-CSF but not by M-CSF or Multi-CSF. Finally, the involvement of macrophages and macrophage cell lines in the induced production of these CSFs as well as their display of specific receptors for the different CSFs is examined.

1986 Biochemistry of macrophages. Pitman, London (Ciba Foundation Symposium 118) p 7-28

The colony-stimulating factors

At least four purified and well characterized colony-stimulating factors (CSFs) are able, to a greater or lesser extent, to stimulate the production of macro-phages from specific precursor cells. These factors are (1) macrophage-CSF (M-CSF) or CSF-1, which is the subject of the paper by E. R. Stanley in this volume; (2) granulocyte–macrophage-CSF (GM-CSF); (3) multipotential-CSF (Multi-CSF) or interleukin 3 (IL-3); and (4) granulocyte-CSF or G-CSF (see Fig. 1 and Table 1).

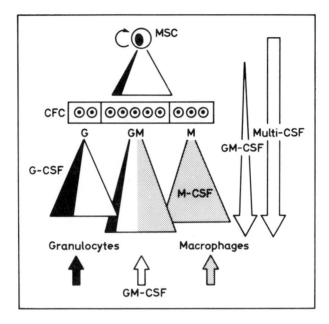

FIG. 1. Spectrum of activity of four purified CSFs within the granulocyte–macrophage cell lineage. Multi-CSF and GM-CSF (unshaded) stimulate all cell compartments although GM-CSF has weaker and incomplete actions on multipotential and stem cells (MSC). G-CSF (dark shading) is predominantly restricted to a subset of granulocytic and bipotential progenitor cells but also allows survival of more primitive cells. M-CSF (stippled shading) is restricted to macrophage-committed or bipotential cells.

TABLE 1 Molecular properties of colony-stimulating factors

	M_r	Disulphides	Core protein M_r	Glycosylated[a]	Receptor M_r[b]
M-CSF	70 000	Inter subunit	14 500	Yes (endo D)	150 000
GM-CSF	23 000	Intra subunit	13 500[c]	Yes (endo F)	50 000
G-CSF	25 000	Intra subunit	<14 000	Yes (endo H)	150 000
Multi-CSF	19 000[d]	Intra subunit	15 000[c]	Yes	50 000
	–30 000				and 70 000

[a] Endoglycosidase specificity for removal of carbohydrate moieties.
[b] By chemical cross-linking.
[c] Based on the deduced sequence from molecularly cloned cDNAs.
[d] The molecule from LB-3-conditioned medium comes in two forms (19 000 and 23 000) while the molecule from WEHI-3B-conditioned medium is 24 000–30 000.

Only M-CSF is restricted in its action almost exclusively to cells of the mononuclear phagocyte cell series. It differs from the other CSFs in being a disulphide-bonded dimer, and since the specificity, structure and action of this molecule are dealt with in detail in the next paper in this volume (Stanley 1986) this paper will deal predominantly with the other three CSFs as they relate to macrophage development.

GM-CSF is a glycoprotein of M_r 23 000 with internal disulphide bonds which has been purified from medium conditioned by lung tissue from endotoxin-injected mice (Burgess & Nice 1985) and more recently from medium conditioned by the continuous T-cell line, LB-3 (R. L. Cutler et al, unpublished). The full amino acid sequence is known for this molecule from cDNA molecular clones (Gough et al 1984) and binding studies have been performed with radioiodinated derivatives (Walker & Burgess 1985). GM-CSF is able to stimulate the production of neutrophilic granulocyte, macrophage and mixed granulocyte–macrophage colonies from mouse bone marrow cells, and the types of colonies developing depend on the concentration of GM-CSF, with lower concentrations favouring macrophage colony development (see Metcalf 1984). In addition, GM-CSF can stimulate the formation of eosinophil colonies from fetal liver progenitor cells (Metcalf & Nicola 1983) and initiate but not complete colony formation by progenitor cells committed to several other haemopoietic cell lineages (see Metcalf 1984). Finally, GM-CSF can stimulate some functional activities in mature granulocytes and macrophages (see Metcalf 1984).

Multi-CSF is a glycoprotein of M_r 19 000–28 000 and also contains internal disulphide bonds. It has been purified from medium conditioned by cells of the myelomonocytic leukaemic line WEHI-3B and termed interleukin 3, P-cell stimulating factor, haemopoietic cell growth factor, burst-promoting activity and mast cell growth factor (see review by Nicola & Vadas 1984). It has also been purified from medium conditioned by lectin-stimulated spleen cells (SCM) (Cutler et al 1985) and from the LB-3 cell line (R. L. Cutler et al, unpublished). The full amino acid sequence is known from cDNA clones (Fung et al 1984, Yokota et al 1984) and binding studies have been performed with radioiodinated derivatives (Palaszynski & Ihle 1984). Multi-CSF shows a very broad haemopoietic specificity and in addition to stimulating colony formation from granulocyte and macrophage progenitors it also stimulates the formation of eosinophil-, megakaryocyte-, erythroid-, mast- and multipotential colonies.

G-CSF is a glycoprotein of M_r 25 000 containing internal disulphide bonds. It has been purified from medium conditioned by lung tissue from endotoxin-injected mice (Nicola et al 1983) but has not yet been molecularly cloned. Binding studies have been performed with radioiodinated derivatives (Nicola & Metcalf 1984, 1985, Nicola et al 1985). At low concentrations G-CSF appears to be an exclusive stimulus for a subset of neutrophilic granulocyte progenitor cells but at higher concentrations it can also stimulate granulocyte and macrophage colony formation as well as initiate colony formation in several haemopoietic cell lineages (Metcalf & Nicola 1983). It is distinguished from the other CSFs by its ability to induce terminal differentiation in the myelomonocytic leukaemic cell line, WEHI-3B, to granulocytes and macrophages (Metcalf & Nicola 1982). Murine G-CSF has a clearly defined human equivalent, CSFβ, and these two molecules and their respective cellular receptors appear to have been strongly conserved during evolution (Nicola et al 1985).

It can be seen that four different and well-defined regulators of haemopoietic cell proliferation and differentiation can each stimulate macrophage progenitor cells to proliferate. This raises several questions. (1) Do these four CSFs act on the same or overlapping sets of macrophage progenitor cells? (2) Are the overlapping actions of the CSFs mediated by common or separate cellular receptors? (3) Do the various progenitor cells produce the same or different types of differentiated macrophages? (4) When and where are the four different CSFs produced in the body and is their production coordinated? (5) Do the CSFs have differential actions on the survival, proliferation, differentiation and functional activation of macrophages or their progenitors?

Most of these questions cannot yet be definitively answered but some observations have emerged. To some extent at least, it is clear that there exist subsets of macrophage or bipotential granulocyte/macrophage progenitor cells which respond differentially to these CSFs and even to different concentrations of, for example, GM-CSF (see Metcalf 1984). However, it is also clear that many, probably most, macrophage progenitors can respond to proliferative stimulation by more than one CSF. This has been established by clone transfer experiments which indicated that clones initiated with G-CSF, GM-CSF or Multi-CSF and subsequently transferred to M-CSF could develop as macrophage colonies (see Metcalf 1984). Nevertheless, the action of these CSFs, especially on biopotential granulocyte–macrophage progenitors is not always the same. Results from experiments in which combinations of CSFs were used to stimulate bone marrow cultures, and an analysis of the effects of different CSFs on paired daughter cells, have indicated that different CSFs can affect the differentiation outcome of bipotential progenitor cells (see Metcalf 1984).

Each of the four CSFs appears to have a unique and private receptor with no direct cross-reactivity with other CSFs (Das et al 1980, Palaszynski & Ihle 1984, Nicola & Metcalf 1984, Walker & Burgess 1985). However, there is increasing evidence that the expression of these private receptors can be modulated by other CSFs (F. Walker et al, unpublished) as well as other classes of haemopoietically-active compounds (Guilbert & Stanley 1984).

Whether some of the apparent CSF cross-reactivities of CSFs can be explained by such receptor modulations remains to be established.

Little effort has been made to determine whether macrophages produced by the action of different CSFs are equivalent in differentiation state and in functional activities but this is an important question worth further study. Also, relatively little is known about the sites of production and action of the CSFs. Multi-CSF has not been detected in the serum but after endotoxin injection relatively rapid and large rises are seen in the circulating levels of G-CSF and a form of GM-CSF or M-CSF that is recognized by anti-L-cell M-CSF sera (Das et al 1980, Stanley 1979). However, whether these circulating CSFs have an effect on populations of bone marrow cells or are restricted in their action to activating tissue granulocytes and macrophages is not clear. Similarly, it is not known what forms of CSF are important in the bone marrow microenvironment.

In this context a number of workers have derived cloned stromal cell lines from mouse marrow populations. These have a fibroblast-like or pre-adipocyte morphology and are capable of the constitutive production of a CSF which from its biological actions appears to be M-CSF (see review by Metcalf 1984). This suggests strongly that M-CSF may be produced locally within the marrow, and other studies have shown that mouse marrow cells are able to produce GM-CSF and G-CSF. More recently, cloned stromal cell lines have been developed with multiple actions on stem and various progenitor cells (C. L. Li & G. R. Johnson, unpublished). The active agent appears not to be Multi-CSF and has yet to be characterized.

An interesting situation exists in the fetus, since the major sources of CSF— yolk sac, fetal liver—clearly produce M-CSF, and most progenitor cells in the early fetal liver appear to be macrophage-committed. Thus, in early fetal life, a matching regulator–target cell system exists that is biased towards mac-rophage formation and it is only in later fetal life that granulopoiesis occurs (see Metcalf 1984).

Proliferation and differentiation of granulocyte and macrophage precursors

Murine fetal liver cells can be fractionated by fluorescence-activated cell sort-ing (after labelling with fluorescein-conjugated pokeweed mitogen and rhoda-mine-labelled anti-myeloid antibodies) to produce cell populations enriched for progenitor cells (Nicola et al 1981). This population of cells consists of essentially pure basophilic blast cells with a total cloning efficiency of 30–80%. Fig. 2 shows that, in liquid suspension cultures, the cells undergo an exponen-tial growth phase after a lag period when stimulated by a variety of CSFs

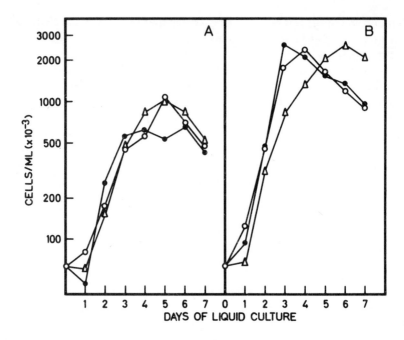

FIG. 2. Cell kinetics of purified murine fetal colony-forming cells in liquid cultures stimulated with different conditioned media. (A) O——O, stimulated with L-cell conditioned medium; △——△, stimulated with PMUE; ●——● stimulated with yolk sac conditioned medium. (B) O——O, stimulated with SCM; (●——●) stimulated with SCM plus PMUE; △——△, stimulated with mouse lung conditioned medium. Only viable non-adherent cells were counted. Fifty thousand purified cells were seeded in each liquid culture. Note the log scale for cell number.

of different origins. With three different sources of M-CSF (Das et al 1980) (L-cell conditioned medium, pregnant mouse uterus extract [PMUE] or yolk sac conditioned medium), all pre-titrated in agar cultures and used at a concentration giving maximal colony formation, the cell growth curves were very similar. Total cell numbers increased about 20-fold over a five-day period and then plateaued or slightly decreased. With pokeweed mitogen-stimulated spleen-conditioned medium (SCM) (a source of Multi-CSF and GM-CSF) total cell numbers increased to a higher level (about 60-fold) and addition of M-CSF did not increase the rate of cell production or the maximal numbers of cells achieved. Similar cell numbers were achieved with mouse lung-conditioned medium (a source of GM-CSF and G-CSF) but it took longer to achieve maximal cell numbers (Fig. 2). In all cases the cell doubling time during the exponential phase was 12–13 h. This suggests that a smaller subset of progenitor cells is stimulated by M-CSF than by Multi-CSF or GM-CSF. Analysis of the morphology of cells produced also indicated that M-CSF may have stimulated a more restricted set of progenitor cells than Multi-CSF and GM-CSF since many more granulocytes were seen in the latter cultures (Nicola & Metcalf 1982). In similar cultures, G-CSF stimulated even fewer progenitors and these were almost exclusively granulocyte-restricted (Metcalf & Nicola 1983).

In tests designed to determine how long these purified blast cells retained their clonogenicity and what kinds of differentiation commitment were occurring under the influence of different CSFs, we used different CSFs to initiate liquid cultures and at daily intervals samples of cells were removed and cloned in semi-solid agar cultures containing other CSFs (Fig. 3). It can be seen from Fig. 3 that PMUE-stimulated liquid cultures initially contained similar numbers of clonogenic cells detected in agar cultures stimulated with PMUE or SCM. However, by day 4 of liquid culture many more clones developed in PMUE-stimulated agar cultures than in SCM-stimulated agar cultures.

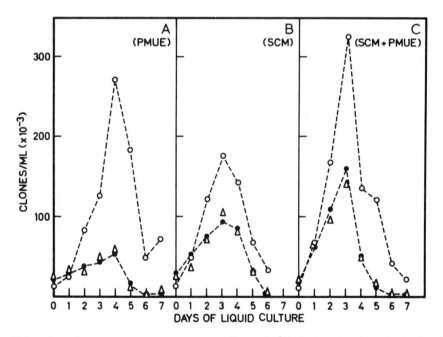

FIG. 3. Clone-forming cell production in liquid cultures of purified colony-forming cells stimulated with different conditioned media. Fifty thousand purified cells were seeded per liquid culture and stimulated with (A) PMUE, (B) SCM or (C) both PMUE and SCM. At daily timepoints, a sample of cells was removed from the liquid cultures and seeded at 2000 cells/plate in agar cultures stimulated with different conditioned media. Seven days later, clones developing in agar cultures stimulated with PMUE (O-----O), SCM (●-----●) or SCM + PMUE (△-----△) were enumerated.

Initially, this was ascribed to the expansion in liquid cultures of cells responsive
only to PMUE. However, addition of SCM to PMUE-stimulated agar cultures
reduced the number of clones developing to the number seen in cultures
stimulated with SCM alone (Fig. 2A). Moreover, liquid cultures stimulated
with SCM alone or a combination of SCM + PMUE produced the same pattern
of responsiveness of the clonogenic cells as seen with PMUE-stimulated cultures (Fig. 2B,C). Finally, Fig. 4 shows that various conditioned media containing M-CSF, Multi-CSF, GM-CSF and G-CSF could all, to a greater or lesser
extent, stimulate the formation of clonogenic cells which responded in agar
to PMUE (or other sources of M-CSF) but were specifically inhibited by
SCM. The clones forming in agar cultures stimulated with PMUE (or L-cell
conditioned medium or yolk sac-conditioned medium) varied in size and,
in particular, were of progressively smaller size the longer the duration of

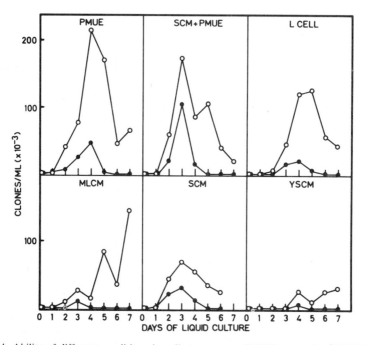

FIG. 4. Ability of different conditioned media to generate PMUE-responsive/SCM inhibitable
colony- and cluster-forming cells. Fifty thousand purified cells were seeded per liquid culture
stimulated with the indicated conditioned media. At daily time-points samples of cells were
removed from each culture and seeded at 2000 cells/plate in agar cultures stimulated with PMUE
or with PMUE + SCM. Seven days later the difference in clones (PMUE-stimulated clones minus
PMUE + SCM-stimulated clones) was determined. The figures show the calculated number of
such colony-forming cells (●——●) or total clone-forming cells (○——○) in each type of primary
liquid culture. MLCM, mouse lung conditioned medium. YSCM, yolk sac conditioned medium.

the initial primary liquid cultures. Stained cultures revealed that clones invariably consisted of monocytoid cells only, and the cells were tightly packed in the clones, with little evidence that they could migrate in agar.

It appeared then that by day 3–4 of liquid culture, under the influence of several different types of CSF, blast cells were differentiated to a cell type that could proliferate under the influence of M-CSF but was specifically inhibited from proliferating by a substance in SCM. Reference to Figs. 1 and 3 indicates that at day 4 in liquid cultures stimulated with PMUE up to 30–40% of the cells shared this property, and since most cells in these liquid cultures had the morphology of monocytes this cell type can be identified as a monocyte.

It should be pointed out that the inhibitor present in SCM is very specific in its action on this monocytic progenitor cell. The SCM preparations used as inhibitors were in fact selected to be maximal stimuli for blast cell proliferation in the liquid cultures (Fig. 2) and for colony formation in agar. In fact the same preparation of SCM showed similar dose-response curves for, on the one hand, stimulation of bone marrow colony formation and, on the other, for inhibition of monocyte progenitor cell proliferation (results not shown). SCM is known to contain interferon-γ and interferons are known to selectively inhibit proliferation of some macrophage progenitors (Hale & McCarthy 1982). It is therefore likely, though not proven, that interferon is the specific inhibitor detected in these experiments and that its inhibitory action on macrophage proliferation is restricted not to the earliest stages of macrophage development (blast cells) but to later developmental stages. In fact differential growth and serum requirements for progenitors of bone marrow macrophages relative to the more mature types in blood and the peritoneum have been described by Yen & Stewart (1982), indicating separate levels of proliferative control in the macrophage cell lineage.

Proliferation and differentiation of myelomonocytic leukaemic cells

We have used as a model the transplantable leukaemic cell line WEHI-3B D$^+$ to study the ability of the four CSFs to regulate cell multiplication and differentiation in leukaemias. The tissue culture-adapted WEHI-3B D$^+$ no longer requires exogenous CSF to stimulate cell proliferation and it grows as a population of blast cells with the potential to differentiate into both granulocytes and macrophages (Metcalf & Nicola 1982). Somewhat surprisingly, M-CSF and Multi-CSF, both of which have the capacity to stimulate normal progenitor cells to form differentiating granulocytes and macrophages, have no discernible effects on WEHI-3B D$^+$ cells. GM-CSF has a relatively weak differentiation-inducing activity on these cells while G-CSF has a relatively strong differentiation-inducing activity. Again it is surprising that, whereas the differentiating action of low concentrations of G-CSF on normal progenitor cells is predominantly to stimulate granulocyte formation, the action on WEHI-3B D$^+$ cells is predominantly to induce differentiation to macrophages (Table 2). Only higher concentrations of G-CSF induce the leukaemic cells to form maturing granulocytes. The reason for this concentration-dependent difference in action on normal versus leukaemic cells is unclear but it may imply that the action of G-CSF on cells which bear receptors for it is to activate a predetermined differentiation programme rather than to direct a granulocytic differentiation pathway. Consistent with this, G-CSF can also stimulate proliferation and differentiation of some bipotent and macrophage-committed progenitor cells at higher concentrations (Metcalf & Nicola 1983), and some normal monocyte–macrophages as well as some macrophage cell lines bear specific receptors for G-CSF (see later).

TABLE 2 Types of differentiation induced in WEHI-3B D$^+$ colonies by purified G-CSF[a]

Dilution of G-CSF	% Differentiated colonies[b]	% Colonies composed of[c]				
		U	U + M	U + M + G	U + G	G
1:1	100	0	48	40	7	5
1:2	52	4	71	14	7	4
1:4	29	48	37	4	9	2
1:8	18	46	32	4	14	4
1:16	8	73	27	0	0	0
1:32	5	86	12	0	2	0
Saline	3	93	7	0	0	0

[a] In each case at least 60 sequential colonies were removed at day 7 of culture and stained (data from Metcalf & Nicola 1982).
[b] Colonies with a dispersed morphology.
[c] U, undifferentiated cells; M, macrophages; G, granulocytes (myelocytes to polymorphs).

Specific receptors exist for G-CSF on WEHI-3B D$^+$ cells and on normal murine bone marrow cells (Nicola & Metcalf 1984, 1985) and these are not directly competed for by any of the other CSFs or unrelated growth factors. Interestingly, cells of the differentiation-unresponsive subline WEHI-3B D$^-$, which arose spontaneously from the D$^+$ line, have no or grossly reduced numbers of detectable G-CSF receptors (Nicola & Metcalf 1984). In normal murine tissues, autoradiographic analysis has shown that a proportion of blast cells and all cells of the neutrophilic granulocytic series have receptors for G-CSF. At least a proportion of bone marrow monocytes and macrophages, but not erythroid or lymphoid cells, also show small numbers of receptors (Nicola & Metcalf 1985). Even on the cells with the most abundant G-CSF receptors (WEHI-3B D$^+$, granulocytes) the number of receptors is relatively small (a few hundred) and the binding kinetics are unusual, with a very fast 'on' constant and a very slow 'off' constant. Consistent with the observation of small numbers of G-CSF receptors on a proportion of macrophages, at least two myelomonocytic or macrophage cell lines (WEHI-3B D$^+$ and J774) display specific G-CSF receptors (Table 3, Fig. 5).

G-CSF and its receptor appear to have been strongly conserved across species, with the murine molecule and the human homologue, CSFβ, competing equally well for binding to human or murine receptors (Nicola et al 1985). In the human, CSFβ is also primarily a granulocytic colony-stimulating factor, in contrast to CSFα (Nicola et al 1979), and specific receptors for G-CSF (presumably CSFβ receptors) exist mainly on normal promyelocytes and to a lesser extent on other granulocytic cells. In addition, cells from all patients with acute myeloid leukaemia (M1, M2, M3, M4 and M5) and with chronic myeloid leukaemia also display specific receptors for G-CSF (Nicola et al 1985).

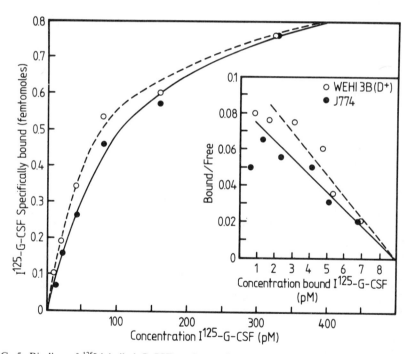

FIG. 5. Binding of ^{125}I-labelled G-CSF to the myelomonocytic leukaemic cell line WEHI-3B D$^+$ and the monocyte/macrophage cell line J774. Specific binding of ^{125}I G-CSF to 2×10^6 cells in a reaction volume of 120 μl. Inset: Scatchard analysis of the binding data indicating similar receptor numbers and apparent affinity on the two cell types.

TABLE 3 CSF production and CSF receptors on monocyte/macrophage cell lines

Cell line	Description	Endotoxin	CSF produced (units/10⁶ cells)[a]				Receptors/cell			
			GM-CSF	G-CSF	M-CSF	Multi-CSF	GM-CSF	G-CSF	M-CSF	Multi-CSF
WEHI-3B D⁺	Myelomonocytic leukaemia	−	0	0	200	1500	450	700	ND[b]	0
		+	ND	ND	ND	ND				
J774	Monocytic	−	80	50	0	0	350	700	19000	ND
		+	160	160	0	0				
WR19	Monocyte/macrophage leukaemia	−	0	400	0	0	200	100	0	ND
		+	0	8000	0	0				
RAW264	Monocyte/macrophage leukaemia	−	0	160	0	0	200	0	ND	0
		+	0	4000	0	0				
R309	Monocyte/macrophage leukaemia	−	0	400	0	0	400	0	ND	ND
		+	0	8000	0	0				
WEHI-274	Monocyte/macrophage leukaemia	−	7000	0	0	0	ND	0	ND	ND
		+	8000	0	0	0				
WEHI-265	Monocyte/macrophage leukaemia	−	0	0	0	0	ND	0	ND	ND
		+	0	4000	0	0				
Peritoneal macrophage	Resident	−	0	3000	0	0	ND	ND	7000	ND
		+	70	10000	0	0				

[a] GM-CSF assayed by the ability to stimulate proliferation in the FDCP but not 32D cl.3 cell lines, Multi-CSF by the ability to stimulate proliferation of 32D cl.3 cells, G-CSF by the ability to induce differentiation in WEHI-3B D⁺ cells and M-CSF by colony formation after chemical fractionation. The data are in part from Metcalf & Nicola (1985a).

[b] Not done.

G-CSF, and to a lesser extent GM-CSF, can be used to suppress the leukae-mogenicity of WEHI-3B D⁺ cells. These molecules are not anti-proliferative—indeed they may slightly enhance the early proliferation of WEHI-3B cells—but exert their suppressive effects by increasing the probability of cell differen-tiation at the expense of self-renewal at each cell division. The end-result is that the percentage of proliferative cells generated is eventually reduced to zero, with a progressive rise in the number of non-dividing granulocytes and macrophages (Metcalf & Nicola 1982). In principle, G-CSF does not seem to have any unique property (except its cellular specificity), compared to other CSFs, that influences cell differentiation, and it may be that other leukaemic cell lines could be triggered into terminal differentiation pathways by other CSFs.

Production of CSFs by macrophages

It has been demonstrated that mouse macrophages can synthesize and release GM-CSF and G-CSF and that Kupffer cells and macrophages can produce erythropoietin (see Metcalf 1984). It appears, however, that macrophages do not synthesize Multi-CSF or M-CSF. In the human, it has been suggested that macrophages do not themselves synthesize human GM-CSF but release a product that induces T-cells or endothelial cells to make GM-CSF (Bagby et al 1983). In the mouse it seems clear, however, that macrophages do synthe-size CSF and that this production is increased by endotoxin and tumour pro-moters (Burgess & Nicola 1984) but decreased by lactoferrin (Broxmeyer et al 1980). Peritoneal macrophages synthesize large amounts of G-CSF when stimulated by endotoxin (Metcalf & Nicola 1985b). It can be seen from Table 3 that most macrophage cell lines produce G-CSF and this is inducible by endotoxin, while only a few produce GM-CSF. On the other hand most macro-phage cell lines have receptors for GM-CSF while only a few have receptors for G-CSF. It would be interesting to determine whether the cell lines reflect a heterogeneity present in normal macrophages.

The production by macrophages of some CSFs obviously raises some ques-tions about haemopoietic regulation. Since mature macrophages can produce CSFs able to stimulate macrophage proliferation, how is progressive expansion of macrophage populations prevented? A number of factors probably prevent this from happening. First, resting macrophages produce very little CSF unless they are stimulated by endotoxin, and they do not produce M-CSF or Multi-CSF. Second, tissue macrophages are isolated from the bone marrow and it is not clear whether the CSFs produced by these cells reach the marrow environment to stimulate the earliest macrophage progenitor cells. The role of this CSF may be to activate granulocytes and macrophages in the tissues.

Finally, as mentioned above, mechanisms exist for switching off CSF production and there is some evidence that 'activated' macrophages (e.g. after endotoxin treatment of thioglycollate induction) become refractory to further CSF production.

In addition there are some interesting examples of 'regular cascades' where one CSF affects the production of another CSF by macrophages. It is probable that Multi-CSF and M-CSF can stimulate the production of G-CSF by peritoneal macrophages (Metcalf & Nicola 1985b). It also appears that GM-CSF can stimulate the production of erythropoietin by fetal liver Kupffer cells (Metcalf & Nicola 1984). The biological significance of these effects is not clear but they do point out the need for the action of a CSF in cultures of unfractionated cells to be assessed carefully if direct and indirect effects are to be distinguished.

Conclusions and outstanding problems

Four well-defined CSFs have each been shown to be able to stimulate *in vitro* the production of macrophages from progenitor cells. All appear to be able to stimulate the survival of macrophage progenitor cells, their proliferation and their differentiation. In addition at least two, M-CSF and GM-CSF, stimulate functional activities in mature cells although this has not been tested for the other two. It remains to be established whether different types of macrophage progenitor cells respond differently to these four CSFs, whether the macrophages stimulated to develop by each CSF are functionally equivalent, how the production and compartmentalization of each CSF is arranged *in vivo*, and what contribution the production of CSFs by macrophages themselves makes to haemopoiesis *in vivo*.

Acknowledgements

The experimental work described here was supported by The National Health and Medical Research Council, Canberra, Australia; The National Institutes of Health, Bethesda, MD (Grants CA-22556 and CA-25972); the Carden Fellowship Fund of the Anti-Cancer Council of Victoria, Australia; and the J. D. and L. Harris Cancer Fund.

REFERENCES

Bagby GC, McCall E, Bergstrom KA, Burger D 1983 A monokine regulates colony-stimulating activity production by vascular endothelial cells. Blood 62:663-668

Broxmeyer HE, De Sousa M, Smithyman A, Ralph P, Hamilton J, Kurland JI, Bognacki J 1980 Specificity and modulation of the action of lactoferrin, a negative feedback regulator of myelopoiesis. Blood 55:324-333

Burgess AW, Nice EC 1985 Purification of murine granulocyte–macrophage colony-stimulating factor. Methods Enzymol, in press

Burgess AW, Nicola NA 1984 Effects of 12-0-tetradecanoyl phorbol-13-acetate (TPA) on the proliferation of granulocyte–macrophage colony-forming cells. Blood 61:575-579

Cutler RL, Metcalf D, Nicola NA, Johnson GR 1985 Purification of a multipotential colony stimulating factor from pokeweed mitogen-stimulated mouse spleen cell conditioned medium. J Biol Chem 260:6579-6587

Das SK, Stanley ER, Guilbert LJ, Forman LW 1980 Discrimination of a colony stimulating factor subclass by a specific receptor on a macrophage cell line. J Cell Physiol 104:359-366

Fung MC, Hapel AJ, Ymer S et al 1984 Molecular cloning of cDNA for murine interleukin 3. Nature (Lond) 307:233-237

Gough NM, Gough J, Metcalf D et al 1984 Molecular cloning of cDNA encoding a murine haemopoietic growth regulator, granulocyte–macrophage colony-stimulating factor. Nature (Lond) 309:763-768

Guilbert LJ, Stanley ER 1984 Modulation of receptors for the colony stimulating factor, CSF-1, by bacterial lipopolysaccharide and CSF-1. J Immunol Methods 73:17-28

Hale ML, McCarthy KF Effect of mouse type I interferon on mouse bone marrow cells and peritoneal exudate cells cultured in vitro. Exp Hematol 10:263-270

Metcalf D 1984 The hemopoietic colony stimulating factors. Elsevier, Amsterdam

Metcalf D, Nicola NA 1982 Autoinduction of differentiation in WEHI-3B leukaemia cells. Int J Cancer 30:773-780

Metcalf D, Nicola NA 1983 Proliferative effects of purified granulocyte colony-stimulating factor (G-CSF) on normal mouse hemopoietic cells. J Cell Physiol 116:198-206

Metcalf D, Nicola NA 1984 The regulatory factors controlling murine erythropoiesis in vitro. In: Young NS et al (eds) Aplastic anemia: stem cell biology and advances in treatment. Liss, New York, p 93-105

Metcalf D, Nicola NA 1985a The role of colony stimulating factors in the emergence and suppression of myeloid leukemia populations. In: Wahren B et al (eds) Biological characterization of tumor cells. Raven Press, New York, p 215-232

Metcalf D, Nicola NA 1985b Synthesis by mouse peritoneal cells of G-CSF, the differentiation inducer for myeloid leukemia cells: stimulation by endotoxin, M-CSF and Multi-CSF. Leukemia Res 9:35-50

Nicola NA, Metcalf D 1982 Analysis of purified fetal liver hemopoietic progenitor cells in liquid culture. J Cell Physiol 112:257-264

Nicola NA, Metcalf D 1984 Binding of the differentiation-inducer, granulocyte-colony-stimulating factor, to responsive but not unresponsive leukemic cell lines. Proc Natl Acad Sci USA 81: 3765-3769

Nicola NA, Metcalf D 1985 Binding of ^{125}I-labeled granulocyte colony-stimulating factor to normal murine hemopoietic cells. J Cell Physiol 124:313-321

Nicola NA, Vadas M 1984 Hemopoietic colony-stimulating factors. Immunol Today 5:76-80

Nicola NA, Metcalf D, Johnson GR, Burgess AW 1979 Separation of functionally distinct human granulocyte–macrophage colony-stimulating factors. Blood 54:614-627

Nicola NA, Metcalf D, von Melchner H, Burgess AW 1981 Isolation of murine fetal hemopoietic progenitor cells and selective fractionation of various erythroid precursors. Blood 58:376-386

Nicola NA, Metcalf D, Matsumoto M, Johnson GR 1983 Purification of a factor inducing differentiation in murine myelomonocytic leukemia cells. Identification as granulocyte colony-stimulating factor (G-CSF). J Biol Chem 258:9017-9023

Nicola NA, Begley CG, Metcalf D 1985 Identification of the human analogue of a regulator
    that induces differentiation in murine leukaemic cells. Nature (Lond) 314:625-628
Palaszynski EW, Ihle JN 1984 Evidence for specific receptors for interleukin 3 on lymphokine
    dependent cell lines established from long-term bone marrow cultures. J Immunol 132:1872-
    1878
Stanley ER 1979 Colony-stimulating factor (CSF) radioimmunoassay: detection of a CSF subclass
    stimulating macrophage production. Proc Natl Acad Sci USA 76:2969-2973
Walker F, Burgess AW 1985 Specific binding of radioiodinated granulocyte macrophage colony
    stimulating factor to hemopoietic cells. EMBO (Eur Mol Biol Organ) J 4:933-939
Yen SE, Stewart CC 1982 Effects of serum factors on the growth of mononuclear phagocytes.
    J Cell Physiol 112:107-114
Yokota T, Lee F, Rennick D et al 1984 Isolation and characterization of a mouse cDNA clone
    that expresses mast cell growth factor activity in monkey cells. Proc Natl Acad Sci USA 81:1070-
    1074

DISCUSSION

Gordon: How can you be sure that macrophage colony-stimulating factor
(M-CSF) is not being produced in the last experiment you discussed? Are you
just assaying the secreted medium?

Nicola: We can't detect any M-CSF in the medium but it is true that the
macrophages could be producing some and using it up as rapidly as they
produce it.

van Furth: You demonstrated that these CSFs are active *in vitro*. Has anyone
demonstrated any effect *in vivo*?

Nicola: I can't answer that. We would like to inject purified CSF into animals
and see what happens but that is very difficult. The half-life of intravenously
injected CSF in mice is in the order of minutes, so to maintain a level that we
know to be effective *in vitro*, we would need milligram amounts which are not
yet available.

Ezekowitz: What are the cells of origin of the various CSFs?

Nicola: T cells can make Multi-CSF and GM-CSF. As far as we know, in
normal tissues T cells are the only source of interleukin 3 or Multi-CSF.
GM-CSF can probably also be produced by macrophages, endothelial cells,
fibroblasts and so on. The fibroblast is the only normal cell type that has been
shown to make M-CSF (Stewart & Lin 1978, Tushinski et al 1982). Macrophages are the only normal cells we know of that make G-CSF, especially
after induction with endotoxin.

Ezekowitz: Is G-CSF just a nutrient factor or can it affect the function of
polymorphs, for example the cooperation of macrophages and polymorphs in
tissues?

Nicola: I don't know about cooperation but highly purified blood neutrophils can be stimulated by G-CSF to act in antibody-dependent cell killing reactions, to ingest bacteria and probably to adhere to tissues (Lopez et al 1983).

G-CSF is completely cross-reactive between mice and humans. We can for example show that purified mouse G-CSF is just as effective in stimulating various functional activities in human blood neutrophils as it is in mouse blood neutrophils (Lopez et al 1983). In addition, it stimulates RNA synthesis and protein synthesis, and prolongs the lifetime of granulocytes *in vitro*.

Hogg: Moore et al (1984) added antibodies to interferon-α and interferon-β to cultures of proliferating bone marrow and got significant enhancement of mononuclear phagocyte proliferation. This suggests that you may be looking at interferon-like inhibiting factors.

Nicola: We have no direct evidence that it is the interferons which inhibited macrophage proliferation in our assay. We should be able to test that.

Hogg: Have you looked at the phenotypic properties of the colonies formed in response to the different CSFs? Walker et al (1981) claimed that a minority of bone marrow-derived macrophage colonies expressed class II molecules, while other colonies were completely negative. It is an attractive idea that different CSFs, although working on the same stem cell, may produce a phenotypically different type of colony.

Nicola: We haven't looked at different phenotypes but it would be very useful if someone would look and see whether macrophages produced by these different CSFs are functionally equivalent or whether subtypes of macrophages are produced.

Stanley: Have you any evidence that the receptors for G-CSF, GM-CSF or Multi-CSF have any ligand-inducible enzyme activities?

Nicola: No, not yet.

Springer: Could you say more about the effects of these factors on the functions of mature cells? Some of the factors have been reported to enhance granulocyte antibody-dependent killing. Weisbart et al (1985) reported that GM-CSF acts as a migration-inhibiting factor for granulocytes and will augment the respiratory burst given by f-Met-Leu-Phe.

Nicola: That was done with human GM-CSF, which has sequence homology with mouse GM-CSF. The original assay was based on migration inhibition. Those workers have also shown that the same molecule enhances the f-Met-Leu-Phe-induced respiratory burst (Weisbart et al 1985). We have been looking at the effect of CSF-stimulation of granulocytes, particularly human granulocytes, on antibody-dependent cell killing, various fluorescence activities, phagocytosis and so on (Vadas & Lopez 1984). We have described two types of human CSF, CSF-α and CSF-β, which appear to be present in most sources of human CSF (Nicola et al 1979). CSF-β is now known to be functionally identical to mouse G-CSF (Nicola et al 1985) and CSF-α is probably the human

GM-CSF that has recently been cloned (Wang et al 1985). Both these molecules stimulate highly purified human neutrophils for antibody-dependent cell killing. Only CSF-α stimulates eosinophils to kill parasites or adhere to them.

The activities ascribed to CSF-α include the production of granulocyte, macrophage and eosinophil colonies in human cultures, whereas CSF-β almost exclusively stimulates granulocytic colonies. In the mouse both GM-CSF and G-CSF stimulate neutrophils. We don't know yet whether Multi-CSF or interleukin 3 stimulate neutrophils or macrophages. There is a fair amount of evidence that M-CSF and GM-CSF stimulate pleiotropic effects in macrophages as well as stimulating plasminogen and activator synthesis and release (Hamilton et al 1980).

Stanley: There is a real problem in resolving primary effects of these growth factors from secondary effects due to their stimulation of the survival of end cells. Direct effects on function are often not clear.

Nicola: Some things happen very rapidly, such as CSF-induced changes in metabolic parameters of eosinophils, where the effect is much more rapid than the rate of death of the cells (Vadas et al 1983). It is, however, a serious problem. In fact in the whole CSF field, since the progenitor cells are dependent on CSF for their survival, people are worried about whether everything else follows as a consequence of that survival.

van Furth: What markers did you use for classifying a cell as a macrophage?

Nicola: We use a non-specific esterase with α-napthylacetate as substrate. All we can say is that they look like monocytes and macrophages.

Dean: You mentioned autofluorescence changes. What kind of fluorophores are you talking about?

Nicola: This is just endogenous autofluorescence at 460 nm and I don't think people are sure what the fluorophores are. It has been suggested that NADPH is responsible for the autofluorescence (Thorell 1981).

Nathan: Interleukin 2, which was once thought to be T-cell-specific, also acts on B cells and perhaps even on other cells. With that in mind, has anyone used purified myeloid CSFs in the improved systems that are now available to see whether they have effects on B cells, T cells or natural killer (NK) cells, either proliferating or differentiating?

Nicola: Not much has been done on endothelial cells, fibroblasts and so on. The original work was with crude spleen-conditioned medium and something in the conditioned medium, thought at that stage to be Multi-CSF, was apparently able to stimulate the production of dispersed colonies which had some of the non-specific killing properties of NK cells (Claesson et al 1982). This is probably an important question for Multi-CSF or interleukin 3 because this has such broad specificities in the whole haemopoietic system that it may also act on other non-haemopoietic cells.

Cohn: In your use of multipotential stem cells as progenitor cells, what type of purity are you talking about? Do you need stromal layers in addition to the different factors?

Nicola: I didn't say much about multipotential stem cells. In the fractionation where we obtained an enriched population of colony-forming cells, at a lower fluorescence cut we can obtain a population of cells enriched in CFU-S and depleted in *in vitro* colony-forming cells. The purity is not very high, only a few per cent, but again it is a population of undifferentiated cells, without any mature cells. Using that population, we have been able to monitor the production of pure colony-forming cells (CFC) over a period of time (Nicola & Johnson 1982). Maximum production of new CFCs occurs at about day 3 to day 5 in that culture system. Of the four CSFs that I discussed today, only Multi-CSF (interleukin 3) was able to stimulate CFC production from this precursor compartment. It produced erythroid-CFC, granulocyte-CFC, macrophage-CFC and mixed-CFC. M-CSF, GM-CSF and G-CSF at that early stage are inactive in producing CFCs from precursor cells whereas Multi-CSF is active. Richard Stanley will probably describe another activity which is not Multi-CSF or interleukin 3 but which may be active even earlier than I have described for interleukin 3 (Jubinsky & Stanley 1985).

Cohn: In that area of so-called committed stem cells, can you differentiate stages of commitment for the factors?

Nicola: There are bipotential cells which can form both granulocytes and macrophages, and there are unipotential cells which appear to be more committed to one cell lineage. I showed a couple of examples of responsiveness to the different CSFs depending on the state of differentiation. Richard Stanley has worked on cells with a very high proliferative potential within the macrophage cell lineage which require factors other than those I described.

Cohn: Do you consider the bipotential cell to be a precursor of the cell which is specifically committed or is it a third pathway?

Nicola: I don't know. The simplest concept would be that multipotential cells give rise to bipotential and then to unipotential cells. But with the high proliferative potential cells there may be an alternative pathway which doesn't go via the bipotential precursor cell but may be direct from a stem cell or progenitor cell which has a very high proliferative capacity and which may be committed exclusively to the macrophage lineage, generating many thousands of cells, all of which will be macrophages.

Werb: M-CSF makes mature or relatively mature macrophages proliferate. Do any of the other factors work on an elicited mature macrophage population?

Nicola: We haven't looked at that. I couldn't find any published reports on whether GM-CSF or Multi-CSF can make elicited macrophages proliferate.

Stanley: We have found that purified GM-CSF stimulates the proliferation of starch-induced peritoneal exudate macrophages, though it is not as effective as

M-CSF (CSF-1) (unpublished work). We have also shown that Multi-CSF (interleukin 3; haemopoietin 2) generates, albeit less effectively, adherent cells from the same cells, or a subpopulation of the same cells, that CSF-1 stimulates to become adherent proliferating mononuclear phagocytes (Bartelmez et al 1985).

van Furth: Is it correct that you only saw proliferation when you used elicited macrophages, not with resident macrophages?

Stanley: We didn't look at resident macrophages in that experiment.

Singer: These are all *in vitro* growth factor effects. Is it possible that *in vivo* a cell–cell interaction directs a greater degree of specificity to macrophage stimulation?.

Nicola: As far as I know, circulating Multi-CSF has never been detected in the serum, whereas G-CSF and something that is immunoreactive with M-CSF antibody are detected in serum and increase several hundredfold after endotoxin injection. One possibility is that the other CSFs don't normally circulate but that their effects are mediated by cell–cell contact, for example in the bone marrow. There are localized pockets of granulopoiesis and erythropoiesis in the bone marrow, and with that cell–cell contact one might expect very rapid induction, for example.

At the Ludwig Institute in Melbourne Gough et al (1985) have been looking at cloned cDNAs from a T-cell line called LB3 and found that LB3 produces two types of message. One message appears to produce a classic secreted protein product, GM-CSF and Multi-CSF. In both cases there is an alternative cDNA which appears to have some of the hallmarks of an integral membrane protein. It certainly has the GM-CSF and Multi-CSF sequence but at its N-terminal end it codes for a hydrophobic region preceded by a sequence containing several charged groups. This is characteristic of a membrane-bound protein. That would be very interesting if, as you suggest, forms of GM-CSF and Multi-CSF produced in the bone marrow are membrane-bound and their effects are localized by cell–cell contact, whereas under other circumstances you can produce a secreted form of CSF which circulates and activates granulocytes and macrophages in the periphery.

Ezekowitz: If you use fluorescence or immunocytochemistry in the bone marrow in places where you expect haemopoiesis to begin, do you see T cells which might be instructing these cells?

Nicola: That is not my area.

Cohn: Differentiating granulocytes normally take about 12 days before the usual pattern of granule formation and nuclear changes is seen. What is the state of differentiation of these cells in culture. Have ultrastructural studies been done?

Nicola: I don't think anyone has looked at that carefully, certainly not in terms of functional activities. It is an important issue. It is a question of whether granulocytes produced by these different CSFs are functionally equivalent and whether they are at equivalent states of differentiation and so on.

Cohn: The nuclear changes are very mature here but there is the question of whether cytoplasm keeps up with this maturation.

Nicola: Most of our work was done in the mouse and in normal stained preparations it is not easy to see large granules. Ultrastructually it should be possible, and some studies have been done (e.g. Shoham et al 1974).

REFERENCES

Bartelmez SH, Sacca R, Stanley ER 1985 Lineage specific receptors used to identify a growth factor for developmentally early hemopoietic cells: assay of hemopoietin-2. J Cell Physiol 122:362-369

Claesson MH, Olsson L, Martinsen L, Brix-Poulsen P 1982 Bone marrow derived diffuse colonies: their cytotoxic potential, morphology, and antigenic phenotype. Exp Hematol (NY) 10:708-721

Gough N, Metcalf D, Gough J, Grail D, Dunn AR 1985 Structure and expression of the mRNA for murine granulocyte-macrophage colony stimulating factor. EMBO (Eur Mol Biol Organ) J 4:645-653

Hamilton JA, Stanley ER, Burgess AW, Shadduck RK 1980 Stimulation of macrophage plasminogen activator activity by colony-stimulating factors. J Cell Physiol 103:435-445

Jubinsky PT, Stanley ER 1985 Purification of hemopoietin 1: A multilineage hemopoietic growth factor. Proc Natl Acad Sci USA 82:2764-2768

Lopez AF, Nicola NA, Burgess AW et al 1983 Activation of granulocyte cytotoxic function by purified mouse colony-stimulating factors. J Immunol 131:2983-2988

Moore RN, Larse HS, Horohov DW, Rouse BT 1984 Endogenous regulation of macrophage proliferative expansion by colony-stimulating factor-induced interferon. Science (Wash DC) 223:178-181

Nicola NA, Johnson GR 1982 The production of committed hemopoietic colony-forming cells from multipotential precursor cells in vitro. Blood 60:1019-1029

Nicola NA, Metcalf D, Johnson GR, Burgess AW 1979 Separation of functionally-distinct human granulocyte-macrophage colony-stimulating factors. Blood 54:614-627

Nicola NA, Begley CG, Metcalf D 1985 Identification of the human analogue of a regulator that induces differentiation in murine leukaemic cells. Nature (Lond) 314:625-628

Shoham D, Ben David E, Rosenszajn LA 1974 Cytochemical and morphological identification of macrophages and eosinophils in tissue cultures of normal human bone marrow. Blood 44:221-223

Stewart CC, Lin H-S 1978 Macrophage growth factor and its relationship to colony stimulating factor. J Reticuloendothel Soc 23:269-285

Thorell B 1981 Flow cytometric analysis of cellular endogenous fluorescence simultaneously with emission from exogenous fluorochromes, light scatter and absorption. Cytometry 2:39-43

Tushinski RJ, Oliver IT, Guilbert LJ, Tynan PW, Warner JR, Stanley ER 1982 Survival of mononuclear phagocytes depends on a lineage-specific growth factor that the differentiated cells selectively destroy. Cell 28:71-81

Vadas MA, Lopez AF 1984 Regulation of granulocyte function by colony stimulating factors. Lymphokine Res 3:45-50

Vadas MA, Varigas G, Nicola NA 1983 Eosinophil activation by colony-stimulating factor in man: metabolic effects and analysis by flow cytometry. Blood 61:1232-1241

Walker WS, Hester RB, Gandour DM, Stewart CC 1981 Evidence of a distinct progenitor for the Ia-bearing (Ia⁺) murine bone marrow-derived mononuclear phagocyte (MNP). In: Forster O, Landy M (eds) Heterogeneity of mononuclear phagocytes. Academic Press, London, p 229-234

Weisbart RH, Golde DW, Clarke SC, Wong GG, Gasson JC 1985 Human granulocyte-macrophage colony-stimulating factor is a neutrophil activator. Nature (Lond) 314:361-363

Wong GG, Witek J, Temple PA et al 1985 Human GM-CSF: molecular cloning of the complementary DNA and purification of the natural and recombinant proteins. Science (Wash DC) 228:810-815

Action of the colony-stimulating factor, CSF-1

E. RICHARD STANLEY

Departments of Microbiology & Immunology, and Cell Biology, Albert Einstein College of Medicine, 1300 Morris Park Avenue, Bronx, NY 10461, USA

Abstract. Colony-stimulating factor 1 (CSF-1) is a glycoprotein growth factor that specifically regulates the survival, proliferation and differentiation of mononuclear phagocytes and their precursors via a cell surface receptor selectively expressed on these cell types. The purified receptor is a single glycosylated polypeptide, M_r 165 000, which exhibits CSF-1-dependent autophosphorylation in tyrosine. CSF-1 alone regulates cells of the mononuclear phagocytic series (CSF-1-dependent colony-forming unit [CFU-C] → monoblast → promonocyte → monocyte → macrophage). However, the presence of a multipotent haemopoietic cell growth factor, haemopoietin-1, permits CSF-1 to stimulate precursors of CFU-C to proliferate and differentiate to macrophages. Precursors of CFU-C possess low levels of the CSF-1 receptor but there is an increase in receptor levels on CFU-C just before their differentiation to adherent, proliferating mononuclear phagocytes. As the timing of this developmentally associated increase in receptor expression coincides with the acquisition of responsiveness to CSF-1 alone, it is an early indicator of determination to the mononuclear phagocytic lineage.

1986 Biochemistry of macrophages. Pitman, London (Ciba Foundation Symposium 118) p 29-41

The colony-stimulating factors (CSFs) regulate the production of mature macrophages and granulocytes from immature cells. The generic name for these growth factors is derived from their action in stimulating individual haemopoietic progenitor cells in culture to form colonies of granulocytes and/or macrophages. One of the CSFs, CSF-1, was defined by its detection in specific radioimmuno- and radioreceptor assays. It was subsequently shown to selectively stimulate the survival, proliferation and differentiation of mononuclear phagocytes (CSF-1-dependent colony-forming cells [CFU-C] → monoblast → promonocyte → monocyte → macrophage). It is found in a wide variety of adult mouse tissues and in the circulation. It is known to be synthesized by cells with fibroblast morphology in the bone marrow and the peritoneal cavity. However, it may well be synthesized by other cell types. CSF-1 is

29

identical to macrophage growth factor and it appears to be the only growth factor specific to mononuclear phagocytes that has been described to date. Results of preliminary *in vivo* studies are consistent with its action as such a growth factor *in vivo* (reviewed in Stanley 1981, Stanley et al 1983).

Structure of CSF-1

CSF-1 has been purified from serum-free medium conditioned by cultured mouse L cells and from human urine (Stanley & Heard 1977, Das et al 1980). It constitutes 10^{-3} of the total protein of L cell-conditioned medium and 10^{-5} of the total protein of normal human urine. The purified CSF-1 is a dimeric glycoprotein of variable M_r (45 000–90 000), composed of two subunits of similar size and charge. The active dimeric form is maintained by disulphide bonds. It is not known whether these bonds are interchain or intrachain or a combination of both types. Mild reduction of CSF-1 even in the absence of dissociating agents results in subunit dissociation and loss of its biological, antibody-binding and receptor-binding activities. Results of studies with endoglycosidases and tunicamycin indicate that the molecule is substantially (40–60%) glycosylated with asparagine-linked 'complex type' oligosaccharides. Neither O-glycosidically linked oligosaccharides, nor N-glycosidically linked oligosaccharides of the high mannose type, were demonstrable. Removal of >80% of the carbohydrate did not result in loss of biological, antibody-binding or receptor-binding activities (Das & Stanley 1982). Thus the carbohydrate moiety does not appear to be necessary for the *in vitro* biological activity of CSF-1. However, it may be important for CSF-1 stability and/or the relative resistance of CSF-1 to attack by proteolytic enzymes.

The molecular weight (M_r) of the polypeptide portion of the subunits of either murine (M_r 66 000) or human (M_r 45 000) CSF-1 was 14 500. Results of partial amino acid sequence determination of L cell CSF-1 (the first 39 amino terminal amino acids and an internal sequence of 23 amino acids) together with fragmentation studies are consistent with a model of CSF-1 composed of two identical subunits. In addition, considerable sequence homology exists between the amino terminal amino acid sequences of murine and human CSF-1 (J. E. Strickler et al, unpublished work 1985).

Interaction of CSF-1 with mononuclear phagocytes

CSF-1 can be radiolabelled with ^{125}I to high specific radioactivity (>300000 c.p.m. per ng) without loss of biological or antibody-binding activity (reviewed in Stanley & Guilbert 1981). The binding reaction between ^{125}I-labelled CSF-1 and murine peritoneal exudate or bone marrow-derived macrophages has been studied in experiments at $0 \, ^\circ C$, pH 7.35. The binding is of high affinity ($K_d \leq 10^{-13}$ M) and is not competed for by other known CSF subclasses, growth factors or hormones. It is saturable within 1 h at a CSF-1 concentration of 2 nM (Guilbert & Stanley 1980). A variety of approaches, including thick-section light autoradiography, temperature jump and pH 4 dissociation experiments, indicate that the bound ^{125}I-labelled CSF-1 is at the cell surface in an unaltered, biologically active state. Kinetic analyses of the binding data at both 4 °C and 37 °C are consistent with the binding of CSF-1 to a single class of binding sites (L. J. Guilbert et al, unpublished work 1985).

[125]I-labelled CSF-1 binding at 4 °C was used to study the distribution, frequency and morphology of binding cells in mouse bone marrow, spleen, blood, peritoneal cavity, alveolar lavage, lymph node and thymus (Byrne et al 1981). These studies indicated that binding is restricted to cells of the mononuclear phagocytic system and that, with the exception of a proportion of alveolar macrophages, virtually all mononuclear phagocytes bind CSF-1, even though in some cases (e.g. resident peritoneal macrophages) binding cells are unable to proliferate in response to CSF-1. In a separate study of ^{125}I-labelled CSF-1 binding by rodent cell lines, binding was also restricted to cells of macrophage or myelomonocytic cell lines (Stanley et al 1984). The CSF-1 binding site is therefore an excellent marker of mononuclear phagocytes, irrespective of their tissue of origin or state of differentiation.

Interaction of ^{125}I-labelled CSF-1 with macrophages at 37 °C is more complex. There is an initial binding reaction ($K_d \sim 0.1$ nM) followed by either dissociation (10%) or internalization (90%) of the bound ligand. Ligand is internalized by receptor-mediated endocytosis. The internalized ^{125}I-labelled CSF-1 is intralysosomally degraded to ^{125}I-labelled tyrosine and released from the cell. The rate of degradation of ^{125}I-labelled CSF-1 is slower in bone marrow-derived macrophages than in peritoneal exudate macrophages and results in a larger accumulation of ^{125}I-labelled CSF-1 in the more primitive bone marrow-derived macrophage population (Stanley & Guilbert 1981, Chen et al 1984, L. J. Guilbert & E. R. Stanley, unpublished work 1985). It is not clear whether increased accumulation of CSF-1 by cells is causally related to an increased proliferative response. However, receptor-mediated endocytosis and intralysosomal destruction of CSF-1 by macrophages is the major mechanism by which CSF-1 is cleared from the circulation (A. Bartocci et al, unpublished work 1985).

The pleiotropic response to CSF-1

CSF-1 generally stimulates the survival, proliferation and differentiation of mononuclear phagocytes. However the response varies with mononuclear phagocyte type. For example, in tissue culture the mature, non-dividing macrophage is only stimulated to survive, whereas the non-adherent CFU-C is stimulated to survive, proliferate and differentiate to adherent proliferating macrophages. Cell biological studies of the action of CSF-1 have mostly been carried out on murine bone marrow-derived macrophages (BMM) (Tushinski et al 1982). BMM are devoid of CSF-1-producing cells (fibroblastoid) and require CSF-1 for survival. Cells can be maintained indefinitely without proliferating if they are cultured with regular medium changes at low concentrations of CSF-1. Most BMM (93–98%) are cycling when cultured in the presence of CSF-1 and about 80% of BMM rendered quiescent by removal of CSF-1 enter DNA synthesis synchronously within 24 h of CSF-1 addition (Tushinski & Stanley 1985).

Addition of CSF-1 to quiescent BMM rapidly causes increased membrane ruffling (at 1–2 min), followed by vacuole formation (within 15 min) (R. J. Tushinski et al, unpublished work 1983). As the vacuoles do not stain with Oil Red O and do not possess demonstrable acid phosphatase, they are probably pinocytic in origin. Within 2 h of CSF-1 addition, the protein synthetic rate is maximally stimulated and this, together with a CSF-1-induced decrease in the rate of intracellular protein degradation, leads to an accumulation of total cell protein which is apparent as little as 2 h after stimulation. The synthetic rate increases linearly with CSF-1 concentration whereas the degradative rate decreases exponentially. As the decrease in degradative rate is small at concentrations above those stimulating BMM survival without proliferation, the inhibition of the protein degradative rate may be an integral part of the mechanism by which CSF-1 induces the survival of BMM (Tushinski & Stanley 1983).

Studies of the regulation of BMM proliferation indicate that the presence of CSF-1 during G_1 phase of the cell cycle is both necessary and sufficient for entry of the cells into S phase and their progression through G_2 and M. Removal of CSF-1 from exponentially growing BMM cultured in medium containing 15% fetal calf serum decreases the rate of DNA synthesis by more than 100-fold. Addition of CSF-1 to these cells causes them to resume DNA synthesis within 10–12 h. The presence of CSF-1 is required for almost the entire lag period for entry of any cells into S phase. After addition of CSF-1 to quiescent BMM, the kinetics of their entry into S phase in the presence and absence of serum is the same (Tushinski & Stanley 1985). Thus, despite evidence that other growth factors (e.g. GM-CSF) can stimulate BMM proliferation, there is no evidence for a dual factor requirement, such as the reported competence and progression functions of platelet-derived growth factor (PDGF) and epidermal growth factor (EGF), respectively, for fibroblastoid cells. CSF-1 possesses both these functions.

The CSF-1 receptor

Kinetic analyses of the binding reaction between ^{125}I-labelled CSF-1 and its cell surface receptor on macrophages at both 4 °C and 37 °C are consistent with the existence of a single class of CSF-1 receptor sites (L. J. Guilbert et al, unpublished work 1985). Chemical cross-linking studies indicate that ^{125}I-labelled CSF-1 bound at the macrophage surface is closely associated with a protein of M_r approximately 165 000, composed of a single polypeptide chain that is not covalently linked to any other protein via disulphide bonds (Morgan & Stanley 1984).

The CSF-1 receptor has been purified (Y. G. Yeung et al, unpublished work 1985) from cells of the J774.2 clone of the J774 mouse macrophage cell line (Diamond et al 1978). Although this line has a relatively low number of receptors per cell ($\sim$20 000) compared with other macrophage cell lines (Morgan & Stanley 1984), it was selected because it can be grown to high cell density in suspension culture. The starting material for the purification is the post-nuclear supernatant fraction obtained after hypotonic swelling and Dounce homogenization of the cells. This membrane preparation (step 1) is concentrated by centrifugation through 15% sucrose (step 2), solubilized (step 3), chromatographed on a CSF-1 affinity column (step 4) and subjected to gel-filtration on Sepharose 6B (step 5). This procedure results in a 7000-fold purification with $\sim$70% recovery of activity. The purification was followed using an ^{125}I-labelled CSF-1 binding assay for the solubilized receptor that is modified from an assay for the solubilized insulin receptor (Cuatrecasas 1972). The purified receptor (step 5) behaves as a single polypetide chain of M_r approximately 165 000 when electrophoresed under reducing conditions on 7% SDS-PAGE and visualized by silver staining. Its apparent M_r is unchanged under non-reducing conditions, indicating that the receptor is a single polypeptide chain. Preincubation of the purified receptor with CSF-1 and subsequent incubation of the complex with [γ-^{32}P]ATP at 4 °C results in phosphorylation of the 165 000 M_r receptor band. Phosphoamino acid analysis of the phosphorylated receptor indicates that the ligand-dependent autophosphorylation is specifically in tyrosine residues. The CSF-1 receptor is therefore similar in properties to the receptors for EGF and PDGF. Because of the close sequence homology between the EGF receptor and the v-erb-B oncogene product, the possible relationship of the CSF-1 receptor to other known oncogenes of the src-related tyrosine kinase family is now being examined.

Biochemistry of CSF-1 action

The mechanisms mediating and coordinating the pleiotropic responses to growth factors are poorly understood. A major problem is determining whether an early event is causally related to a particular biological effect of the growth factor. Because several growth factor receptors are tyrosine kinases, protein phosphorylation is likely to be an important transduction mechanism and we are now investigating this for CSF-1.

In an initial approach to the problem, the CSF-1-dependent increase in protein phosphorylation in isolated membrane preparations was studied. Membrane preparations from three cell populations were incubated at 2 °C with CSF-1 and [γ-^{32}P]ATP. When membrane preparations from cells requiring CSF-1 for growth (BMM, BAC1 cells; Schwarzbaum et al 1984) were studied, there was a CSF-1-dependent increase in the phosphorylation of about 14 proteins. In contrast, the phosphorylation of only three of these proteins was increased in a CSF-1-dependent fashion in membranes from receptor-bearing cells that did not require CSF-1 for growth (J774.2 cells). In each case, one of the proteins phosphorylated possessed the M_r of the CSF-1 receptor (~165 000) (P. T. Jubinsky et al, unpublished work 1985). These phosphorylated proteins are being characterized and identified now. Several approaches are being used to identify which protein phosphorylations are causally related to proliferation.

Action of CSF-1 on precursors of CFU-C

The most primitive haemopoietic cells that are stimulated to proliferate by CSF-1 alone are the CFU-C. However, studies by Bradley, Hodgson and colleagues (Bradley & Hodgson 1979, Bradley et al 1980, Kriegler et al 1982, McNiece et al 1982) indicate that, in the presence of other factors, CSF-1 can stimulate the proliferation of developmentally earlier cells than CFU-C. Thus, despite their inability to respond to CSF-1 alone, precursors to CFU-C must possess CSF-1 receptors. Accordingly, CSF-1 receptor-based methods have been developed to detect and assay growth factors that act on precursors to CFU-C. These procedures involve measuring the increase in the number of CSF-1 receptors in cultures of developmentally early murine bone marrow cells cultured with growth factor preparations (Bartelmez et al 1985).

Two growth factors have been identified by this approach. Haemopoietin-2 (H-2) acts on developmentally earlier cells than CSF-1 alone does and generates cells that respond to CSF-1 alone (Bartelmez et al 1985). However, there is some degree of synergism between H-2 and CSF-1 in the generation of non-adherent mononuclear phagocytes (CFU-C). Purified interleukin-3 (Ihle et al 1982) has similar properties to H-2 and possesses both H-2 and erythroid-burst-promoting activities (reviewed in Bartelmez et al 1985). It is therefore likely that they are identical and that H-2 is a multilineage growth factor.

In contrast to both H-2 and CSF-1, haemopoietin-1 (H-1) alone has no detectable effect on the proliferation and differentiation of primitive haemo-poietic cells. However, in the presence of CSF-1, H-1 stimulates the proliferation and differentiation of developmentally earlier cells than those that respond to either CSF-1 or H-2 alone (Bartelmez & Stanley 1985). Human H-1 has been purified and is a protein of M_r ~17 000 (Jubinsky & Stanley 1985). While pre-CFU-C cultured with CSF-1 plus purified H-1 proliferate and differentiate to macrophages, the proliferation and differentiation of CFU-C and their progeny by CSF-1 is unaffected by H-1. Furthermore, as purified H-1 does not possess erythroid-burst-promoting activity, it is clear that its action in the haemopoietic system is restricted to very early cells. In fact, recent studies indicate that H-1 can synergize with other haemopoietic growth factors, besides CSF-1, to dramatically increase the number of cells forming mixed colonies containing granulocytes, erythroid cells, megakaryocytes and macrophages in semi-solid cultures of primitive cells (E. R. Stanley et al, unpublished work 1985). Thus H-1 clearly regulates the proliferation and differentiation of multipotent cells.

The developmental regulation of the CSF-1 receptor has been studied in cultures of early murine haemopoietic cells incubated with various combinations of H-1, H-2 and CSF-1 (Bartelmez et al 1985, Bartelmez & Stanley 1985). These studies indicate that primitive cells express a low receptor number per cell that dramatically increases (by ~10-fold) on CFU-C just before they differentiate to adherent proliferating mononuclear phagocytes (Fig. 1). The

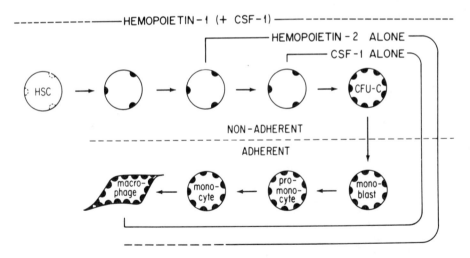

FIG. 1. Postulated expression of the CSF-1 receptor (●) on cells during haemopoiesis, indicating the cell types regulated by the haemopoietins and CSF-1. The presence or absence of the CSF-1 receptor on the haemopoietic stem cell (HSC) has not been established. The effect of H-1 + CSF-1 on adherent cells is indistinguishable from the effect of CSF-1 alone (E. R. Stanley, unpublished work 1984). (Reprinted, with permission, from Bartelmez & Stanley (1985) J Cell Physiol 122:370-378.)

change in receptor density is independent of the growth factor(s) used (CSF-1, H-2, H-1 + CSF-1, H-1 + CSF-1) and of direct effects of these growth factors on receptor levels (e.g. down-regulation). It reflects a developmentally associated increase in the capacity of cells to express the receptor that is correlated with acquisition of responsiveness to CSF-1 alone. As the occurrence of the CSF-1 receptor on later haemopoietic cells is restricted to the mononuclear phagocytic lineage, its increased expression represents a very early marker of determination to this lineage.

Acknowledgements

This work was supported by grants CA26504 and CA32551 from the National Cancer Institute and the AECOM Cancer Centre Core Grant. The author is the recipient of an Irma T. Hirschl Career Scientist Award.

Addendum

Immediately after this meeting, it was shown that the CSF-1 receptor is physio-chemically, immunologically and functionally related to the c-*fms* proto-onco-gene product (Sherr CJ, Rettenmier CW, Sacca R, Roussel MF, Look AT, Stanley ER 1985. The c-*fms* proto-oncogene product is related to the receptor for the mononuclear phagocyte growth factor, CSF-1. Cell 41:665-676).

REFERENCES

Bartelmez SH, Stanley ER 1985 Synergism between hemopoietic growth factors (HGFs) detected by their effects on cells bearing receptors for a lineage specific HGF. Assay of hemopoietin-1. J Cell Physiol 122:370-378

Bartelmez SH, Sacca R, Stanley ER 1985 Lineage specific receptors used to identify a growth factor for developmentally early hemopoietic cells: assay of hemopoietin-2. J Cell Physiol 122:362-369

Bradley TR, Hodgson GS 1979 Detection of primitive macrophage progenitor cells in mouse bone marrow. Blood 54:1446-1450

Bradley TR, Hodgson GS, Bertoncello I 1980 Characteristics of primitive macrophage progenitor cells with high proliferative potential: Their relationship to cells with marrow repopulating ability in 5-fluorouracil treated mouse bone marrow. In: Baum SG et al (eds) Experimental hematology today. Karger, New York, p 284-297

Byrne PV, Guilbert LJ, Stanley ER 1981 The distribution of cells bearing receptors for a colony stimulating factor (CSF-1) in murine tissues. J Cell Biol 91:848-853

Chen BD-M, Kuhn C III, Lin H-S 1984 Receptor-mediated binding and internalization of colony-stimulating factor (CSF-1) by mouse peritoneal exudate macrophages. J Cell Sci 70:147-166

Cuatrecasas P 1972 Isolation of the insulin receptor of liver and fat-cell membranes. Proc Natl
  Acad Sci USA 69:318-322
Das SK, Stanley ER 1982 Structure–function studies of a colony stimulating factor (CSF-1).
  J Biol Chem 257:13679-13684
Das SK, Stanley ER, Guilbert LJ, Forman LW 1980 Discrimination of a colony stimulating
  factor subclass by a specific receptor on a macrophage cell line. J Cell Physiol 104:359-366
Diamond B, Bloom BR, Scharff MD 1978 The F_c receptors of primary and cultured phagocytic
  cells studied with homogeneous antibodies. J Immunol 121:1329-1333
Guilbert LJ, Stanley ER 1980 Specific interaction of murine colony-stimulating factor with mono-
  nuclear phagocytic cells. J Cell Biol 85:153-159
Ihle JN, Keller J, Henderson L, Klein F, Palaszynski E 1982 Procedures for the purification
  of interleukin-3 to homogeneity. J Immunol 129:2431-2436
Jubinsky PT, Stanley ER 1985 Purification of hemopoietin 1: a multilineage hemopoietic growth
  factor. Proc Natl Acad Sci USA 82:2764-2768
Kriegler AB, Bradley TR, Januszewicz E, Hodgson GS, Elms ER 1982 Partial purification and
  characterization of a growth factor for macrophage progenitor cells with high proliferative
  potential in mouse bone marrow. Blood 60:503-508
McNiece IK, Bradley TR, Kriegler AB, Hodgson AS 1982 A growth factor produced by WEHI-3
  cells for murine high proliferative potential GM-progenitor colony forming cells. Cell Biol
  Int Rep 6:243-251
Morgan CJ, Stanley ER 1984 Chemical cross-linking of the mononuclear phagocyte specific
  growth factor CSF-1 to its receptor at the cell surface. Biochem Biophys Res Commun 119:35-41
Schwarzbaum S, Halpern R, Diamond B 1984 The generation of macrophage-like cell lines
  by transfection with SV40 origin defective DNA. J Immunol 132:1158-1162
Stanley ER 1981 Colony stimulating factors. In: Stewart WE, Hadden JW (eds) The lymphokines.
  Humana, Clifton, NJ, p 102-132
Stanley ER, Guilbert LJ 1981 Methods for the purification, assay, characterization and target
  cell binding of a colony stimulating factor (CSF-1). J Immunol Methods 42:253-284
Stanley ER, Heard PM 1977 Factors regulating macrophage production and growth. Purification
  and some properties of the colony stimulating factor from medium conditioned by mouse
  L cells. J Biol Chem 252:4305-4312
Stanley ER, Guilbert LJ, Tushinksi RJ, Bartelmez SH 1983 CSF-1—A mononuclear phagocyte
  lineage-specific hemopoietic growth factor. J Cell Biochem 21:151-159
Stanley ER, Guilbert LJ, Tushinski RJ, Bartelmez SH 1984 Growth factors regulating mononuc-
  lear phagocyte production. In: Volkman A (ed) Mononuclear phagocyte biology. Dekker,
  New York, p 373-387
Tushinski RJ, Oliver IT, Guilbert LJ, Tynan PW, Warner JR, Stanley ER 1982 Survival of mono-
  nuclear phagocytes depends on a lineage-specific growth factor that the differentiated cells
  selectively destroy. Cell 28:71-81
Tushinski, RJ, Stanley ER (1983) The regulation of macrophage protein turnover by a colony
  stimulating factor (CSF-1). J Cell Physiol 116:67-75
Tushinski RJ, Stanley ER 1985 The regulation of mononuclear phagocyte entry into S phase
  by the colony stimulating factor, CSF-1. J Cell Physiol 122:362-369

DISCUSSION

Cohn: You referred to a heavily glycosylated $17\,000\text{-}M_r$ subunit of CSF-1.
Are the other portions of the molecule identical subunits?

Stanley: The molecule is composed of two polypeptide chains of about 14000-M_r that appear to be identical. Each of these chains is glycosylated to the same degree (40–60% of the subunit M_r).

Cohn: And there is covalent linkage?

Stanley: The active dimeric state of the molecule is maintained by disulphide bonds. It is not clear whether these are intra- or inter-chain bonds. However, reduction with 0.1M 2-mercapto ethanol under very mild conditions (pH 8, 20°C, no detergent) results in dissociation of the subunits and loss of biological activity.

Singer: With that high degree of glycosylation the polypeptide subunit may have been a proteolysis fragment, that is part of a polypeptide that was originally an integral protein of the membrane.

Stanley: We are studying that possibility at present. In our laboratory Kelly Price has used the F(ab′)$_2$ fragments of the monoclonal anti-CSF-1 antibody to demonstrate surface immunofluorescence on L cells.

Nathan: Does the protein kinase receptor have GTPase activity? Does it have phosphatidyl inositol kinase activity? And does CSF-1 activate protein kinase C?

Stanley: We haven't tested the purified CSF-1 receptor-kinase for these activities.

Singer: When the *src* oncogene product is activated, a fibroblast that is very flat and sticky can be converted to a round cell that doesn't stick. You seem to be doing the converse, making a non-adherent cell adhere. Could this have something to do with the adherence properties mediated by tyrosine kinases? In preliminary experiments with a monoclonal antibody to phosphotyrosine in a fibroblast culture system and in other cell systems where cell–cell contact is made, we have recently found that this antibody is concentrated at cell junctions where normal cells usually adhere to one another (Maher et al 1985).

Stanley: It is possible that tyrosine phosphorylation is related to the stimulation of macrophage spreading by CSF-1. In our laboratory Rosalba Sacca has recently demonstrated that the addition of CSF-1 to macrophage membrane preparations results in the phosphorylation of several membrane proteins in tyrosine.

Springer: Your 165000-M_r receptor for CSF-1 is similar in M_r to the α chain of Mac-1. It is also increased on macrophages compared to early stem cells, which is similar to the distribution of Mac-1. There seemed to be a band at about 95000 M_r on your gel. Have you checked for a possible identity with Mac-1?

Stanley: Not yet.

Gordon: Another macrophage molecule of 160000 M_r which is remarkably similar in expression is the F4/80 antigen, though ours is a broader band than yours and we use a different labelling system.

Hogg: Waterfield and colleagues (Downward et al 1984) showed that the *erb*-B molecule is part of the EGF receptor, leading to the idea that there is autostimulation via a truncated receptor for receptor adhesion. On your J774 cells which show three bands you have what you think is the receptor. Could the other bands be truncated molecules, analogous to the EGF receptor situation, such that an altered receptor could in some way play a part in the proliferation of these aberrant macrophages?

Stanley: It is conceivable. However J774.2 cells do not require CSF-1 for growth and the three proteins exhibiting increased phosphorylation in J774.2 membrane preparations in response to CSF-1 appear to be a subset of the 14 or so proteins which exhibit CSF-1-dependent increases in phosphorylation in membranes prepared from macrophages requiring CSF-1 for growth.

Ezekowitz: The difference in the kinetics of CSF-1 cycling between the resident cells and the bone marrow cells reminded me of experiments by Besterman et al (1981), who found rapid recycling of fluid-phase reagents by the endosome compartment within 10 to 15 minutes. Does the ligand dissociate at pH 6 or at lower pH values? Alternatively, are there differences in cross-linking of the receptors in the more mature cell which would explain why that needed to be degraded and directed to the lysosome, like the Fc receptors that Melman described?

Stanley: In incubations for 10 minutes at 0°C about 100% of the ^{125}I-labelled CSF-1 bound to the cell surface dissociates at pH 4.0, about 50% at pH 5.0 and none at pH 6.0 (L.J. Guilbert & E.R. Stanley, unpublished work). We have no idea why cells that are apparently more differentiated degrade CSF-1 more rapidly.

Werb: What are the properties of the receptor, in terms of down-regulation, upon treatment with CSF-1 in the two kinds of cells?

Stanley: Down-regulation occurs very rapidly in both cell types. In 1 nM CSF-1, the receptors are almost completely down-regulated. There is no significant difference between the on-rate constant and the off-rate constant of the two different cell types. The difference is solely in the degradation rate constant (L.J. Guilbert et al, unpublished work).

Werb: What is happening when the down-regulated receptors are kept in for 12 hours? The current thinking on EGF is that it doesn't have to go in at all and that a sub-subset of the receptors is important with EGF action, not the most prevalent form that is cleared from the surface when ligand is added.

Stanley: There is no evidence for the same situation with CSF-1. All the evidence is consistent with the existence of a single class of receptor sites at 37°C.

Werb: A small subpopulation of the EGF receptor has a K_d several orders of magnitude higher than the bulk of the EGF receptor, which is a pretty respectable receptor itself.

Stanley: All the data Dr Guilbert and I have assembled are consistent with the existence of a single class of CSF-1 receptor sites on the surface of macrophages.

Cole: The implication is that there must be a distinct increase in the constitutive synthesis of the receptor in the more mature cell. If the receptor on the more mature cell is being destroyed and is not recycling onto the surface, there should be a higher synthetic rate for that receptor if responsiveness is to be maintained.

Stanley: We know little about receptor recycling in the two cell types except that it is relatively low compared with receptor recycling in other systems, e.g. the LDL receptor. The more immature cells accumulate more CSF-1 than the mature cells which degrade it rapidly. However, CSF-1 uptake and degradation studies do not provide information about the destruction or synthesis of the receptor. It is quite possible, therefore, that both cell types have exactly the same rates of receptor synthesis.

Unkeless: Where is haemopoietin-1 made?

Stanley: We have purified it from medium conditioned by the human urinary bladder carcinoma cell line, 5637. It is also found in human placental-conditioned medium and human spleen-conditioned medium. We have no other information on where it is made *in vivo.*

Unkeless: What disorders or diseases might be associated with over-production of these factors?

Stanley: At this point, I'd rather not speculate.

van Furth: In the blood of mice and rabbits we have recently demonstrated, during the early phase of an inflammation, a factor that increases monocytopoiesis (van Waarde et al 1977a,b, Sluiter et al 1983). This factor, FIM, acts only *in vivo*, not *in vitro* It increases the division of promonocytes and monoblasts and the number of promonocytes. It has no chemotactic activity and has no effect on *in vitro* proliferation of bone marrow cells. FIM is not CSF-1, as Richard Stanley has demonstrated with a monoclonal antibody assay. FIM is produced and secreted by macrophages. Recently we demonstrated that it is specific only for mononuclear phagocytes; when we inject serum with FIM we get increased production of monocytes only, not of granulocytes or lymphocytes. FIM is not species-specific. It is not very stable in serum, probably because of proteolysis by enzymes in the serum. It has an M_r of about 20000. It is produced and secreted by macrophages and can be inhibited with protein synthesis inhibitors. It is apparently a factor which is active only *in vivo.* In sum, FIM can be considered as a positive feedback mechanism in the production of macrophage precursors, the monocytes, in the bone marrow.

The activity of FIM seems to be genetically controlled: after an inflammatory stimulus there is an increase in macrophages and monocytes in B10 mice and almost none in CBA mice. We thought that B10 mice might produce FIM while

CBA mice do not, but when we looked for FIM activity with a different method they both made exactly the same amount of FIM.

When we inject serum with a high activity of FIM into B10 mice, they react with an increased production of monocytes, but CBA mice are not responsive (Sluiter et al 1984). Thus macrophages of B10 mice as well as CBA mice produce and secrete FIM, but only in B10 is there a response from monoblasts and promonocytes. We need more purified FIM and a monoclonal antibody to study whether in CBA mice the receptors are lacking or whether an inhibitor is present.

Stanley: We have shown that, *in vitro*, haemopoietin-1 doesn't enhance the effect of CSF-1 on CFU-C or more differentiated mononuclear phagocytes, but we haven't examined its effects *in vivo*.

REFERENCES

Besterman JM, Airhart JA, Woodworth RC, Low RB 1981 Exocytosis of pinocytosed fluid in cultured cells: kinetic evidence for rapid turnover and compartmentation. J Cell Biol 91:716-727

Downward J, Yarden Y, Mayes E et al 1984 Close similarity of epidermal growth factor receptor and v-erb-B oncogene protein sequences. Nature (Lond) 307:521-527

Maher P, Pasquale EB, Wang JYJ, Singer SJ 1985 Phosphotyrosine-containing proteins are concentrated in focal adhesions and intercellular junctions in normal cells. Proc Natl Acad Sci USA, in press

Sluiter W, Elzenga-Claasen I, Hulsing-Hesselink E, van Furth R 1983 Presence of the factor increasing monocytopoiesis (FIM) in rabbit peripheral blood during an acute inflammation. J Reticuloendothel Soc 34:235-252

Sluiter W, Elzenga-Claasen I, van der Voort van der Kley-van Andel A, van Furth R 1984 Differences in the response of inbred mouse strains to the factor increasing monocytopoiesis. J Exp Med 159:524-536

van Waarde D, Hulsing-Hesselink E, Sandkuyl LA, van Furth R 1977a Humoral regulation of monocytopoiesis during the early phase of an inflammatory reaction caused by particulate substances. Blood 50:141-154

van Waarde D, Hulsing-Hesselink E, van Furth R 1977b Properties of a factor increasing monocytopoiesis (FIM) occurring in the serum during the early phase of an inflammatory reaction. Blood 50:727-742

Actin filament architecture and movements in macrophage cytoplasm

JOHN H. HARTWIG

Hematology–Oncology Unit, Harvard Medical School, Cox Building, 6th Floor, Massachusetts General Hospital, Boston, MA 02114, USA

Abstract. Actin filaments are the predominant structural elements in macrophage cortical cytoplasm. These fibres form a unique orthogonal network that fills all lamellae extended from the cell and which, in the cell body, bifurcates to form layers 0.2–0.5 μm thick on the cell top and bottom. Single short filaments, 0.1 μm in length, intersect in space in either T-shaped or X-shaped overlaps to form this ultrastructure. Network assembly and pseudopod extension occur when actin filaments within the network elongate. This filament growth is driven by a large storage pool of actin bound to the sequestering protein, profilin. Elongation is regulated by acumentin, gelsolin and possibly severin, proteins that bind to the end of the filaments, preventing the addition of actin monomers to the filaments. The cytosolic concentration of calcium controls whether filaments assemble or disassemble. Filaments can assemble when the filament ends are not blocked by gelsolin, a condition predicted to occur when the calcium concentration is < 0.1 μm. Orthogonality results when actin filaments are cross-linked by molecules of actin-binding protein.

1986 Biochemistry of macrophages. Pitman, London (Ciba Foundation Symposium 118) p 42-53

Actin is one of the most abundant and conserved of cellular proteins. This globular protein reversibly assembles into filaments that are believed to give shape to cytoplasm, particularly the cell cortex in which most of these filaments reside. By interacting with a number of additional proteins, actin filaments might generate bulk movements of cytoplasm, such as the extension and retraction of pseudopodia. Evidence is increasing that the assembly and organization of actin in macrophages is regulated by a number of actin regulatory proteins (Table 1). Biochemical studies have led to hypotheses that aim to explain the function of actin in cell movement. Here I review how these proteins might interact to generate propulsive cell movements, and I speculate on how cytoplasmic movement is ultimately controlled by membrane receptors.

TABLE 1 Macrophage actin regulatory proteins used in propulsive cell movements

Class	Protein	Structure (kDa)	Function
Filament cross-linking	Actin-binding protein	2×270	Formation of 3-D orthogonol actin network in cell cortex
	α-Actinin	2×100	Promotes the lateral association of actin filaments
Regulation of filament length and assembly	Gelsolin	91	Severs actin filaments at calcium concentration $>0.1\,\mu M$. Remains attached to end of filament having the fastest growth rate, after severing, in a calcium-insensitive fashion
	'Severin'	42	Calcium-reversible binding to the same filament end as gelsolin. Binding promoted by μM calcium
	Acumentin	65	Binds to the opposite end of actin filaments, i.e. end not bound by gelsolin or severin. Limits filament disassembly
Stabilize actin monomers	Profilin	15	Binds actin monomers inhibiting self-nucleation

The three-dimensional organization of actin filaments in macrophage cytoplasm

Actin filaments in macrophage cortical cytoplasm are organized in a three-dimensional network (Hartwig & Stossel 1985). The structure of this network can be revealed by detergent permeabilization of the cells. Figure 1A shows a branching network of actin filaments in the periphery of a macrophage cytoskeleton. Filaments in the network have two features. They are short, of the order of 100 nm in average length, and they intersect with striking perpendicularity.

Two actin filament cross-linking proteins have been purified from macrophages: actin-binding protein (ABP) and α-actinin. Three sets of observations indicate that ABP is responsible for the orthogonality of actin filaments in the cell. First, the bulk of actin cross-linking activity in macrophage extracts is accounted for by ABP (Brotschi et al 1978). Second, actin assembled in the presence of ABP *in vitro* forms a gel composed of perpendicular filament branches (Fig. 1B). Last, ultrastructural studies with anti-ABP IgG and gold particles coated with anti-IgG demonstrate that ABP is located at points of filament intersection in the cell cortex (Fig. 1C). ABP is an extended homo-dimer composed of subunits of 270 kDa. In the electron microscope, individual

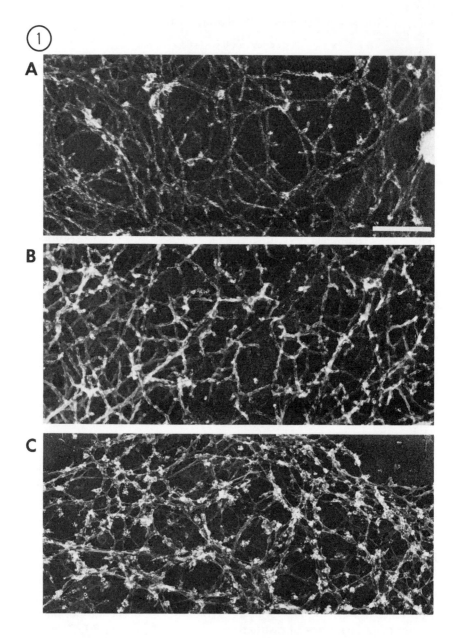

FIG. 1. Comparison of actin filament structure in macrophage cortical cytoplasm (A) with actin filaments assembled in the presence of actin-binding protein (ABP) (B) and ultrastructural localization of ABP in the cortical cytoplasm of a macrophage (C). All samples were prepared for

molecules are flexible strands 3–5 nm in diameter, 160 nm in length, which have binding sites for actin located near their ends (Hartwig & Stossel 1981). Although α-actinin cross-links actin filaments *in vitro*, it does not cause actin to gel at 37 °C, the temperature at which macrophages function (Bennett et al 1984). We have no idea yet of its function *in vivo*.

Activation of cellular movements

Two possible pathways for regulating cytoplasmic actin filament structure have been defined: (1) the mobilization of ionized calcium and (2) protein phosphorylation by protein kinase C. Both are activated when receptors on the cell surface encounter their ligands.

The better understood of the two pathways is calcium mobilization. Binding of chemotactic agents such as fMet-Leu-Phe (Pozzan et al 1983) or the Fc region of IgG, a mediator of phagocytosis (Young et al 1984), to their receptors leads to rapid and reversible increases in cytosolic calcium to micromolar levels (high calcium). Calcium is mobilized from internal pools of unknown composition and from the medium bathing the cells, apparently by moving down a concentration gradient through calcium channels. The mechanism by which the high concentration of calcium is cleared from the cytoplasm after stimulation also remains to be clarified, but it may involve its extrusion through calcium pumps in the plasma membranes (Lew & Stossel 1980). The activation of leucocyte movement with chemotactic agents increases the cellular content of actin filaments (White et al 1982, Krishna & Varni 1982, Howard & Meyer 1984), a finding consistent with the idea that actin assembly provides the mechanical force for cell movement. Furthermore, since actin assembly is inhibited in the presence of cytochalasins, filaments elongate from their high affinity ends. The cytochalasins inhibit actin filament assembly at their fast-growing ends (see below).

The role of inositol phospholipid turnover in cells has only recently been clarified (for review, see Berridge & Irvine 1984). It involves the activation and/or release of a membrane-associated kinase, protein kinase C. Protein kinase C is believed to phosphorylate cytoplasmic proteins, thereby modifying

---

the electron microscope by glutaraldehyde fixation, dehydration in ethanol, critical-point drying in CO_2, and metal coating with platinum and carbon.
A and C: Spread macrophages were treated with 0.75% Triton X-100 in an isotonic buffer containing 10 mM EGTA for 2 min before fixation.
B: Actin was assembled on an electron microscope grid with ABP at a molar ratio of 1 ABP: 50 actin monomers. C: ABP was localized by incubating detergent permeabilized cells with goat anti-ABP IgG and gold particles coated with rabbit anti-goat IgG. The bar represents 100 nm.

their behaviour. One example of a leucocyte movement that may be activated by the inositol pathway is C3-coated particle ingestion (D. Stendahl & P. D. Lew, personal communication), a process that occurs without measurable increases in cytosolic calcium concentrations. Furthermore, cellular activation by phorbol myristate acetate has been demonstrated to occur through the direct activation of kinase C, while cytoplasmic calcium in cells is decreased below basal levels (DiVirgilio et al 1984). It has been recently demonstrated that phorbol esters also cause a net increase in f-actin content in leucocytes (White et al 1984). Therefore, a second, calcium-independent, mechanism exists that can affect the state of cellular actin assembly.

Propulsive cell movements

To understand the regulation of actin filament assembly in cells it is first necessary to review briefly the mechanism by which pure actin assembles (Fig. 2). This involves two main steps. The first step, which is rate-limiting, is the self-aggregation of two or three actin monomers into stable complexes called nuclei. In a second, more rapid, step filaments elongate as monomers assemble onto the ends of the nuclei. These are polarized structures and monomers do not add at equal rates to the two filament ends. One end, with a higher affinity for monomer, grows faster than the other end. This fast-growing end corresponds to the 'barbed end' of filaments that have been labelled with the myosin fragment, heavy meromyosin.

A large fraction of actin, approximately 30–40% of the total cellular actin, exists as monomers in complex with a protein called profilin. This large pool of actin is stable because profilin inhibits the aggregation of actin into short oligomers or nuclei which can serve as sites for filament growth. Filament assembly occurs from the profilin–actin complex only in the presence of actin nuclei, and only the high affinity ends of nuclei or larger actin oligomers (filaments) are capable of abstracting actin from profilin. Monomers dissociating from the filament ends can be trapped by uncomplexed profilin, a condition that occurs slowly when the high affinity filament end is capped *in vitro* (DiNubile & Southwick 1985). In cells, such disassembly may occur even more slowly because of the presence of acumentin, a protein that binds to the slow-growing ends of actin filaments, inhibiting monomer release at this end (Southwick & Hartwig 1982, DiNubile & Southwick 1985).

To maintain a profilin–actin pool, resting cells prevent the exposure of fast-growing actin filament ends. Two proteins have been purified from macrophages that bind to the fast-growing filament end of actin, thereby preventing monomer additions at this end. They are gelsolin (Yin et al 1981) and a recently discovered 42 kDa protein (Southwick & DiNubile 1984). As indicated in Table 1, both of these proteins require micromolar levels of calcium for binding to actin. However, once gelsolin has bound to filament ends *in vitro*, it remains associated even in the presence of EGTA (Bryan & Kurth 1984, Janmey et al 1985). Complex formation has also been demonstrated in platelets *in vivo* which, on stimulation with thrombin to increase cytosolic calcium, have the bulk of their cellular gelsolin converted into stable gelsolin–actin complexes (Kurth & Bryan 1984). Therefore, the monomeric actin pool

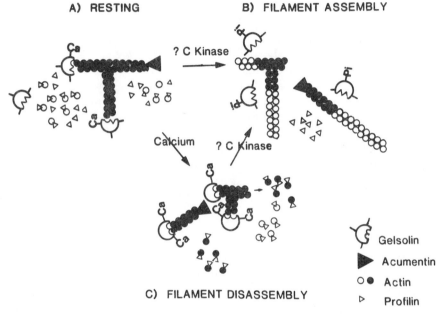

FIG. 2. Regulation of filament assembly and disassembly by macrophage proteins and its hypothetical control by ionized calcium and protein kinase C.

A: *Resting state of cell.* It is assumed that in a resting state all actin filaments comprising the cortical filament network are cross-linked by ABP molecules and are capped at the fast-growing end by gelsolin while the slow-growing end is stabilized by acumentin. A pool of profilin–actin complexes exists as well as free molecules of profilin.

B: *Filament assembly.* For filaments to elongate, gelsolin must be dissociated from the (+) filament end. Free (+) ends will dissociate profilin–actin complexes, resulting in net filament assembly. Activation of gelsolin to dissociate may be mediated by protein kinase C. The modified gelsolin is indicated by the addition of Pi- (phosphate). Phosphorylation of gelsolin molecules capping the (+) filament ends would result in the dissociation of gelsolin.

C: *Filament disassembly.* A large excess of free profilin was generated when filaments were assembled in B above. After activation, the stimulus for assembly diminishes, allowing free profilin to compete successfully with acumentin for monomers at the low affinity filament end. This process is calcium-triggered and two calcium molecules are bound per gelsolin molecule, indicated by the addition of Ca to gelsolin. Increases in cytosolic calcium activate gelsolin to fragment actin filaments and cap the high affinity ends of these fragments.

in resting macrophages could remain stable because gelsolin can form a calcium-insensitive complex on the fast-growing end of actin filaments. In marked contrast to platelets, however, the bulk of cellular gelsolin is free in the cytoplasm of macrophages. Therefore, this population of gelsolin can respond to increased cytoplasmic calcium by fragmenting actin filaments and binding to the high affinity ends of the fragmented filaments (Fig. 2). The role in this process of the 42 kDa protein, a molecule which also binds to the high affinity filament ends, is not yet clear.

If actin filaments in macrophage cytoplasm can become irreversibly capped in the presence of high cytosolic calcium, how do agents such as fMet-Leu-Phe, which increase cytoplasmic calcium, mediate filament assembly? Two possibilities exist: (1) gelsolin-capped filament ends could become unblocked, and/or (2) additional protein(s) could nucleate filament assembly by exposing sites equivalent to the fast-growing end of actin filaments, since actin assembly, as mentioned above, is cytochalasin-sensitive. Of the two mechanisms, the former is the more likely, since macrophages are able to maintain high levels of uncomplexed gelsolin. Moreover, it has recently been observed that after stimulation of macrophages with fMet-Leu-Phe to mobilize calcium, the stable gelsolin–actin complex that is formed rapidly reverses (C. Chaponnier, personal communication), indicating that a mechanism exists in macrophages to dissociate actin–gelsolin complexes (Fig. 2). One possibility is the phosphorylation of gelsolin by protein kinase C. Phosphorylation of gelsolin would cause it to dissociate from actin. This would make free fast-growing filament ends available, thereby generating actin filament growth from the profilin–actin pool. Once assembled, new filaments could become integrated into the cortical actin network by associating with ABP. Such dissociation of gelsolin from the fast-growing filament ends when phosphorylated would also provide an explanation for the calcium-independent activation of actin assembly when leucocytes are exposed to phorbol esters (Fig. 2).

Acknowledgements

This work was supported by NIH grant HL 27971 and a grant from the Council for Tobacco Research.

REFERENCES

Bennett JP, Zaner KS, Stossel TP 1984 Isolation and some properties of macrophage α-actinin: evidence that it is not an actin gelling protein. Biochemistry 23:5081-5086
Berridge MJ, Irvine RF 1984 Inositol triphosphate, a novel second messenger in cellular signal transduction. Nature (Lond) 312:315-321

Brotschi EA, Hartwig JH, Stossel TP 1978 The gelation of actin by actin-binding protein. J Biol Chem 253:8988-8993

Bryan J, Kurth MC 1984 Actin–gelsolin interactions. Evidence for two actin-binding sites. J Biol Chem 259:7480-7487

DiNubile MJ, Southwick FS 1985 Effects of macrophage profilin on actin in the presence and absence of acumentin and gelsolin. J Biol Chem 260:7402-7409

DiVirgilio F, Lew PD, Pozzan T 1984 Protein kinase C activation of physiological processes in human neutrophils at vanishingly small cytosolic Ca^{2+} levels. Nature (Lond) 310:691-693

Hartwig JH, Stossel TP 1981 The structure of actin-binding protein molecules in solution and interacting with actin filaments. J Mol Biol 145:563-581

Hartwig JH, Stossel TP 1985 The 3-D organization of actin filaments in motile cytoplasm. J Cell Biol 101:275a

Howard TH, Meyer WH 1984 Chemotactic peptide modulation of actin assembly and locomotion in neutrophils. J Cell Biol 98:1265-1271

Janmey PA, Chaponnier C, Lind SE, Zaner KS, Stossel TP, Yin HL 1985 Interactions of gelsolin and gelsolin:actin complexes with actin. Effects of calcium on actin nucleation, filament severing and end blocking. Biochemistry 24:3714-3723

Krishna KM, Varani J 1982 Actin polymerization induced by chemotactic peptide and concanavalin A in rat neutrophils. J Immunol 129:1605-1607

Kurth M, Bryan J 1984 Platelet activation induces the formation of a stable gelsolin–actin complex from monomeric gelsolin. J Biol Chem 259:7473–7479

Lew PD, Stossel TP 1980 Calcium transport by macrophage plasma membranes. J Biol Chem 255:5841-5846

Pozzan T, Lew PD, Wollheim CB, Tsien RY 1983 Is cytosolic ionized calcium regulating neutrophil activation? Science (Wash DC) 221:1413-1415

Southwick FS, DiNubile MJ 1984 Macrophages contain a fragmin/severin-like protein. J Cell Biol 99:308a

Southwick FS, Hartwig JH 1982 Acumentin, a protein in macrophages which caps the 'pointed' end of actin filaments. Nature (Lond) 297:303-307

White JR, Naccache PH, Sha'afi RI 1982 The synthetic chemotactic peptide formyl-methionyl-leucyl-phenylalanine causes an increase in actin associated with the cytoskeleton in rabbit neutrophils. Biochem Biophys Res Commun 108:1144-1149

White JR, Huang C-K, Hill JM Jr, Naccache PH, Becker EL, Sha'afi RI 1984 Effect of phorbol 12-myristate 13-acetate and its analogue 4-phorbol 12,13-didecanoate on protein phosphorylation and lysosomal enzyme release in rabbit neutrophils. J Biol Chem 259:8605-8611

Yin HL, Hartwig JH, Maruyama K, Stossel TP 1981 Ca^{2+} control of actin polymerization. Interaction of macrophage gelsolin with actin monomers and effects on actin polymerization. J Chem Biol 256:9693-9697

Young JD, Ko SS, Cohn ZA 1984 The increase in intracellular free calcium associated with IgGγ2b/γ1 Fc receptor–ligand interactions: role in phagocytosis. Proc Natl Acad Sci USA 81:5430-5434

DISCUSSION

Singer: How does this work fit in with the idea that local changes in ATP and ADP concentration can have an effect on actin assembly and disassembly?

Hartwig: There is a controversy about that. Actin assembly seems to require ATP but the rate of hydrolysis of ATP is not completely related in time-scale to assembly at the end of the filament. Some people believe the filament is capped with ATP–actin and that the interior of the filament contains ADP– actin. So when a filament is cut in the ADP region, a rapid total disassembly of the filament occurs because there are no longer any ATP caps to keep the filament stable at the ends. But I don't think there are any data on the rates of actin disassembly in cells *in vivo*. *In vitro*, where one may have a complete ATP filament, one does not see a rapid disassembly and reassembly to a given state: the filament simply disassembles to the cut state and stays there.

Singer: In connection with microtubule assembly, GTP–GDP conversion is mediated by calcium, so it is possible that calcium might affect ATP–ADP conversion too.

Hartwig: It is a possibility but there is no evidence yet. The rate of actin incorporation in monomers is incredibly fast. In pulse chase studies with labelled actin, the actin becomes associated with the filaments within seconds of coming off the ribosome, though that says nothing about disassembly.

Cohn: Do there have to be attachments with membranes, or do the membranes conform to the structure of the underlying matrix?

Hartwig: In the simple propulsive type of movement I talked about, attachments with membranes are not needed. Clearly, however, there are attachments of actin filaments with membranes. If one wants to put retractive force on membrane there must be attachments. The clearest example of that is in platelets with glycoprotein G1b which acts as an attachment protein between platelets and transmits retractive force between platelets.

In platelets there is evidence suggesting that the attachment of f-actin to G1b occurs through actin-binding protein (ABP). Immunoprecipitation studies show co-precipitation of the receptor and ABP. We don't yet know the stoichiometry of this interaction but there seems to be a site on ABP molecules for binding the receptor. A number of other proteins are also likely candidates for attaching actin to membrane. These include the non-erythroid spectrins, a group of unambiguous membrane-associated proteins, and vinculin, which may interact with other membrane molecules and actin filaments.

Singer: There is a temporal problem, as you said. Different steps occur at different times along the way and it isn't clear how they are all integrated. For example an important element in cell movement, but one that doesn't show up until later than the time range of seconds that you are talking about, is the insertion of new membrane mass into the leading edge of the cell. That is, there is not only an internal force-generating system propelling the cytoplasm but also new membrane mass has to be inserted into the leading edge. A macrophage treated with monensin becomes immobile, presumably not because of any effect on the actin structure, which looks the same, but rather because monensin inhibits the incorporation of new membrane mass derived from the Golgi. Insertion of new membrane mass probably takes some minutes. The time-scale here is a very critical factor in the succession of events leading to motility.

Hartwig: Insertion at the front edge of these cells is an attractive idea. Some of the published work is not totally convincing and there is some evidence, at least in fibroblasts, that insertion occurs at the very edges of the ruffles. I don't think there is any evidence in other cells that is believable.

Cohn: Would you expect something similar to happen with particle ingestion?

Hartwig: Your work (Young et al 1984) indicates that Fc-mediated phagocytosis occurs similarly, since that seems to lead to an increase in cytoplasmic calcium. We haven't looked at any other events except phorbol ester stimulation of these cells. We had hoped that when we stimulated with phorbol this would result in C kinase-mediated phosphorylation of gelsolin, which would inactivate it and allow filament assembly. That is clearly not the case: no phosphate is incorporated into gelsolin. Even more curious is that phorbol makes the complex formation between gelsolin and actin totally irreversible. We see complete complexing of gelsolin in 0–5 min, the sort of time-scale that one sees for actin assembly. There is no inactivation of complex formation under these conditions so we have very little idea how that is occurring.

One possibility is that the treatment of cells with phorbol ester is leading to the formation of other active metabolites. The evidence is still very preliminary but Lassing & Lindberg (1985) have shown that phosphatidylinositol 4,5-biphosphate can cause the profilin–actin complex to dissociate, which could lead to filament assembly in cells. How one would integrate that with the other macrophage actin regulatory proteins is very hard to know at this point, particularly under conditions where gelsolin is complexed and one would expect it to be capping filaments as they start to form. We have no idea what is going on with the protein C kinase pathway or inositol turnover.

Nathan: Doesn't a calcium-independent stimulus lead to assembly of the same meshwork that you showed us for f-Met-Leu-Phe? If so, doesn't that challenge the whole hypothesis of the involvement of increased intracellular calcium?

Hartwig: It is naive to say that if phorbol esters are present no calcium is released. There might be a localized release so that you would not see it. The fact that gelsolin becomes complexed suggests that there may be a calcium flux. Phorbol, however, does not activate the pathway which causes gelsolin to dissociate from the filament end.

Tremendous pseudopods form and extend in these phorbol-treated cells, which become incredibly filled with a meshwork very similar to the one that develops in spreading cells, at least in high concentrations.

Nathan: Is the requirement of gelsolin for calcium to cap the filament end different from its requirement to bind along the filament? This seemed to be an essential part of your hypothesis about how a calcium flash gets filaments to fragment and then reassemble.

Hartwig: I don't think there is any change in affinity of gelsolin for calcium. Calcium binding leads to filament breakage by a totally unknown mechanism and then to capping of the filament ends. I think this has more to do with the fact that there are two sites for actin on gelsolin. When gelsolin is completely saturated with calcium it has two sites for actin monomers, whereas in EGTA it has only one site for actin. The net affinity in EGTA is therefore lower than in calcium for actin filaments. It is about 10^{-10} M in the presence of calcium and an order of magnitude less with EGTA.

Aderem: Is the Ca^{2+} released when the gelsolin–actin complex disassembles?

Hartwig: Free gelsolin in micromolar calcium binds two calcium molecules. When EGTA is added, one calcium remains irreversibly bound. This calcium ion is always bound and when calcium is added again the second site is resaturated. Once you have made a complex you have presumably, by a tertiary conformation of molecules, trapped calcium, at least *in vitro*. In the cell it seems likely that this calcium ion is somehow being removed because there is complete dissociation of the complex.

Singer: Have you an antibody that inhibits the binding of gelsolin to actin?

Hartwig: I wish we had. As I mentioned, Dr Helen L. Yin and her collaborators have shown, by limited proteolysis of gelsolin, that two actin-binding domains, one calcium-insensitive and one calcium-sensitive (Kwiatkowski et al 1984) exist in the native protein. The smallest fragment that binds actin EGTA is a 14 kDa peptide. Dr Yin is now using this fragment to make monoclonal antibodies. None of the monoclonals we have now inhibit gelsolin functions.

Singer: Presumably if you microinject such an antibody into macrophages, you might specifically inhibit motility?

Hartwig: It is a little hard to microinject a macrophage.

Werb: How many of these reactions occur at 2°C or 4°C as well as at 37°C, in terms of cross-linking or uncross-linking? It is pretty clear that with frustrated phagocytosis some actin foci form at the sites of ligand–receptor interaction.

Hartwig: Actin assembly occurs in the cold but at a slower pace. The actin filament cross-linking ability of α-actinin is much tighter in the cold. But it depends how you assay. The binding affinity of α-actinin to actin goes up in the warm. If you use a gelation assay as a valid test for cross-linking then it is promoted by low temperatures. However, I think that is simply an effect of temperature on actin filament length and not to do with interaction of α-actinin and actin. Further, in the cold, the cytoplasmic calcium concentations are probably perturbed, and many reactions activated by calcium may affect cellular function and actin structure.

Werb: In macrophages the phorbol diester promotes spreading. In fibroblasts it does exactly the opposite. Could that be due to the accessory proteins such as gelsolin and ABP being present in different cells at very different ratios? What are the ratios, at least in the macrophage?

Hartwig: Fibroblasts have stress fibres, don't they.

Werb: The stress fibres disappear.

Hartwig: If the cell is going to move it has to get rid of the stress fibres first. So if one waits long enough, do they orient and start moving? I think they do if you don't give them so much phorbol that you kill them.

In macrophages about 1% of the total cell protein is gelsolin and about 10% is actin, with a molar ratio of about 1:25, so there is quite a bit of this protein in the cell. It is interesting that only a small amount, between 5 and 30%, of the total gelsolin goes into the cytoskeleton. This works out to one gelsolin molecule for every 0.5 μm of filaments, which is of the order of the observed length of filaments in the cytoskeleton. Which is to say, there is theoretically enough gelsolin in the cytoskeleton to cap every filament.

Werb: What about ABP and the other proteins?

Hartwig: ABP is there in a lower molar ratio of about 1:100 (ABP:actin). Acumentin constitutes about 5% of the total cell protein, a high 1:2 molar ratio to actin. I don't think anybody has ever completely figured out how much profilin is in cells, particularly the amount of free profilin.

Cohn: Obviously a great deal of soluble gelsolin is present. If you calculate the amount that is bound, how much does this work out at?

Hartwig: The resting amount of bound gelsolin varies. About 20 to 30% is soluble and always bound to actin. When macrophages are stimulated with f-Met-Leu-Phe that figure goes up to 100% (1 mole of actin to 1 mole of gelsolin), then returns to 30% as the calcium concentration comes back to the basal level. Under specific conditions one can wash off all the actin except what is specifically bound to the gelsolin and get a precise count.

Singer: The subtlety of that is that in a uniform solution, the f-Met-Leu-Phe is all around the cell. In a gradient presumably only the forward end of the cell would be affected.

Hartwig: Yes. That fits into the much more complicated mechanics of cell movement to which you referred earlier. We are nowhere near understanding chemotaxis.

REFERENCES

Kwiatkowski DJ, Mole JE, Yin HL 1984 Plasma gelsolin contains two actin binding sites, one calcium sensitive and one calcium insensitive. J Cell Biol 99:306a

Lassing I, Lindberg U 1985 Specific interaction between phosphatidylinositol 4,5 bisphosphate and profilactin. Nature (Lond) 314:472-474

Young JD-E, Ko SS, Cohn ZA 1984 The increase in intracellular free calcium associated with IgGγ2b/γ1 Fc receptor-ligand interactions: role in phagocytosis. Proc Natl Acad Sci USA 81:5430-5434

Localization and function of tissue macrophages

SIAMON GORDON*, PAUL R. CROCKER*, LYNN MORRIS*, SZU HEE LEE*, V. HUGH PERRY[†] and DAVID A. HUME[a]

*Sir William Dunn School of Pathology and [†]Experimental Psychology, University of Oxford, South Parks Road, Oxford OX1 3RE, UK

[a]Present address: John Curtin School of Medical Research, Garran, A.C.T. 2606, Australia

Abstract. The rat monoclonal antibody F4/80 defines a plasma membrane glycoprotein of about 160 kilodaltons that is expressed by mature mouse macrophages. The antigen has been used to define macrophage distribution within the mouse (normal adult, embryo, infection models) by cytochemistry and quantitative immunochemical analysis. Macrophages migrate into fetal and adult haemopoietic and other tissues in an ordered sequence. The surface properties of 'fixed' macrophages isolated from various organs (bone marrow, liver, spleen) are distinct from those of circulating monocytes or free cells (peritoneal and pleural cavities, alveolar) and may play a role in local adhesion and trophic interactions with other cells.

1986 Biochemistry of macrophages. Pitman, London (Ciba Foundation Symposium 118) p 54-67

Antigen F4/80 is a pan-macrophage marker (Austyn & Gordon 1981) expressed by monocytes and macrophages in many tissues of the mouse. The epitope defined by rat monoclonal F4/80 is relatively stable to glutaraldehyde perfusion fixation and embedding, so immunocytochemical studies with the avidin–biotin–peroxidase method have revealed its presence on the plasma membrane of macrophages in many sites with high selectivity and good preservation of morphology. F4/80-positive cells are rounded ('monocyte-type') or stellate and include most members of the mononuclear phagocyte system defined by other criteria in haemopoietic and lymphoid organs (Hume et al 1983a), as well as cells in skin (Langerhans cells), the central nervous system (microglia) (Hume et al 1983b), gut (Hume et al 1984a), kidney (Hume & Gordon 1983), endocrine organs (Hume et al 1984b) and elsewhere (Hume et al 1984c). Apart from immature precursors (Hirsch et al 1981), there may be F4/80-negative macrophages in adult spleen (Witmer & Steinman 1984) and gut-associated lymphoid tissue (D. A. Hume, unpublished). Osteoclasts and Steinman–Cohn dendritic cells from spleen lack F4/80, but it is not clear whether they represent distinct lineages of bone marrow origin. Extensive studies of isolated cells and those in normal adult, fetal and reactive tissues have failed to reveal F4/80 labelling of cells which are not macrophages. Generally, studies with other specific antibodies have given similar results, although these macrophage antigens have sometimes not been detected on cells in certain tissues (e.g. Kupffer cells [Flotte et al 1983], microglia) or from other species (e.g. human Langerhans cells). These differences may be technical (antigen lability) or due to differential expression of markers and thus a reflection of heterogeneity among macrophages, resulting from cell maturation or modulation in their local environment, or both. A recent study by Perry et al (1985) has shown a similar distribution of three different macrophage antigens on microglia (F4/80, Mac-1: Springer et al 1979; type 3 complement receptor, CR3; and 2.4G2 [IgG1/2b Fc receptor]: Unkeless 1979), providing further evidence for the use of F4/80 as a valid probe for detecting macrophages in tissues. Lee et al (1985) have taken advantage of the specificity of F4/80 antibody to develop a quantitative adsorption immunoassay for measuring the F4/80 content of tissues without cell isolation and thus for estimating macrophage numbers in various organs directly. Results were in excellent agreement with those obtained by immunocytochemistry and confirmed that gut, liver, bone marrow, spleen and kidney are major sites of macrophage distribution.

These studies give rise to many interesting questions. How and when do macrophages enter tissues? How do they respond to their local environment? What is their function in different sites? In this paper we review some of our current experiments designed to study these problems. Experimental details will be reported in full elsewhere.

Macrophage distribution in adult mice

In the normal adult mouse, macrophages in tissues originate mostly from bone marrow precursors via delivery of blood monocytes. In the mouse, the spleen also retains haemopoietic activity, so it contains locally derived immature stages of macrophage development as well as blood-derived macrophages (van Furth & Diesselhoff-den Dulk 1984). The extent to which proliferation of macrophages continues in other sites such as lung, peritoneal cavity and liver has not been fully determined, although some evidence would support significant local production under steady-state conditions (Volkman et al 1984). During inflammation and many infections there can be massive increased recruitment, enhanced production in the bone marrow and an increase in macrophage turnover (Spector & Ryan 1970).

Studies of antigen F4/80 localization in normal adult mice show a pattern of distribution of 'resident' macrophages according to a likely route of migration from blood. F4/80-positive cells are found within vessels, adhering to vascular endothelium, as sinusoid-lining cells (e.g. liver, adrenal), in pericapillary sites (e.g. gut, brain) or in an interstitial location. An association with epithelia can also be discerned (Hume et al 1984a). F4/80-positive cells, often characteristically stellate, occur beneath epithelia, outside the basement membrane (e.g. kidney, gut) or between cells of simple epithelia (e.g. within duct epithelium of salivary glands), or they penetrate complex epithelia (Langerhans-type cells in basal layer of skin, cervix; throughout the full thickness of transitional epithelium of bladder). Macrophages can migrate as 'free' cells across epithelia and mesothelia into serosal cavities, the alveolar space and into secretions. This distribution implies that (a) there are mechanisms enabling monocytes to adhere to endothelium and leave the circulation normally, without obvious inflammatory stimuli, (b) cells migrate until they become arrested in specific sites, and (c) tissue macrophages become involved in diverse local interactions, e.g. with connective tissue matrix and many different cell types, e.g. in epidermis and brain.

After the initial period of macrophage recruitment during development (to be considered further below), macrophages persist in certain sites (e.g. retina, central nervous system) throughout adult life. It is not clear whether they are continuously replaced from blood at low levels or by local production, whether migration from blood occurs randomly or at selected sites, and how rapidly resident macrophages turn over. Macrophages recruited to sites of inflammation and infection are less mature, retain the ability to proliferate, and display phenotypic changes characteristic of 'activated' cells such as enhanced respiratory burst activity. These cells become localized in focal lesions (e.g. in mycobacterial granulomata [S. Rabinowitz, unpublished]) or exhibit an apparently normal distribution within tissues (e.g. Kupffer cells in malaria [S. H. Lee, unpublished]). Recruitment during inflammation probably involves different chemotactic agents from those active during normal development and is associated with pronounced changes in vascular permeability and marked regional differences in localization.

Both quantitatively and qualitatively it is likely that these recently recruited macrophages contribute more to cell-mediated immunity than resident cells; the functions of the resident tissue macrophages are less clear. Apart from first-line host defence (e.g. along portals of entry), we suspect that these cells perform important local functions in different tissues, perhaps of a trophic nature. Macrophages are able to produce a large variety of secretory products and express surface molecules which endow them with the potential to interact with many different cells and molecules in their local environment. However, these properties have been defined on peritoneal, blood or bone marrow culture-derived macrophages and there is very little information concerning the phenotype of tissue macrophages, which are considerably more difficult to isolate. Studies with resident macrophages from bone marrow, liver and spleen have revealed several novel features which distinguish some 'fixed' from 'free' macrophages and make it likely that resident macrophages perform important regulatory functions in haemopoietic and lymphoid tissues in addition to their phagocytic activity. Little is known about tissue macrophages in other sites.

Resident macrophages in bone marrow stroma

Labelling of active femoral marrow *in situ* revealed F4/80-positive cells with long processes at the centre of haemopoietic islets, as well as small numbers of developing monocytes (Hume et al 1983a). Mature macrophages identified in marrow on morphological grounds were thought to participate mainly in phagocytosis, e.g. of erythrocyte nuclei, but other possible macrophage functions within the stromal microenvironment have received little experimental support. Mature macrophages in bone marrow are associated with erythroid and myeloid cells, but other stromal cells, e.g. alkaline phophatase-positive fibroblastoid cells may also play a role in haemopoiesis (Westen & Bainton 1979). The long-term bone marrow culture system devised by Dexter (1982) to retain haemopoietic activity *in vitro* contains an adherent stromal layer which is rich in macrophages, but in addition contains fibroblasts ('blanket cells'), adipocytes and other cells. F4/80-positive macrophages in these cultures are also associated with developing myeloid and erythroid cells (P. Simmonds, unpublished).

In order to define the function of stromal macrophages we have used collagenase digestion to isolate haemopoietic clusters from mouse bone marrow (P. Crocker, unpublished). These contain central F4/80-positive macrophages with extended plasma membrane processes which are intimately associated with erythroid and myeloid cells. The clusters adhere to glass via their central macrophages, which can be stripped free of other cells for further characterization. Few alkaline phosphatase-positive cells are present in these preparations. The central mature macrophages also express other macrophage markers (Fc and mannosyl, fucosyl receptors), and, unlike resident peritoneal macrophages, they express Ia antigen but no Mac-1 antigen. In addition they express a novel receptor which produces rosetting of sheep erythrocytes (see below). The resident bone marrow macrophages show evidence of phagocytic activity (e.g. erythrocyte debris in vacuoles), but haemopoietic cells clustered on their surface proliferate vigorously. The nature of the macrophage/haemopoietic cell interaction is under study.

Macrophage ontogeny and role in fetal haemopoiesis

During fetal life haemopoietic activity appears sequentially in a well-ordered process in yolk sac (day 8) and liver (day 11) before localizing in spleen (day 15) and bone marrow (day 17). It is assumed that stem cells migrate to each site, but little is known about the role of the microenvironment in this remarkable process. The stroma may also regulate the nature of haemopoiesis, especially erythropoiesis, which differs in the yolk sac and subsequent stages (Labastie et al 1984). Studies with antibody F4/80 (G. Shia, unpublished; L. Morris, unpublished) reveal stellate macrophages with striking erythroid clusters from the fetal liver stage of haemopoiesis, but not in yolk sac. These stromal-type F4/80-positive macrophages in fetal liver appear one to two days before overt signs of erythrocyte production. In the yolk sac, monocyte-like F4/80-positive macrophages appear *after* erythroid stages, at day 9–10, and without morphological evidence of specific association with haemopoietic cells. Since immature macrophage progenitors lack F4/80 antigen it seems likely that the yolk sac cells are the first mature macrophages found in the embryo, presumably derived from the same stem cells as give rise to the erythroid series, but not able to function as stromal cells. Since F4/80-positive macrophages are able to produce erythropoietin, e.g. under hypoxic conditions (I. Rich, personal communication), it is possible that stromal-type macrophages control terminal erythroid differentiation in liver, but not yolk sac, where this does not occur.

How then do stromal macrophages arise in fetal liver? Presumably by migration of progenitors or their products from the yolk sac via early vascular channels. F4/80-positive macrophages also appear widely in the mesenchymal tissue of the embryo from day 10, especially at sites of active tissue remodelling (G. Shia, unpublished), and become evident in developing non-haemopoietic organs such as gut and kidney. The recruitment of monocytes into retina (Hume et al 1983b) and the central nervous system (Perry et al 1985) has been defined in some detail. After phagocytosis of senescent neurons and axons generated by programmed cell death, the F4/80-positive cells differentiate into extensively arborized microglia. These studies raise intriguing questions regarding migration of macrophages in the embryo and the role of the local environment in sites such as the central nervous system during microglial maturation and in liver, where macrophages 'transform' into Kupffer cells as hepatic haemopoiesis ceases. The nature and sources of the molecules which control macrophage recruitment and growth during development are obscure.

The phenotype of tissue macrophages from adult mice

In addition to studies on bone marrow resident macrophages, there is new information on expression of various antigens, receptors and secretory products by macrophages isolated from liver, spleen and epidermis. There are also data on the alteration in tissue phenotype brought about *in vivo* by infections such as *Plasmodium yoelii* (S. H. Lee, unpublished) and *in vitro* by lymphokines such as interferon-γ. A detailed consideration of these findings is beyond the scope of the present discussion, but some interesting features are beginning to emerge.

(a) Resident tissue macrophages differ from circulating monocytes and 'free' macrophages from serosal cavities in several respects. Particularly striking is the appearance of a receptor which binds unopsonized sheep erythrocytes (E_R) (P. Crocker, unpublished), and which may be representative of novel macrophage tissue–adhesion binding sites. The E_R has been found on resident macrophages isolated by collagenase digestion from bone marrow, lymph nodes, liver and spleen. Collagenase-treated monocytes and peritoneal or pleural macrophages do not display this receptor. The E_R is present on macrophages recruited to liver by *Plasmodium yoelii* infection, presumably by induction on monocytes which adhere to liver sinusoids and differentiate into 'Kupffer cells'. The E_R of resident tissue macrophages mediates binding, rather than ingestion of erythrocytes, but ingestion can be activated on tissue macrophages by infection. It is not known whether the E_R or a different agglutinin plays a role in phagocytosis and/or clustering of murine myeloid and erythroid cells around resident bone marrow macrophages. Since macrophages which pass through tissues (e.g. alveolar and peritoneal cells) lack the E_R, two major classes of mature macrophages may be determined by the expression of this receptor, namely those which are retained within tissues (E_R-positive) and those which are free to leave (E_R-negative).

(b) Resident macrophages isolated from bone marrow (P. Crocker, unpublished) and liver (S. H. Lee, unpublished) express very low levels of or lack the CR3 Mac-1 antigen, unlike monocytes and peritoneal macrophages. This observation is interesting since the CR3 is thought to participate with lectin-like receptors such as the mannosyl, fucosyl receptor in macrophage adhesion to various cellular targets (Ezekowitz et al 1984). After isolation, resident macrophages express Mac-1 antigen on further cultivation. It is not known whether the Mac-1 antigen is initially absent, blocked by ligand or, indeed, down-regulated. These findings, however, underline the importance of variable marker expression by macrophages *in situ* and in culture. An important role for the native environment in contrast to culture conditions has also been demonstrated in recent studies with epidermal Langerhans cells which are thought to lose macrophage markers (F4/80) as they 'differentiate' into 'dendritic cells' in culture (Schuler & Steinman 1985).

(c) Resident macrophages in different organs also differ from one another. It has long been suspected that alveolar macrophages, for instance, differ in several respects from peritoneal macrophages. The role of the local environment in these and other phenotypic differences has not been defined. The extent to which haemopoiesis is present (bone marrow > spleen > liver) and resultant maturation differences must be taken into account in evaluating such heterogeneity.

(d) The expression of 'activation' markers by 'resident' macrophages and their response to activating agents (lymphokines, interferon-γ) is of considerable interest. Resident bone marrow macrophages express Ia, but no respiratory burst activity (P. Crocker, unpublished), whereas Kupffer cells are in a sense 'deactivated' and selectively refractory to lymphokine priming of respiratory burst activity (D. A. Lepay & R. M. Steinman, personal communication). In contrast, spleen macrophages from normal mice display higher levels of fibrinolytic and respiratory burst activity than resident peritoneal macrophages (S. H. Lee, unpublished), perhaps reflecting the presence of an immature population in that organ. Possibly, lack of respiratory burst protects selected tissue sites from oxidative injury.

Conclusions

Regulation of the macrophage phenotype is more complex than was initially thought. Tissue macrophages interact with different components which could profoundly alter their phenotype. In turn, the function of tissue macrophages may involve homeostatic and trophic interactions with other cells which go beyond traditional views of macrophage function in host defence. Macrophages, even if derived from a common circulating pool, are remarkably adaptable to particular local stimuli and are able to express a variety of novel features in responding to their local environment. These features include synthesis and secretion of trophic and growth factors (e.g. interleukin 1) and plasma membrane receptors which could regulate endocytosis and cell interactions in various sites, including haemopoietic and lymphoid tissues, brain, gut and endocrine organs. The isolation and characterization of macrophages from these diverse sources and elucidation of their function *in situ* will be a formidable task for the future.

Acknowledgements

Work in the authors' laboratory was supported by a grant from the Medical Research Council, UK. L.M. is a Wahl scholar, Republic of South Africa. We thank Christopher Graham and Gilbert Shia for their collaboration and Pam Woodward for typing the manuscript.

REFERENCES

Austyn JM, Gordon S 1981 F4/80, a monoclonal antibody directed specifically against the mouse macrophage. Eur J Immunol 11:805-815

Dexter TM 1982 Stromal cell associated haemopoiesis. J Cell Physiol (suppl) 1:87-94

Ezekowitz RAB, Sim R, Hill M, Gordon S 1984 Local opsonisation by secreted macrophage complement components. Role of receptors for complement in uptake of zymosan. J Exp Med 159:244-260

Flotte TJ, Springer TA, Thorbecke GH 1983 Dendritic cell and macrophage staining by monoclonal antibodies in tissue sections and epidermal sheets. Am J Pathol 111:112-124

Hirsch S, Austyn JM, Gordon S 1981 Expression of the macrophage-specific antigen F4/80 during differentiation of mouse bone marrow cells in culture. J Exp Med 154:713-725

Hume DA, Gordon S 1983 The mononuclear phagocyte system of the mouse defined by immunohistochemical localisation of antigen F4/80. Identification of resident macrophages in renal medullary and cortical interstitium and the juxtaglomerular complex. J. Exp Med 157:1704-1709

Hume DA, Robinson AP, MacPherson GG, Gordon S 1983a The immunohistochemical localisation of antigen F4/80. The relationship between macrophages, Langerhans cell, reticular cells and dendritic cells in lymphoid and hematopoietic organs. J Exp Med 158:1522-1536

Hume DA, Perry VH, Gordon S 1983b The histochemical localisation of a macrophage-specific antigen in developing mouse retina. Phagocytosis of dying neurons and differentiation of microglial cells to form a regular array in the plexiform layers. J Cell Biol 97:253-257

Hume DA, Perry VH, Gordon S 1984a The mononuclear phagocyte system of the mouse defined by immunohistochemical localisation of antigen F4/80. Macrophages associated with epithelia. Anat Rec 210:503-512

Hume DA, Halpin D, Charlton H, Gordon S 1984b The mononuclear phagocyte system of the mouse defined by immunohistochemical localisation of antigen F4/80. Macrophages of endocrine organs. Proc Natl Acad Sci USA 81:4174-4177

Hume DA, Loutit JF, Gordon S 1984c The mononuclear phagocyte system of the mouse defined by immunohistochemical localisation of antigen F4/80. Macrophages of bone and associated connective tissue. J Cell Sci 66:189-194

Labastie M-C, Thiery J-P, Le Douarin NM 1984 Mouse yolk sac and intraembryonic tissues produce factors able to elicit differentiation of erythroid burst-forming units and colony-forming units, respectively. Proc Natl Acad Sci USA 81:1453-1456

Lee S-H, Starkey P, Gordon S 1985 Quantitative analysis of total macrophage content in adult mouse tissues. Immunochemical studies with monoclonal antibody F4/80. J Exp Med 161:475-489

Perry VH, Hume DA, Gordon S 1985 Immunohistochemical localization of macrophages and microglia in the adult and developing mouse brain. Neuroscience 15:313-326

Schuler G, Steinman RM 1985 Murine epidermal Langerhans cells mature into potent immunostimulatory dendritic cells in vitro. J Exp Med 161:526-546

Spector WG, Ryan GB 1970 The mononuclear phagocyte in inflammation. In: van Furth R (ed) Mononuclear phagocytes. Blackwell Scientific, Oxford, p 219-232

Springer T, Galfre G, Secher D, Milstein C 1979 Mac-1: a macrophage differentiation antigen identified by a monoclonal antibody. Eur J Immunol 9:301-306

Unkeless JC 1979 Characterization of a monoclonal antibody directed against mouse macrophage and lymphocyte Fc receptors. J Exp Med 150:580-596

van Furth R, Diesselhoff-den Dulk MMC 1984 Dual origin of mouse spleen macrophages. J Exp Med 160:1273-1283

Volkman A, Chang N-CA, Strausbach PH, Morahan PS 1984 Maintenance of resident macrophage populations in monocyte depleted mice. In: Volkman A (ed) Mononuclear phagocyte biology. Dekker, New York, p 419-437

Westen H, Bainton DF 1979 Association of alkaline-phosphatase-positive reticulum cells in bone marrow with granulocytic precursors. J Exp Med 150:919-937
Witmer MD, Steinman RM 1984 The anatomy of peripheral lymphoid organs with emphasis on accessory cells; Light-microscopic immunocytochemical studies of mouse spleen, lymph node, and Peyer's patch. Am J Anat 170:465-481

DISCUSSION

Werb: When do you first see macrophages or F4/80-positive cells relative to the development of blood vessels and epithelial precursors such as salivary glands?

Gordon: Their initial distribution seems to coincide in time with the appearance of small vessels. We haven't looked at that in sufficient detail yet.

I didn't say much about the appearance of macrophages in non-haemopoietic sites in the embryo. We have looked at that in the kidney, the gut and various other sites of more active morphogenesis and tissue remodelling. Clearly macrophages are involved. They enter the mesenchyme and they are there at the time one would expect them to be, because of their phagocytic activity.

Other problems remain to be looked at. For example these macrophages seem to be excluded from certain sites and then they penetrate or enter others. We need to learn a lot more about what recruits them into these sites, what determines their longevity, and so on.

Schreiber: Is the sheep erythrocyte receptor a distinct receptor or does the macrophage secrete a component such as neuraminidase which subsequently alters the sheep erythrocyte surface and induces rosetting through another type of receptor?

Crocker: The E receptor on the macrophage binds after gentle fixation with paraformaldehyde. It is therefore unlikely that secretion is involved.

Hogg: Can you demonstrate that the E receptor is biosynthesized?

Crocker: It is difficult to do those experiments. On glass coverslips receptor expression drops so much over time that re-expression after trypsinization is minimal. We need to find a system where we can show induction of E receptor and then do the same type of experiment.

Hogg: In humans the sheep red cell receptor is expressed on T cells. It seems to be a very important receptor in the initial events of T cell activation. A trivial explanation would be that you are looking at adsorbed T cell molecules.

Crocker: It is possible but unlikely, for a number of reasons. First, mouse thymocytes don't bind under the same conditions. Secondly, the binding is calcium- and magnesium-independent whereas the human T receptor is not (Jondal et al 1972). Thirdly, it is not inhibited by metabolic inhibitors which inhibit T cell receptor binding, and fourthly binding to macrophages is lost after neuraminidase treatment of erythrocytes, which enhances binding to human T cells.

Springer: The human E rosette receptor is not dependent on divalent cations, according to Weiner et al (1973), so the information on this is conflicting. Have you tested whether monoclonal antibodies to the E rosette receptor, namely those to T11 and LFA-2, bind to your cells?

Crocker: We cannot test for the presence of the murine equivalent of the human T cell E receptor since the antibodies you mention were made in mice.

Springer: Have you looked at the analogous cell in the human?

Crocker: We haven't done any work yet on humans.

Dean: Have you done cross-linking studies to demonstrate exactly how many molecules on the two different cell surfaces are specifically in juxtaposition with each other?

Crocker: No.

Humphrey: What did you mean by fixed macrophages, Dr Gordon?

Gordon: The E receptor is expressed mainly by macrophages obtained by collagenase digestion from haemopoietic and lymphoid tissues and not by circulating monocytes or 'free' macrophages in serosal cavities. The possible role of E receptor in local interactions between macrophages, neighbouring cells and matrix needs further investigation.

Humphrey: Are you defining those macrophages which survive whole-body irradiation, and are presumably not dependent on replenishment from the bone marrow?

Gordon: Not yet.

Humphrey: Professor van Furth published a paper recently in which he described local production as well as bone marrow derivation of macrophages present in the spleen (van Furth & Diesselhof-den Dulk 1984).

van Furth: The cells that divide locally originated from the bone marrow as well.

Gordon: In the adult bone marrow there are two populations of macrophages: the resident population that I talked about and newly forming monocytes which are obviously immature. There is hardly any haemopoietic activity in the adult liver, resident-type population. In the mouse spleen there is a mixed bag, with significant local production and a resident population. One therefore has to consider maturity differences together with population heterogeneity.

van Furth: How accurately can the number of cells be quantitated by extraction? We counted the cells by isolation and also used a cytomorphometric method to quantitate the binding of F4/80 to mononuclear phagocytes (Nibbering et al 1985). The results show that although most cells are F4/80-positive (Table 1, column 1), the amounts of monoclonal antibody bound to the various macrophages differ a great deal (Table 1, column 2). The low values for the

Kupffer cells are probably due to the method of isolation (Crofton et al 1978). When we now apply the same type of calculation as used by Lee et al (1985), the calculated J774.1 equivalents per tissue differ from the total number of macrophages that we isolated from these tissues (Table 1, columns 3 and 4) and the values also differ from those found by Lee et al (column 5). I am afraid that this indirect approach— comparing the amount of F4/80 bound to macrophages and J774 cells—is not accurate. Even counting the number of macrophages isolated by mechanical methods and enzyme digestion from tissues will give an underestimation, but in my opinion the results are close to the real values.

TABLE 1 (*van Furth*) **Calculations on the total number of cells**

Cells	Swiss mice				C57BL/6 mice
	Percentage F4/80- positive cells	F4/80 binding per cell	Calculated J774.1 equivalents per tissue $(\times 10^7)$	Total number of cells isolated per tissue $(\times 10^7)$	Calculated number of J774.2 equivalents per tissue[a] $(\times 10^7)$
Blood monocytes	94	57.0	0.20	0.15	
Kupffer cells	44	9.2	0.08	0.91	1.6
Spleen macrophages	79	19.4	0.14	0.40	0.5
Lung macrophages	100	41.7	0.20	0.21	0.07
Peritoneal macrophages	100	66.7	0.36	0.24	
J774.1 cells	100	44.9			

[a] From Lee et al (1985).

*Gordon:*We are measuring antigen content and I expressed all these in J774 equivalents. I am not suggesting that every macrophage has a constant amount of F4/80. We know that the amount of antigen is modulated and varies a great deal with maturity. We also know that if macrophages are activated, for example with BCG, the amount per cell drops as well. Our results give average values for a population of cells which varies in heterogeneity in organs such as spleen and liver.

We are aware of all these complications, but we tried to estimate macrophage content without any bias about kinetics or labelling patterns. There are clearly macrophages that will not label or turn over very actively, which one neglects if one just looks at population kinetics. Our results indicate an estimate of about 1×10^8 for the total number of J774 equivalents in a mouse. Organ content is clearly subject to environmental factors such as gut flora and filtered air.

Nathan: It is now clear that reactive oxygen intermediates are mutagenic and carcinogenic under some circumstances. It is a neat idea that macrophages that may be so intimately involved with cells of high mitotic turnover, such as in the marrow or the epithelial lining of the gut, may be suppressed in their potential to secrete such products.

Gordon: We haven't isolated the gut macrophages. We don't know whether the resident macrophages in bone marrow fail to react to interferon-γ in the way the Kupffer cells do. Haemopoietic cells which associate with stromal macrophages can proliferate or be ingested, indicating a delicate control of cell–cell interactions.

Stanley: Do resident cells in the bone marrow associate with fibroblast-like cells *in situ*?

Crocker: Of clusters isolated by digestion about 30% show endogenous reactivity to alkaline phosphatase, which is a marker of fibroblastoid cells in mouse bone marrow (Westen & Bainton 1979). About 80% have F4/80 reactivity, so there is a subpopulation of clusters which has both resident macrophages and fibroblastoid cells.

Unkeless: There are periodic reports on receptors for IgM on macrophage populations. Have you looked at these so-called fixed macrophages, or could those earlier results be explained by the presence of an erythrocyte receptor?

Crocker: This is possible. We included IgM as one of the controls for complement receptor determination. There was the same degree of binding as with unopsonized erythrocytes.

Singer: Why do these cell clusters withstand collagenase treatment?

Crocker: The E receptor itself is resistant to collagenase treatment but is destroyed by trypsin. It is possible that the E receptor interacts with haemopoietic cells in the formation of clusters.

Humphrey: Haemopoietic clusters are characteristic of healthy bone marrow smears but the macrophage in the middle usually has some fat in it. Were yours full of fat?

Crocker: By phase contrast microscopy of living or fixed cells there is no evidence of fat accumulation.

Cohn: A fair amount of iron is stored in the bone marrow. Did you see any of that?

Crocker: We haven't looked at that by the Prussian blue reaction but in Giemsa-stained preparations we can see haemosiderin-like material similar to that seen in stromal spleen macrophages.

Nicola: Can macrophages that reside in the bone marrow be made to proliferate *in vitro*?

Crocker: In *in vitro* labelling studies with 2-h or 16-h pulses with tritiated thymidine we have seen no evidence for turnover of that population. In experiments with crude conditioned media, such as lung- or L-cell-conditioned media, there was no thymidine incorporation after exposure for 24 or 48 h. As yet we have no evidence that they can be stimulated to proliferate *in vitro*.

Nicola: So is it possible, without first expanding them in culture, to get enough cells to seed with fresh bone marrow and try to determine the full range of haemopoietic activities?

Crocker: This is possible, although the present yield of less than 10^5 macrophages per two femora would make such studies difficult.

Gordon: One interesting question is whether those cells are locally derived or whether they are circulating monocytes that come back to the marrow.

Nathan: You referred to erythrocytes, and you have shown what look like myeloid cells. Could there be significant numbers of T or B cells or NK cells?

Gordon: In bone marrow most of them look like erythroid or myeloid cells and there are a few monocytes too. We haven't looked in detail at the lymphoid tissues.

Nathan: Maybe the lymphoid cells that are an important constituent of marrow are not collagenase-resistant.

Gordon: There aren't many T cells in normal marrow to start with.

Springer: You said that so far F4/80 has not stained any cell that is not a macrophage. What is your definition of a macrophage?

Gordon: We have done careful studies with microglia to show that the same population expresses three different antigens (F4/80, Mac-1 and 2.4G2).

Springer: F4/80 antigen is on Langerhans cells and dendritic cells, which are non-phagocytic cells. By definition, one would expect a mononuclear phagocyte to be phagocytic. The definitions of 'macrophage' and 'mononuclear phagocyte' have never been entirely clear to me and often seem *ad hoc*.

Gordon: Schuler & Steinman (1985) have shown that Langerhans cells when isolated lose their F4/80 antigen and become a population that has mixed leucocyte reaction (MLR)-stimulating activity. Spleen dendritic cells lack F4/80. We suspect that some mononuclear phagocytes are F4/80-negative, e.g. the precursors do not have detectable antigen. Steinman has reported that macrophages in the marginal zone of the spleen lack F4/80. In gut-associated lymphoid tissue there may be cells that also don't label. F4/80 is therefore an almost 'pan-macrophage' maker.

Moore: Are murine NK cells negative for F4/80?

Gordon: We haven't looked yet.

Stanley: In your staining of Kupffer cells for F4/80 in sections of liver are you able to state that endothelial cells are definitely not stained?

Gordon: Absolutely. We are very interested in that endothelial cell population. They are not like other endothelial cells. They have Fc receptors and mannosyl receptors.

Springer: So far the resident stromal cells are positive for some of the markers we associate with macrophages and negative for other markers found on virtually all macrophages, including Mac-1. Have you looked for markers characteristic of other cells such as endothelial cells or epithelial cells?

Gordon: We haven't screened adequately outside the macrophage phenotype. We don't have good markers for mouse endothelial cells. The one we tested was a beautiful macrophage marker.

REFERENCES

Crofton RW, Diesselhoff-den Dulk MMC, van Furth R 1978 The origin, kinetics and characteristics of the Kupffer cells in the normal steady state. J Exp Med 148:1-17

Jondal M, Holm G, Wigzell H 1972 Surface molecules on human T and B lymphocytes. 1. A large population of lymphocytes forming nonimmune rosettes with sheep red cells. J Exp Med 136:207-215

Lee SH, Starkey PM, Gordon S 1985 Quantitative analysis of total macrophage content in adult mouse tissues. J Exp Med 161:465-489

Nibbering PH, Leijh PCJ, van Furth R 1985 A cytophotometric method to quantitate the binding of monoclonal antibodies to individual cells. J Histochem Cytochem 33:453-459

Schuler G, Steinman RM 1985 Murine epidermal Langerhans cells mature into potent immunostimulatory dendritic cells in vitro. J Exp Med 161:526-546

van Furth R, Diesselhoff-den Dulk MMC 1984 Dual origin of mouse spleen macrophages. J Exp Med 160:1273-1283

Weiner MS, Bianco C, Nussenzweig V 1973 Enhanced binding of neuraminidase-treated sheep erythrocytes to human T lymphocytes. Blood 42:939-946

Westen H, Bainton DF 1979 Association of alkaline phosphatase positive reticulum cells in bone marrow with granulocytic precursors. J Exp Med 150:919-932

Macrophage antigens and the effect of a macrophage activating factor, interferon-γ

NANCY HOGG, YOGI SELVENDRAN, GRAEME DOUGHERTY & CATHERINE ALLEN

Macrophage Laboratory, Imperial Cancer Research Fund, Lincoln's Inn Fields, London, WC2A 3PX, UK

Abstract. Molecules characteristic of mononuclear phagocytes have been identified using monoclonal antibodies (MAb). MAb 3.9 reacts with a 150/95 000 dalton heterodimer which is found exclusively on monocytes and macrophages and appears to be the third member of the lymphocyte function-associated (LFA) family of molecules. In contrast, the reactivity of MAb 24, which bonds to a 175 000 dalton protein, is most highly expressed on the macrophages in lymphoid tissue. Both 3.9 and 24 detect the interdigitating cells in the T cell areas of these tissues, which strongly suggests that this cell type belongs to the macrophage family. A third MAb, 10.1, reacts selectively with a set of macrophages outside lymphoid tissue, particularly on Kupffer cells, alveolar macrophages and microglia. Thus subsets of tissue macrophages are proving easy to identify whereas it appears that circulating monocytes are not easily subdivided. None of the MAbs detected either Langerhans' cells, dendritic reticulum cells of B cell areas, or osteoclasts, indicating that these cells are not mononuclear phagocytes. As a first step towards identifying macrophage molecules which have a biological function, we have investigated the effect of macrophage-activating factor, interferon-γ, on the expression of macrophage membrane molecules. There was greatly increased expression of only two out of ten molecules detected with anti-myeloid antibodies.

1986 Biochemistry of macrophages. Pitman, London Ciba Foundation Symposium 118) p 68-88

In order to identify cells belonging to the mononuclear phagocyte family and to understand the molecular events involved in their activities, we have characterized monoclonal antibodies (MAbs) which are specific for cells of this lineage (Table 1). Using these MAbs we have looked for evidence for monocyte and macrophage heterogeneity.

Lack of evidence for monocyte subsets

It has been a matter of interest whether there are distinct subsets of monocytes comparable to the T4 and T8 subsets of human T cells, whether monocytes

TABLE 1 Monoclonal antibodies (MAb) reacting with monocytes and/or macrophages

MAb	Mol mass (kDa)	Specificity	Reference
3.9	150/95	Pan monocyte/macrophage p150,95 molecule	N. Hogg et al (1985, unpublished) Sim et al (1985, unpublished)
UCHM1	52	Monocytes	Hogg et al (1984a)
44	170/95	Monocytes, granulocytes C3bi receptor, CR3 (CD18)	Reinherz et al (1985)
24	175	Monocytes Macrophages in lymphoid tissue	Hogg & Selvendran (1985)
10.1	??	Monocytes Macrophage-selected locations	Unpublished
E11	220	C3b receptor, CR1	Hogg et al (1984b)
52	35/28	Class II molecules	Unpublished

perform different functions as they mature, whether local environmental factors act on a common pool of cells to generate a required function, or a combination of these possibilities. A number of our MAbs, UCHM1, 44, 3.9 and E11, reacted with most monocytes (Hogg et al 1984a,b, Hogg et al 1985, in preparation). On the other hand, two other MAbs, 24 and 10.1 reacted with about 50% of monocytes but with wide variations in levels of expression (Hogg & Selvendran 1985, N. Hogg et al, unpublished). Dimitriu-Bona et al 1983) have also reported MAbs of this latter type. It can be argued that this behaviour is more characteristic of antigens which alter in expression as cells mature or are exposed to activation signals. This finding and those by others (for review see Todd & Schlossman 1984) lead to the suggestion that monocytes are a single class of cells which alter their phenotype according to local influences or move into tissues to become tissue macrophages under the influence of stimuli that are still unidentified. Whether activated circulating monocytes are able to revert to the common phenotype when biological signals are removed is at present unknown.

Tissue macrophages

Although it has been difficult to detect monocyte subsets, we and others have found it relatively easy to detect antigenic differences between tissue macrophages (Hogg & Selvendran 1985, N. Hogg et al 1985 unpublished, Hancock et al 1983, Radzun & Parwaresch 1983, Biondi et al 1984). This is not surprising, given the contrasting milieu in which different macrophages are located. We have characterized three MAbs which react well with human tissue macrophages.

The first, MAb 3.9, has been shown by extensive testing on primary cells, cell lines and tissues to react specifically with monocytes and most macrophages, and it can be considered to be a panmonocyte and macrophage marker. A small percentage of cells with the density of neutrophils also label with MAb 3.9. They have not yet been further characterized. Fig. 1a illustrates the reactivity of MAb 3.9 with macrophages in tonsil, as shown by the indirect immunoperoxidase staining technique. MAb 3.9 immunoprecipitates a heterodimer of 150 000 and 95 000 daltons. These same polypeptides are precipitated by two MAbs specific for the β chain common to the three molecules belonging to the human leucocyte differentiation antigen family (Sanchez-Madrid et al 1983), which suggests that MAb 3.9 has specificity for the unique α chain of the third member of this family, the p150,95 heterodimer (R. Sim et al, unpublished work 1985). Less is known about the p150,95 molecule than about the two other members of this family, named the lymphocyte function-associated 1 (LFA-1) molecule and the CR3 molecule which is the receptor for the complement component C3bi. All three of these molecules are found on macrophages, Both the LFA-1 and CR3 molecules participate in adhesive interactions between, respectively, leucocytes (LFA-1) and myeloid cells and their substrates (CR3), so it can be speculated that the macrophage-specific function of the p150,95 molecule will require an adhesion or binding step.

Two other MAbs are more selectively expressed on tissue macrophages. Thus, MAb 24 is expressed chiefly in lymphoid tissue and skin (Hogg & Selvendran 1985), whereas MAb 10.1 is expressed on macrophages outside the lymphoid system, particularly in liver, lung and on brain microglia. Using these MAbs and several others with broader anti-myeloid reactivity we have attempted to identify tissue macrophages.

Langerhans' cells, dendritic reticulum cells and osteoclasts are not macrophages

Because of the lack of identifying features specific to macrophages there has been controversy about which tissue cells are members of the mononuclear phagocyte family. In particular, there has been controversy about the origins of Langerhans' cells found in a suprabasal position in the epidermis of skin and identified by expression of class II and T6 molecules (Rowden et al 1977, Fithian et al 1981). Using immunoperoxidase staining of fresh tissue sections, we found that none of eight MAbs with varying anti-myeloid activity, including the six MAbs listed in Table 1, reacted with these cells. Positively staining cells were found positioned at the interface between dermis and epidermis and in abundance surrounding hair follicles and sweat glands. This evidence suggests that Langerhans' cells are not macrophages. Alternatively, it is not

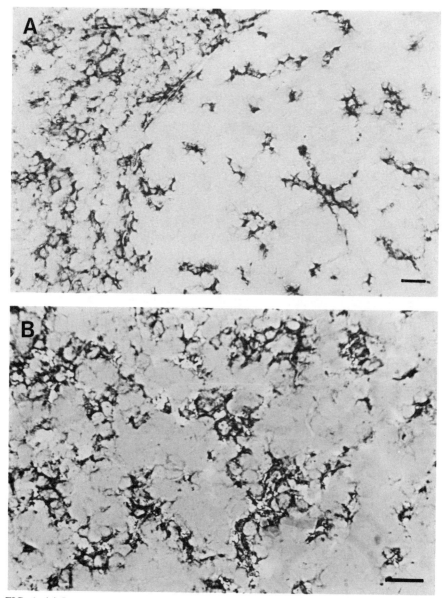

FIG. 1. (A) Immunoperoxidase reaction of MAb 3.9 on human tonsil, showing, on the right, part of a germinal centre containing scattered macrophages; in centre view, the marginal zone area with macrophages aligned along the edge of the germinal centre and, on the left, the T cell area with macrophages of 'interdigitating' morphology. Scale bar, 5 μ. (B) Higher magnification view of MAb 3.9-positive cells with interdigitating appearance seen in the paracortical or T cell area of a lymph node. Scale bar, 5 μ.

impossible that the particular microenvironment in which Langerhans' cells are located causes the down-regulation of many macrophage-specific epitopes and expression of the OKT6 marker which is characteristic of these cells and cortical thymocytes. Analysis of Langerhans' cells in culture would provide a more sensitive analysis of this possibility. The relationship between skin macrophages lining the epidermis and the 'indeterminate' cells, which are dendritic-like cells identified by electron microscopy, is unclear (Rowden et al 1977). These cells possess few of the Birbeck granules which characterize Langerhans' cells but they express class II molecules. Whether they are macrophages, as seems likely, would have to be resolved by immunoelectron microscopy. These findings contradict the studies in the mouse where the well-characterized MAb, F4/80, has been shown to react with murine Langerhans' cells (Hume et al 1983). This may be a genuine difference between mouse and humans. However, mouse epidermis consists of only one cell layer, whereas in humans the epidermis is many layers thick. One possibility might be that the macrophage-positive murine Langerhans' cell is equivalent to the human macrophage positioned at the epidermal/dermal interface, with the human Langerhans' cell representing a specialized cell not seen in the mouse. It has been suggested that this suprabasal population is absent from thin-skinned, furred animals (Balfour et al 1981).

Other cells which failed to label with macrophage specific MAbs were dendritic reticulum cells of B cell germinal centres identified by their CR1 receptors (Hogg et al 1984a). This is consistent with recent proof that these cells are not of haemopoietic origin (Humphrey et al 1984). In addition, none of the MAbs reacted with osteoclasts (M. Horton, personal communication). Thus, in humans, neither Langerhans' cells nor osteoclasts nor dendritic reticulum cells appear to originate from the mononuclear phagocyte lineage.

Are the interdigitating reticulum and lymphoid dendritic cells also macrophages?

There has also been controversy about the lineage of other cells—the interdigitating reticulum cell (IDRC), seen in lymphoid tissue and identified by electron microscopy (Hoffman-Fezev et al 1978), and the lymphoid dendritic or Steinman cell, also isolated from lymphoid tissue and identified by its potent accessory cell activity (Steinman et al 1979). MAbs 3.9 and 24 both reacted with cells of interdigitating or dendritic appearance found in the T cell areas of lymphoid tissue. Fig. 1b shows the characteristic appearance of these cells found in the paracortical or T cell area of a reactive lymph node labelled with MAb 3.9. By means of a double-labelling technique designed to permit simultaneous labelling of a single sample by two MAbs of the same mouse immunoglobulin class, MAb 3.9 and 24 were both shown to overlap completely in their binding to these interdigitating type cells. The double-labelling method is outlined in Table 2 (Hogg et al 1985, unpublished). This finding raised questions about the relationship between these macrophages detected with MAbs 3.9 and 24 and dendritic cells which express high levels of class II molecules but otherwise have shown little phenotypic similarity to macrophages (Van Voorhis et al 1983). We asked whether there were cells in the T cell areas of lymphoid tissue which did not bear macrophage markers but expressed class II molecules and would thus be candidate Steinman dendritic cells. Using the above-mentioned double-labelling technique with MAb 3.9 or 24 plus MAb 52, which is specific for class II molecules, we were unable to detect cells which were MAb 3.9- or 24-negative but class II-molecule-positive. In other words, we were unable to detect cells of dendritic appearance which expressed class II molecules but did not express macrophage molecules. In contrast, many macrophages in T cell areas expressed class II molecules. We concluded that the former cells, if present, must be very few in number compared with macrophages; alternatively, the human dendritic cell found in T cell areas is a macrophage.

TABLE 2 Double-labelling method for monoclonal antibodies

Add sequentially, washing between each step:

(1) First monoclonal antibody
(2) Anti-mouse immunoglobulin coupled to alkaline phosphatase
(3) Second monoclonal antibody directly biotinylated
(4) Vectastain—avidin, biotinylated peroxidase
(5) Develop peroxidase conjugate—diaminobenzidine, H_2O_2
(6) Develop alkaline phosphatase conjugate—naphthol-AS phosphate, Fast Blue

In only one tissue were 'dendritic' cells seen which expressed class II molecules but not macrophage epitopes. Dermatopathic lymphadenopathy is a chronic skin inflammation which leads to greatly enlarged paracortical areas of the draining lymph nodes and large numbers of IDRC (Rausch et al 1977). Double labelling with either MAbs 3.9 or 24 and MAb 52 showed two types of cells—some macrophage-positive cells, many of which failed to express substantial amounts of class II molecules, and other cells of dendritic appearance which were class II-molecule-positive and macrophage-negative. These latter cells were possible candidates for the macrophage-negative dendritic cell. However, we wished to test the possibility that the macrophage-negative cells were Langerhans' cells in passage to or from the skin. Double labelling with MAbs specific for macrophages and T6 molecules (which react with Langerhans' cells) demonstrated that a large proportion of T6-positive cells were present which did not label with macrophage antibodies. Although we did not simultaneously test for the T6 marker and class II molecules, the presumption is that these two antigens coexist on the same cell. Therefore, the conclusion is that many of the class II-molecule-expressing dendritic cells seen in dermatopathic lymphadenopathy are Langerhans' cells.

The effect of interferon-γ on macrophage molecules

An objective in these studies has been to identify macrophage molecules which have a biological function, particularly in the immune response. As a first approach, we have investigated the effect of a macrophage-activating factor, interferon-γ, in recombinant form (rIFN-γ), on the expression of macrophage membrane molecules. In a standard experiment the human monocyte cell line, U937, or the promyelocyte cell line, HL60, was incubated with 100 units/ml of IFN-γ for 18 h. There was greatly increased expression of the two molecules recognized by MAbs UCHM1 and 10.1 (Table 3). This increase was already evident at 4 h after rIFN-γ treatment, with maximum levels being reached at 18 h. Moreover it could be accomplished with rIFN-γ at 1 U/ml and was specific to IFN-γ. Treatment of the cells with rIFN-γ from 10–1000 U/ml had no effect on the expression of the UCHM1 and 10.1 molecules or any others tested. Eight other myeloid molecules were not altered in levels of expression. These included the leucocyte differentiation molecules,

TABLE 3 Alteration in the expression of macrophage antigens after exposure of U937 and HL60 to interferon-γ[a]

Monoclonal antibody	Antigen expression	
	−IFN-γ	+IFN-γ[b]
(A) U937 (n = 4)		
10.1	29 ± 8	92 ± 22
UCHM1	28 ± 8	100 ± 35
E11 − αCR1	21 ± 7	25 ± 12
44 − αCR3	16 ± 1	20 ± 6
3.9 − αp150,95	21 ± 3	22 ± 3
(B) HL60 (n = 3)		
10.1	0[c]	41 ± 1
UCHM1	0	58 ± 6
E11, 44, 3.9	0	0

[a] Antigen expression recorded as the Fluorescence Activated Cell Sorter window in which 50% of the total population of cells gave a positive fluorescence signal.
[b] Cells were exposed to rIFN-γ 100 units/ml for 18 hours.
[c] Positive cells were scored in these samples but the expression of antigen was too low to record as in (a).

CR3 and p150,95, and CR1, the complement receptor for C3b. The failure of CR1 to alter was also observed in the mouse by Vogel et al (1983). Other molecules such as class II molecules (Virelizier et al 1984) and the Fc receptor for human IgG1 (Perussia et al 1983a) have been shown to increase after IFN-γ treatment but these effects are not seen until 8–12 h and later. Thus the increase in UCHM1 and 10.1 molecules is a very early and discrete response to IFN-γ, and the suggestion here would be that these two molecules have a role in IFN-γ-mediated activation of mononuclear phagocytes.

These two MAbs, UCHM1 and 10.1, appear to have little in common. It can be said that neither is a large protein and neither is normally seen in lymphoid tissue where IFN-γ-mediated events might have been expected to occur, particularly as activated T cells are a known source of IFN-γ. It can be speculated that IFN-γ-mediated activation occurs within the circulation, acting principally on monocytes rather than on macrophages. Some of the changes mediated by IFN-γ can be described as activating events, others are also characteristic of more mature macrophages. This again raises the issue of the distinction between activation and maturation and the relationship between the two. Macrophage functions which are known to increase after rIFN-γ treatment are tumour cell cytolysis, antibody-dependent cell-mediated cytotoxicity and phagocytic activity (Perussia et al 1983b, Mannel & Falk 1983). Whether the molecules detected by MAbs UCHM1 and 10.1 play any part in these activities remains to be tested.

REFERENCES

Balfour BM, Drexhage HA, Kamperdijk EWA, Hoefsmit ECM 1981 Antigen-presenting cells, including Langerhans' cells, veiled cells and interdigitating cells. In: Microenvironments in haemopoietic and lymphoid differentiation. Pitman, London (Ciba Found Symp 84) p 281-301

Biondi A, Rossing TH, Bennett J, Todd RF 1984 Surface membrane heterogeneity among human mononuclear phagocytes. J Immunol 132:1237-1243

Dimitriu-Bona A, Burmester GR, Waters SJ, Winchester RJ 1983 Human mononuclear phagocyte differentiation antigens. Patterns of antigenic expression on the surface of human monocytes and macrophages defined by monoclonal antibodies. J Immunol 130:145-151

Fithian E, Kung P, Goldstein G, Rubenfeld M, Fenoglio G, Edelson R 1981 Reactivity of Langerhans' cells with hybridoma antibody. Proc Natl Acad Sci USA 78:2541-2546

Hancock WW, Zola H, Atkins RC 1983 Antigenic heterogeneity of human mononuclear phagocytes: immunohistologic analysis using monoclonal antibodies. Blood 62:1271-1279

Hoffmann-Fezev G, Gotze D, Rodt H, Thierfelder S 1978 Immunohistochemical localization of xenogeneic antibodies against Ia^k lymphocytes on B cells and reticular cells. Immunogenetics 6:367-377

Hogg N, Selvendran Y 1985 An anti-human monocyte/macrophage monoclonal antibody, reacting most strongly with macrophages in lymphoid tissue. Cell Immunol 92:247-253

Hogg N, Ross GD, Jones DB, Slusarenko M, Walport M, Lachmann PJ 1984a Identification of an anti-monocyte monoclonal antibody that is specific for membrane complement receptor type one (CR1). Eur J Immunol 14:236-243

Hogg N, MacDonald S, Slusarenko M, Beverley PCL 1984b Monoclonal antibodies specific for human monocytes, granulocytes and endothelium. Immunology 53:753-767

Hume DA, Robinson AP, MacPherson GG, Gordon S 1983 The mononuclear phagocyte system of the mouse defined by immunohistochemical localization of antigen F4/80. J Exp Med 158:1522-1536

Humphrey JH, Grennan D, Sundaram V 1984 The origin of follicular dendritic cells in the mouse and the mechanism of trapping immune complexes on them. Eur J Immunol 14:859-864

Mannel DN, Falk W 1983 Interferon-γ is required in activation of macrophages for tumor cytotoxicity. Cell Immunol 79:396-402

Perussia B, Dayton ET, Lazarus R, Fanning V, Trinchieri G 1983a Immune interferon induces the receptors for monomeric IgG1 on human monocytic and myeloid cells. J Exp Med 158:1092-1113

Perussia B, Dayton ET, Fanning V, Thiagarajan P, Hoxie J, Trinchieri G 1983b Immune interferon and leukocyte conditioned medium induce normal and leukemic myeloid cells to differentiate along the monocytic pathway. J Exp Med 158:2058-2080

Radzun HJ, Parwaresch MR 1983 Differential immunohistochemical resolution of the human mononuclear phagocyte system. Cell Immunol 82:174-183

Rausch E, Kaiserling E, Goos M 1977 Langerhans' cells and interdigitating reticulum cells in the thymus-dependent region in human dermatopathic lymphadenitis. Virchows Arch B Cell Pathol 25:327-343

Reinherz EL et al (eds) Leucocyte typing II. Springer-Verlag, Berlin, in press

Rowden G, Lewis MG, Sullivan AK 1977 Ia antigen expression on human epidermal Langerhans cells. Nature (Lond) 268:247-248

Sanchez-Madrid F, Nagy JA, Robbins E, Simon P, Springer TA 1983 A human leukocyte differentiation antigen family with distinct α-subunits and a common β-subunit. J Exp Med 158:1785-1803

Steinman RM, Kaplan G, Witmer MD, Cohn ZA 1979 Identification of a novel cell type in peripheral lymphoid organs of mice. V: Purification of spleen dendritic cells, new surface markers and maintenance in vitro. J Exp Med 149:1-16

Todd RF, Schlossman S 1984 Utilization of monoclonal antibodies in the characterization of monocyte-macrophage differentiation antigens. In: Immunology of the reticuloendothelial system: a comprehensive treatise. Plenum, New York, vol. 6, p 87

Van Voorhis WC, Steinman RM, Hair LS et al 1983 Specific antimononuclear phagocyte monoclonal antibodies. Application to the purification of dendritic cells and the tissue localization of macrophages. J Exp Med 158:126-145

Virelizier JL, Perez N, Arenzana-Seisedos F, Devos R 1984 Pure interferon gamma enchances class II HLA antigens on human monocyte cell lines. Eur J Immunol 14:106-108

Vogel SN, English KE, Fertsch D, Fultz MJ 1983 Differential modulation of macrophage membrane markers by interferon: analysis of Fc and C3b receptors, Mac-1 and Ia antigen expression. J Interferon Res 3:153-160

DISCUSSION

Gordon: Have you compared the expression of interferon-γ-treated monocytes with that of untreated monocytes? One of the interesting problems is whether the monocyte is already in a sense an activated cell, and you only talked about HL60.

Hogg: I talked about the U937 cell line which resembles immature monocytes and HL60, the promyelocyte cell line. We are doing the same experiments now with purified monocytes. It is too early to say whether we will have the same findings as with the cell lines.

Gordon: I agree with what you said about the mouse Langerhans cells. The cells we talked about were in the basal layer of the epidermis. There are other macrophages underneath. In sections taken *en face* we can see that they all interdigitate with epidermal cells. I agree there are species differences.

Springer: Mouse Langerhans cells are Mac-1 negative. With a number of markers they seemed to us to be distinct from most cells in the mononuclear phagocyte series (Haines et al 1983). They resembled the interdigitating cell or the lymphoid dendritic cell in the T cell area.

Hogg: We think the interdigitating cells are macrophages!

Springer: We have also been studying an antibody to the same 150,95000 heterodimer (Springer & Anderson 1985) as you studied with MAb 3.9. It was the most striking tissue macrophage-specific antibody found at the Second International Leukocyte Workshop. Tissue macrophages are clearly stronger for p150,95 than for Mac-1 or OKM1.

Hogg: Looking at tissue sections, we find that most tissue macrophages express very little of the CR3 receptor recognized by Mac-1 or OKM1.

Springer: Tissue macrophages are not negative but express lower amounts for Mac-1. The reverse is true for blood monocytes: they are quite high for Mac-1 and OKM1 and low for p150,95.

Hogg: I would agree with that.

Springer: Granulocytes are weakly positive for p150,95. If we induce them with f-Met-Leu-Phe, p150,95 expression increases by about sixfold. So granulocytes have this marker and it is not a macrophage-specific marker. The antigen is also found on hairy leukaemia cells of the B lineage. A normal B cell that expresses this antigen hasn't yet been identified but the molecule may also be expressed on a very small subset of normal B cells.

Hogg: We have screened lots of B cell lines and have not had a positive. I have not yet had the opportunity to screen any hairy cell leukaemias. Stimulating granulocytes might resolve the problem of very low labelling of these cells.

Springer: It is very hard to pick up specific staining above the relatively high granulocyte autofluorescence unless you induce with a chemoattractant.

Ezekowitz: Have you looked at whether 10.1 might be an Fc receptor, although that probably doesn't fit in with the distribution?

Hogg: No, but perhaps the particular tissue localization which we observe has something to do with activation by IFN-γ.

Ezekowitz: The kinetics looked liked Fc receptor activity induced by IFN-γ.

Hogg: Fc receptor activity appears at between 8 and 12 hours, whereas these effects are a lot earlier than that.

Cohn: Obviously the stainability of these cells in the tissues depends on the number of copies on the cell surface. Your antibodies are supposedly macrophage-specific, so how many copies are present when you work with isolated cells?

Hogg: The number has not been rigorously quantitated. We are screening for whether the antibodies are specific or reactive with other cell types. They react with various proportions of monocytes and MAb 3.9 reacts in more or less the same way with most monocytes. As Tim Springer has suggested, there seem to be fewer of those molecules on the monocytes than there are in the tissue macrophages. With MAb 24 and 10.1 the expression is highly variable on circulating monocytes but more constant in the tissues we look at. We don't know whether those markers are directed against maturational molecules or whether the variation that we see in humans is the result of some sort of activation effect over which we have no control.

Cohn: If you isolated more mature macrophage populations would they stain?

Hogg: It is difficult to extract tissue macrophages. In alveolar washes those cells show very heterogeneous staining, even with MAb 24. But again it is very difficult to get normal cell populations in humans. Most of the cells we look at are the result of some sort of complication. In the alveolar washes there are cells that look just like newly arrived monocytes and there are big tissue macrophages that seem to have been there for quite a long time.

Cole: One source of human tissue macrophages is breast milk. We have used breast milk macrophages quite successfully for metabolic labelling and for RNA extraction. We don't know how activated these cells are, but tissue macrophages spread more rapidly after adherence.

Schreiber: Have you had an opportunity to look at cells from patients undergoing clinical trials with IFN-γ?

Hogg: Such a study has just started.

Gordon: You found macrophages in the T cell areas, which is different to our experience in normal mice. Were your patients normal?

Hogg: That spleen was a normal spleen and we consistently see that picture. Because of wishing to know the phenotypic characteristics of dendritic cells and which accessory cells interact with T cells in a normal immune response *in situ*, we looked at a lot of samples. Surprisingly, not many cells with dendritic morphology in the T cell areas have class II molecules, which are the credentials the cells need for interaction with T cells.

Nathan: Why aren't you seeing at least a few activated T cells, which are Ia-positive, among all the B cells?

Hogg: The B cells in particular are very blue in those sections and they have a lot more class II molecules on them than the T cells do. The T cells are recognizable but they don't express many class II molecules compared with the other cell types.

Nathan: How can you conclude that all the blue cells are 3.9 cells?

Hogg: By their morphology. We do not see large cells of interdigitating or dendritic appearance which lack macrophage markers.

van Furth: How did you prepare the bone when you looked at osteoclasts? If certain surface or other characteristics are negative, we think this might be due to the preparation of the cell.

Hogg: Mike Horton at St Bartholomew's Hospital looked at his preparations of human osteoclasts with our antibodies. They were unfixed cells.

Gordon: Everybody seems to be finding that most of the macrophage antigens are not on osteoclasts, but J. O'D. McGee at Oxford has an anti-macrophage antibody that stains osteoclasts (personal communication).

Hogg: Mike Horton looked at all the anti-myeloid antibodies from the Second International Human Leukocyte Differentiation Antigen Workshop in Boston. None of them reacted with his osteoclast preparations (personal communication).

van Furth: His findings may be in agreement with the work of Dr Els Burger, who showed that osteoclasts originate by fusion of dividing mononuclear phagocytes. In that study bone marrow cells grown *in vitro* were co-cultured with fetal bone (Burger et al 1982). When the mononuclear phagocytes were irradiated no osteoclasts were formed. Thus, osteoclasts are formed by cells that divide at least once.

Dean: Have you tried to see how many proteins on the cell surface have their expression changed by IFN-γ? Double-labelling biosynthetic experiments would give an alternative approach to getting monoclonals against just the components you think are most interesting.

Hogg: At the moment we are raising monoclonals directly against IFN-γ-activated cells and doing a differential screen, looking at those molecules which are expressed on activated cells and those that are not expressed on non-activated cells, or the reverse. Some molecules decrease on activated cells. The value of monoclonal antibodies is that they frequently enable one to ask questions about the function of the recognized molecule. To get the total picture of the numbers of cell molecules which alter after IFN-γ activation, the most fruitful approach would be to construct a cDNA library from IFN-γ-activated cells, then screen activated and non-activated cells. This work is being done at the Imperial Cancer Research Fund in the laboratories of Ian Kerr and George Stark.

Dean: How many change their expression?

Hogg: It is too early to know how many monoclonal antibodies we have with distinct specificities to molecules altered by IFN-γ but from the cloning results obtained at the Imperial Cancer Research Fund, it looks as if there are lots of differences.

Springer: A number of different sublines of U937 behave differently in culture. You may have one that is different to the one we and others have been looking at. With PMA we see fairly good induction of Mac-1 and the p150,95 molecule.

Hogg: With PMA we get induction of all the MAbs reacting with macrophages! We don't get that with IFN-γ.

Gordon: It is important to use the right control for that experiment. The cell lines might be defective with regard to the expression of particular markers.

Hogg: U937 is supposed to be an immature or monoblastic type of cell. If we are looking at differentiation, as opposed to activation, perhaps we are seeing the induction of more mature molecules. That is why it will be interesting to do the same experiments with monocytes, which are more differentiated than either of the cell lines used.

Cole: In terms of regulation in response to IFN-γ, U937 does not synthesize or secrete functionally or immunochemically detectable factor B, nor does it have detectable factor B RNA. In our experiments on macrophage maturation, U937 was not very useful.

Springer: We have a good internal control for activation of genes in U937. When we induce with PMA it is very clear that the LFA-1 α subunit is not increased, but Mac-1 and p150,95 α subunits increase dramatically.

REFERENCES

Burger EH, van der Meer JWM, van de Gevel JS, Gribnau JC, Thesingh CW, van Furth R 1982 In vitro formation of osteoclasts from long-term cultures of bone marrow mononuclear phagocytes. J Exp Med 156:1604-1614

Haines KA, Flotte TJ, Springer TA, Gigli I, Thorbecke GJ 1983 Staining of Langerhans cells with monoclonal antibodies to macrophages and lymphoid cells. Proc Natl Acad Sci USA 80:3448-3451

Springer TA, Anderson DC 1985 Antibodies specific for the Mac-1, LFA-1, p150,95 glycoproteins or their family, or for other granulocyte proteins. In: Reinherz EL et al (eds) Leucocyte typing II. Springer-Verlag, Berlin, in press

General discussion 1

Humphrey: My clinical interest in macrophages was stimulated by a man who was referred at the age of 37 to Hammersmith Hospital with a history since the age of 25 years of repeated bacterial and fungal infections and generalized verrucosis. He was one of four brothers and a sister, three of whom had died of infections. They all had the Pelger-Hüet anomaly in their myeloid cells, and myeloid leukaemia. His blood contained no monocytes. The family was described by Kaur et al (1972).

Although the patient's lymphocytes responded normally to phytohaemagglutinin or to allogeneic lymphocytes *in vitro*, they failed to transform in the presence of purified protein derivative (PPD) or *Candida* antigens. He did not show delayed-type hypersensitivity when his skin was tested with these antigens, nor could he be sensitized to dinitrochlorbenzene. It was as though he had no effector cells for evoking delayed-type responses.

In due course he died, and at autopsy his spleen and his lungs showed plenty of typical acid phosphatase-positive macrophages, containing iron, pigment and microorganisms (aspergillus and atypical mycobacteria). So despite the absence of circulating monocytes the resident tissue macrophages were present and not obviously defective (H. Valdimarsson, personal communication).

It may be important to know whether macrophage populations, even within a single tissue, have different lifespans and different capacities. As an example I would like to describe a population of macrophages in the marginal zone of the white pulp in the mouse spleen and in the marginal sinus, septa and medulla of peripheral lymph nodes. We became interested in them because in the mouse they appear exclusively to capture certain thymus-independent (TI) antigens which could be visualized by attaching a fluorescent label (Humphrey & Grennan 1981). A similar population is present in the rat spleen (Gray et al 1984), and they can also be distinguished by a monoclonal antibody which reacts with them quite specifically (E. van Vliet et al, unpublished). We had prepared bone marrow chimeras by reconstituting parental-strain mice with F1 hybrid stem cells, and we used biotinylated monoclonal antibodies specific for H2 of either of the parental strains to identify later whether any given cell was derived from the host or the donor. Marginal zone macrophages in the spleen could be distinguished by means of FITC-labelled hydroxyethyl starch, which they retained exclusively, whereas other macrophages could be recognized by faintly autofluorescent pigment (probably lipofuscin). Spleen cell suspensions were prepared, using collagenase and Dispase so as to release all the macrophages, at various intervals after establishing the chimeras.

By one month all the lymphocytes and the red pulp macrophages were derived from the bone marrow donor. However, marginal zone macrophages were replaced by donor cells much more slowly—at about 25% per month (Humphrey & Sundaram 1985). So there is surely a population of macrophages with different properties and a different replacement rate, even though they ultimately derive from bone marrow precursors. These experiments were done for a different purpose, and unfortunately we did not examine tissue histiocytes or Kupffer cells at the same time. So we have nothing useful to say about their turnover rates, though other evidence suggests that this is relatively slow.

Nevertheless, Ralph van Furth has produced convincing evidence for a steady production of monocytes from bone marrow precursors in mice. They undergo various forms of differentiation which we have been hearing about, and some evidently persist longer than others. What puzzles me is what happens to them in the end. Some are coughed up or lost as pulmonary macrophages, some emigrate through the intestinal wall and through the renal papillae, and some stay around as fixed macrophages for a long time. But what is the ultimate fate of the monocytes generated daily? I have never found a satisfactory answer to this question.

I would like to return to the role of the marginal zone macrophages, which in mice and rats selectively retain TI antigens, which are generally poorly digestible carbohydrate polymers with multiple repeated epitopes, continuously released at low concentration into the bloodstream. Some have additional macrophage-stimulating activity (e.g. bacterial lipopolysaccharides), and are taken up by macrophages generally, but those which I am concerned with are the T1-2 antigens such as haptenated Ficoll, hydroxyethyl starch or linear dextran, and bacterial capsular polysaccharides.

Ian MacLennan's group in Birmingham have produced quite strong evidence that in the rat the cells which respond are a subset of B cells in the marginal zone of the spleen which characteristically bear surface IgM but not IgD, and are relatively sessile, i.e. they do not recirculate as do other B cells. They are also selectively eliminated by a single dose of cyclophosphamide, and such treatment temporarily abrogates the antibody reponse to these T1-2 immunogens (Gray et al 1984). Both this group (Gray et al 1985) and we (Amlot et al 1985) have shown that in adult rats and mice, if the spleen is removed, the response to T1-2 immunogens is greatly and lastingly impaired. The architecture of the spleen appears to be needed, since spleen cell suspensions are unable to restore responsiveness to splenectomized mice, although the appropriate B cells are present in the cell suspensions. It seems as though the initiation of the antibody response to T1-2 immunogens depends on interaction between the B cell subpopulation and the antigen presented by the marginal zone macrophage.

Once the response is under way, however, removal of the spleen has little or no effect.

Interestingly, splenectomy has similar results in humans. Amlot & Hayes (1985) recently published a study of the anti-DNP response to DNP-Ficoll administered either before or after splenectomy and found that the response was grossly impaired in patients whose spleen had been removed up to four years previously, although if the interval was more than four years they gave normal responses when re-immunized 6–28 months later. These observations show that immunization with pneumococcal vaccine, for example, should be done before rather than after the spleen is removed, if this is possible.

van Furth: In a 25-g mouse 1.5×10^6 monocytes leave the circulation every day (van Furth et al 1973). We have calculated the turnover in animals whose cells were labelled with [^{3}H]thymidine. The mean turnover time of macrophages in the tissues is one to two weeks. However, these values are means: we don't know whether tissue macrophages are a homogeneous population or whether there are macrophages that stay much longer (or shorter) in the tissues. We can't differentiate between these cells.

Humphrey: You know where they go but you don't know where they die.

van Furth: The turnover figures mean that the cells have to leave that tissue compartment. Whether they die locally or go to local lymph nodes or to the gut or somewhere else I don't know. We haven't yet been able to isolate enough cells from the gut to do kinetic studies. A number of these cells may just be on their way out, as has been postulated for granulocytes.

Gordon: The cells I am talking about are in the lamina propria. We have not examined F4/80 antigen in faeces.

Cohn: The question John Humphrey has raised is very important. There are probably very large numbers of fixed macrophages with long lifespans. The question is how to measure the turnover rate, particularly in an extravascular compartment. Two labels seem essential; a nuclear label for continuous labelling of the bone marrow and a stable cytoplasmic label. For that you would have to evoke some sort of inflammatory or immune response in the tissue, which by itself might influence the turnover rate.

Humphrey: I once thought I had a stable label. It was a synthetic branched-chain polypeptide, (T,G)-poly Pro-poly L, made by Michael Sela, composed entirely of D-amino acids, and totally resistant to enzymic digestion. When labelled in the tyrosine with ^{125}I it could be incubated with mouse urine and faeces for a week without being degraded. Since it was taken up very well by macrophages *in vivo* I thought it would be an ideal stable marker. However if peritoneal macrophages which had taken it up were washed and reinjected into the peritoneal cavity of fresh mice, and the peritoneal content was removed and examined one day later, some 10% of the label was no longer cell-associated even though it was still in macromolecular form. It seemed that the macrophages which took the polypeptide up also continuously released it, even though they could not.degrade it. Perhaps radiolabelled gold would stay put and be a more stable marker?

Cohn: Colloidal gold should be a stable marker. That might show you whether these cells die locally and are then reingested by other cells which replace them.

Humphrey: But then you have to do electron microscopy.

Cohn: Yes, and autoradiography too. Nobody seems to want to do the experiment!

Werb: The macrophage turnover numbers are a bit strange here. Ralph van Furth says that about a million cells are made a day and Siamon Gordon says the figure is 10^8.

van Furth: I was talking about circulating monocytes. All monocytes in the circulation are renewed every day, roughly, and there are about one and a half million cells in the circulation. In the steady state the same number of monocytes come into the circulation and go out.

Werb: But there is a total of 10^8 and at a million per day that is 100 days to renew the total body pool of macrophages.

Cohn: That would represent 1% of the population but within that there must be heterogeneity, with cells of longer life and cells of shorter life.

van Furth: The liver has about 1×10^7 Kupffer cells (Crofton et al 1978) and the gut has more, probably 1 or 2×10^7 macrophages.

Werb: It is still pretty high.

Springer: To adapt the saying about old soldiers, it sounds as if macrophages don't die, they just fade away. Perhaps they are phagocytosed very rapidly, and one can't fix this event in time in thin sections.

Is it known where granulocytes go? Their turnover is 10^9 per kilogram per day. For a 30-g mouse that would be 30×10^6 cells per day, or 30 times as much as for the monocyte.

Cohn: We know as much about the granulocyte graveyard as we do about monocytes.

Springer: There are many more granulocytes than monocytes, so if one could see where they go one would see this for a granulocyte first.

Humphrey: A long time ago Sam Clark Jr and I injected fluorescent bovine serum albumin into rabbits in order to study its elimination from the circulation. This was exponential until immune complexes were formed. Then the complexes could be visualized initially in granulocytes, and at least some of these granulocytes were detectably phagocytosed by Kupffer cells in histological sections. Once granulocytes have ingested complexes, or even been mildly maltreated, their half-life in the circulation is shortened. For example when granulocytes are concentrated for transfusion, by being collected on nylon wool packs and then eluted off, it is the general experience that they do not remain in the circulation of the recipient as well as granulocytes collected on a cell separator. Even adherence to nylon wool is enough to alter their subsequent ability to remain in the circulation. Another factor which affects granulocyte circulation is endotoxin. Otto Westphal told me that 0.03 μg of Neopyrexal (a highly purified lipopolysaccharide from *S. abortus equi*) administered intravenously to humans would increase the blood granulocyte level three- to fourfold within four hours, without producing any fever or unpleasant effects. We tried it on ourselves and confirmed what he said—though by the next day my plasma C-reactive protein level had risen from being undetectable to 10 μg/ml.

We thought this rise in granulocytes might provide a measure of bone marrow reserve, but an alternative possibility was that the increased granulocyte count was due not to increased rate of output but to a change in the rate of emigration of granulocytes from the bloodstream into the tissues. Two of my colleagues had their granulocytes labelled with indium-101 and reinfused into themselves. When the label was disappearing at a steady exponential rate they were injected with Neopyrexal. Over the next three or four hours the granulocyte count rose but the rate of disappearance of the indium label from the circulation was much slower. This indicated that the emigration of granulocytes from the circulation into the tissues was temporarily held up, so that the balance between entry and leaving was altered and the result was a transient increase in granulocyte concentration within the bloodstream. So the method did not seem to provide a useful measure of bone marrow reserves and was not pursued.

Gordon: It might be interesting to focus on the emigration problem. When there is a large resident population interstitially in tissues, the cells are outside the circulation. In fetal mice there are clearly mechanisms for monocytes to leave without an obvious inflammatory stimulus. John Hartwig told us something about motility and we have to think about other chemotactic systems. Does anyone have any suggestions about the mechanisms of normal emigration? Is there a distinction between macrophage and granulocyte emigration on the one hand and T cell emigration on the other hand? The blood–brain barrier is patent for a few days after birth and cells go into the central nervous system easily, but presumably it is not easy afterwards.

Cohn: Ralph van Furth's studies on the steady-state kinetics of cohorts of labelled monocytes suggest that loss from the circulation is very random. Nothing against that has been reported since then. Depending on the rate of turnover, there must be a very tightly regulated system of replenishment of tissue resources. The stimulus for that is quite unclear. Pathological conditions of inflammation might provide a second set of stimuli. Even with microglia it is not clear that there is not a slow turnover rate through the blood–brain barrier, through the leptomeninges.

Gordon: Another problem is that cells that don't leave the circulation may line, say, the sinusoidal epithelium at selected sites. Those cells are obviously not circulating but they would look as though they were disappearing if one just monitored the peripheral blood, yet they are not extravascular either.

Cohn: There is obviously a marginated pool of granulocytes. The situation for monocytes is not quite so clear.

van Furth: Recently we reinvestigated the issue of a marginating pool of monocytes. We came to the conclusion that in mice about 50 to 60% of the total number of monocytes are in the marginating pool.

Gordon: Yes, but one wonders what is attracting them. Is it an arachidonic acid metabolite or a fibronectin product?

Nathan: Carp (1982) showed that many mitochondrial proteins are *N*-formylated and act as chemotactic factors just as synthetic *N*-formylated peptides do. So here is at least one well-defined example where there is a ligand receptor system in the normal host where tissue breakdown products could be chemotactic.

Cohn: Could chemotactic complement products be produced locally with tissue cell turnover?

Schreiber: They probably wouldn't be very extensive. Complement levels would be limiting in the tissues, and what was there would be tightly controlled by the complement regulatory proteins.

Gordon: We don't know how much complement is produced locally by the tissue macrophages.

Werb: Virtually every breakdown product of the extracellular matrix proteins is chemotactic. Some are there in very respectable amounts and a number of them are reasonably specific for monocytes as opposed to granulocytes. During morphogenesis that is certainly one thing that is going on. It may be a random process that allows cells to go into tissues. It is really a question of what keeps them there. When sites of inflammation clear up, a lot of inflammatory cells disappear and there is some evidence that some of them go elsewhere. What keeps them there may be more important than what makes them emigrate in the steady state.

Ezekowitz: Egress from the bone marrow might be different from egress from the bloodstream. Do cells have to cross an endothelial barrier when they leave the bone marrow?

Crocker: Weiss (1983) has suggested that it is a closed system, such that haemopoietic compartments are sealed off from the vascular sinuses by intact endothelium. However, it has been shown that carbon particles injected into animals can be taken up within those compartments, suggesting that pores exist within the 'endothelial barrier' (Hudson & Yoffey 1963).

Ezekowitz: Jordan Pober has looked at the effect of IFN-γ on endothelium in culture. There was a striking induction of pores. The tight alignment of junctions also seemed to fall away in response to certain agents, including IFN-γ and lipopolysaccharides.

van Furth: The pores are so small that monocytes and granulocytes wouldn't go through. They would only go through the junctions.

Ezekowitz: You mean the disrupted junctions?

Springer: I'll be presenting some information later about the importance of the Mac-1 family of glycoproteins in causing monocytes or granulocytes to leave the circulation. In patients with deficiencies in these proteins, both monocytes and neutrophils are unable or greatly depressed in their ability to cross the endothelial barrier. However, they have no problem getting out of the bone marrow into the circulation, so apparently the bone marrow endothelium is a barrier of a different nature.

Don Anderson has examined thin sections from inflammatory sites in his patients (Anderson et al 1985). The absence of neutrophils is very striking but there are lymphocytes, plasma cells and eosinophils. This implies that the emigration mechanism for eosinophils is different from that for neutrophils and monocytes. It also supports the idea that lymphocytes use different mechanisms, which of course isn't surprising because lymphocytes recirculate through lymph nodes whereas monocytes and granulocytes don't.

Werb: E. Butcher at Stanford has an antibody, MEL-14, which competes with the protein on lymphocytes that binds to high endothelial venules (Gallatin et al 1983, Reichert et al 1984). Now they have found a much lower level on monocytes, although they don't see the monocytes sticking in the section assay.

Springer: The antigen is on granulocytes too but presumably this is not a physiological mechanism because granulocytes don't use high endothelial venules to go into lymph. It is a very interesting observation but it is not sufficient by itself to explain the cell specificity of migration into lymph nodes.

Werb: But at the sites of inflammation the endothelial cells look like those in high endothelial venules. I don't know if they are antigenically similar but they become morphologically similar.

Crocker: Recent work has shown that in conjunction with IFN-γ interleukin 1 can influence the cytoskeleton of endothelial cells (Montesano et al 1985). This may be one mechanism by which the monocyte, having adhered to endothelium, is able to facilitate its own egress from the circulation. It could be particularly relevant during inflammatory and immunological stimuli.

Cohn: There seems to be some dialogue between monocytes and endothelial cells. Dr Pawloski has shown that the mere attachment of monocytes seems to be selective for endothelial cells. It triggers prostacycline synthesis and excretion by endothelial cells, so there might be changes in the size of the lumen and in the contractility of small vessels. Some of this appears to be related to the production of leukotriene C by the monocyte, which will cause endothelial cells to excrete prostacycline by itself at about 10^{-9}M.

Ezekowitz: In the egress of polymorpholeucocytes from the bloodstream, where local factors may act on endothelial cells, how high is the concentration of the factor in that local environment? And how important are the rapidity of blood flow and the affinity of the receptors for those factors on endothelial cells? Is the inference that they act if they are present where the blood flow is sluggish?

Cohn: Flow probably plays a role there. Once cells attach to endothelium of postcapillary venules, there is apposition of surfaces and perhaps vectorial transport of materials which would be at a much higher concentration locally.

REFERENCES

Amlot PL, Hayes AE 1985 Impaired human antibody response to the thymus-independent antigen, DNP-Ficoll, after splenectomy. Lancet 1:1008-1012

Amlot PL, Grennan D, Humphrey JH 1985 Splenic dependence of the antibody response to thymus-independent (T1-2) antigens. Eur J Immunol 15:508-511

Anderson DC, Schmalstieg FC, Finegold MJ et al 1985 The severe and moderate phenotypes of heritable Mac-1, LFA-1, p150,95 deficiency: their quantitative definition and relation to leukocyte dysfunction and clinical features. J Infect Dis, in press

Carp H 1982 Mitochondrial N-formylmethionyl proteins as chemoattractants for neutrophils. J Exp Med 155:264-275

Crofton RW, Diesselhoff-den Dulk MMC, van Furth R 1978 The origin, kinetics and characteristics of the Kupffer cells in the normal steady state. J Exp Med 148:1-17

Gallatin WM, Weissman IL, Butcher EC 1983 A cell-surface molecule involved in organ-specific homing of lymphocytes. Nature (Lond) 304:30-34

Gray D, McConnell I, Kumaratne DS, MacLennan ICM, Humphrey JH, Bazin H 1984 Marginal zone B cells express CR1 and CR2 receptors. Eur J Immunol 14:47-52

Gray D, Chassoux D, MacLennan ICM, Bazin H 1985 Selective depression of thymus-independent anti-DNP antibody responses induced by adult but not neonatal splenectomy. Clin Exp Immunol 60:78-86

Hudson G, Yoffey JM 1963 Reticulo-endothelial cells in the bone marrow of the guinea-pig. J Anat 97:409-416

Humphrey JH, Grennan D 1981 Different macrophage populations distinguished by means of fluorescent polysaccharides. Recognition and properties of marginal-zone macrophages. Eur J Immunol 11:221-228

Humphrey JH, Sundaram V 1985 Origin and turnover of follicular dendritic cells and marginal zone macrophages in the mouse spleen. Plenum Press, New York (8th Germinal Centre Conference), in press

Kaur J, Catovsky D, Valdimarsson H, Jennson O, Spiers ASD 1972 Familial acute myeloid leukaemia with acquired Pelger-Hüet anomaly and aneuploidy of C group. Br Med J 4:327-331

Montesano R, Orci L, Vassalli P 1985 Human endothelial cultures: phenotypic modulation by leukocyte interleukins. J Cell Physiol 122:424-434

Reichert RA, Gallatin WM, Butcher EC, Weissman IL 1984 A homing receptor-bearing cortical thymocyte subset: implications for thymus cell migration and the nature of cortisone-resistant thymocytes. Cell 38:89-99

van Furth R, Diesselhoff-den Dulk MMC, Mattie H 1973 Quantitative study on the production and kinetics of mononuclear phagocytes during an acute inflammatory reaction. J Exp Med 138:1314-1330

Weiss L 1983 The bone marrow. In: Weiss L (ed) Histology. Cell and tissue biology, 5th edn. Elsevier, Amsterdam, p 498-509

Heterogeneity of human and murine Fc_γ receptors

JAY C. UNKELESS

The Rockefeller University, Laboratory of Cellular Physiology and Immunology, 1230 York Avenue, New York City, NY 10021, USA

Abstract. Human leucocytes express at least two different Fc receptors specific for IgG ($Fc_\gamma R$). A low avidity receptor ($Fc_\gamma R_{lo}$) is found on tissue macrophages, neutrophils and NK cells. This receptor is recognized by monoclonal antibody 3G8, which does not react with a high avidity Fc receptor ($Fc_\gamma R_{hi}$) found on blood monocytes and macrophages. We have been interested in the physiological function of these two receptors, which have been shown to differ by more than 200-fold in avidity. Since $Fc_\gamma R_{hi}$ is virtually saturated by IgG present in the serum, we felt that it would not function efficiently for clearance of immune complexes, whereas $Fc_\gamma R_{lo}$ binds monomer very poorly. Immunoperoxidase staining with MAb 3G8 of frozen sections reveals the presence of $Fc_\gamma R_{lo}$ on Kupffer cells and in the red pulp of the spleen. Evidence will be presented demonstrating that infusion of MAb 3G8 into chimpanzees dramatically alters clearance times of autologous erythrocytes opsonized with chimpanzee IgG. These results suggest that $Fc_\gamma R_{lo}$ is primarily responsible for immune complex clearance *in vivo*, and that MAb 3G8 may be of clinical use in the treatment of certain autoimmune diseases.

1986 Biochemistry of macrophages. Pitman, London (Ciba Foundation Symposium 118) p 89-101

Fc receptors for IgG ($Fc_\gamma R$) perform a critical role as a link between the humoral and effector arms of the body's immune defences. Fc_γ receptors are present on a variety of cell types including B and T lymphocytes, NK cells, monocytes, macrophages and polymorphonuclear leucocytes. The binding of immune complexes to $Fc_\gamma Rs$ results in prompt and dramatic sequelae, including release of neutral and acidic hydrolases, metabolites of arachidonic acid such as prostaglandins and leukotrienes, and, in suitably activated macrophages, activated oxygen intermediates. It is easy to understand the need for $Fc_\gamma Rs$ on cells such as macrophages and polymorphonuclear leucocytes that react to the presence of immune complexes by phagocytosis of the particle and release of mediators of inflammation. However, the function of these receptors on lymphocytes is not well understood.

The ease with which $Fc_\gamma Rs$ could be detected by formation of rosettes with IgG-sensitized erythrocytes obscured the complexity of the receptors. It was, therefore, not until the application of competitive binding assays and the development of monoclonal antibodies that the extent of $Fc_\gamma R$ heterogeneity became apparent in the murine system. The first indication that there was more than one receptor came from studies (Unkeless & Eisen 1975) in which the trypsin sensitivity of murine IgG2a binding to mouse macrophages was demonstrated. In contrast, the binding site for rabbit immune complexes on macrophages is strikingly resistant to trypsin degradation. Walker (1976) then demonstrated that murine IgG2a and aggregated IgG2b did not compete for binding. A series of experiments by Diamond et al (1978), Diamond & Scharff (1980), and Diamond & Yelton (1981) in which aggregated IgG of different subclasses was used to compete for the binding of erythrocytes opsonized with monoclonal antibodies of different subclasses defined the independent binding loci for IgG2a, IgG2b/IgG1 and IgG3.

Another approach to the analysis of receptor heterogeneity has been to isolate monoclonal antibodies directed against the Fc_γ receptor. The first such MAb, 2.4G2, was derived from a fusion in which rats were immunized with murine macrophage cell lines, and the hybrid cell supernatants were screened for the ability to inhibit binding of IgG-sensitized erythrocytes to mouse macrophages (Unkeless 1979). The Fab fragment of MAb 2.4G2 blocked the binding to murine macrophages of IgG2b and IgG1 immune complexes but did not inhibit the binding of monomeric IgG2a. Two polypeptides with broad electrophoretic mobility of 60000 and 47000 M_r were isolated from the J774 mouse macrophage cell line by affinity chromatography on 2.4G2 Fab-Sepharose (Mellman & Unkeless 1980). Of great interest was the observation that the purified protein in the absence of detergent retained binding activity for Fc domains of IgG2b, IgG2a and IgG1, but did not bind to IgG3 or to immobilized $F(ab')_2$ complexes. The subclass specificity was lost under these conditions, but in the presence of Nonidet P-40 binding was restricted to murine IgG2b and IgG1 (I. S. Mellman & J. C. Unkeless, unpublished work).

The epitope recognized by MAb 2.4G2 is distributed on a variety of murine cells, including B cells, some T cells, neutrophils, monocytes and macrophages. Further confirmation of the independence of the $Fc_{\gamma2b/\gamma1}R$ and the $Fc_{\gamma2a}R$ on macrophages came from studies of Fc receptor mutants of the J774 murine macrophage cell line (Unkeless et al 1979). These mutants were largely deficient in the ability to bind IgG2b-sensitized erythrocytes, lacked the epitope recognized by MAb 2.4G2, but bound IgG2a normally. Recent evidence, however, suggests that although Fc_γ receptors on murine macrophages and lymphocytes share the epitope recognized by MAb 2.4G2 they may differ in specificity. Lane & Cooper (1982) demonstrated that IgG binding proteins isolated from murine macrophage cell lines by affinity chromatography on

IgG1- or 2.4G2-Sepharose were the same, and were altered slightly in M_r and pI from IgG2a binding proteins isolated from the same cells. However, the L1210 B cell line differed from macrophages in that all subclasses (including IgG2a) were bound poorly as monomers, and all subclasses competed with each other for binding. Furthermore, affinity chromatography on IgG-Sepharose coupled with different subclasses of IgG yielded the same protein (Lane et al 1982).

These results have been confirmed and extended by Teillaud et al (1985), who have examined the binding of Ig to myeloma and hybridoma cells. The binding of immune complexes of IgG2a, IgG2b, and IgG1 subclasses was inhibited by immune complexes of all three subclasses. The Fc$_\gamma$ receptor of X63Ag8.653 cells was trypsin-resistant, and binding of all three subclasses was inhibited by MAb 2.4G2 F(ab')$_2$. The most interesting finding, however, was that heat-aggregated M311 protein, a mutant IgG2b lacking most of the C$_H$3 domain, did not inhibit the binding of IgG2a-, IgG2b- or IgG1-sensitized erythrocytes to X63Ag8.653 cells although M311 aggregates blocked the binding of IgG1- and IgG2b-coated erythrocytes to the J774 macrophage cell line. This demonstrates a different specificity of the Fc$_\gamma$ receptors on the B cells compared to the macrophage—although the Fc receptors on the two cell types bear the same MAb 2.4G2 epitope. Similar conclusions concerning the lack of specificity of B cell receptor were reached by N. Phillips (personal communication) who observed that B cell proliferation of F(ab')$_2$ anti-μ haptenated with arsonate was inhibited by IgG2a, IgG2b, and IgG1 anti-arsonate MAbs, and that the inhibition was relieved by addition of MAb 2.4G2.

We have also found differences between Fc$_\gamma$ receptor on BCL$_1$ cells and J774 cells using monoclonal antibodies (E. Pure & J. Unkeless, unpublished work). MAb 6B7C is directed against the same antigen as MAb 2.4G2, as determined by sequential immunoprecipitation experiments, but the two reagents do not compete for binding to J774 cells, demonstrating that two different epitopes are involved. However, although MAb 6B7C binds to J774 cells nearly as well as MAb 2.4G2 does, 6B7C does not bind to the surface of BCL$_1$ cells. The question that must be raised is whether these differences are due to different gene products that share the epitope defined by MAb 2.4G2, or whether the alterations of specificity are due to subtle post-translational differences.

Given the probable presence of multiple Fc$_\gamma$ receptors on murine cells, one would like to understand more fully the physiological role these receptors play. Clearly, it would be expected that Fc$_\gamma$ receptors are involved in the clearance of immune complexes from the circulation. Indeed, Kurlander et al (1984) found that 2.4G2 IgG or Fab at μg/g doses *in vivo* in mice effectively blocked the clearance of circulating immune complexes, without affecting the clearance of monomeric IgG. The role that the Fc$_{\gamma2a}$R and the Fc$_{\gamma3}$R play in macrophage physiology is not clear. Ralph et al (1980) found that all subclasses of IgG mediate macrophage phagocytosis and lysis of erythrocytes. However, Matthews et al (1981) and Herlyn & Koprowski (1982) both found that the IgG subclass effective in suppression of tumour growth in mice is IgG2a, suggesting a special role for the macrophage high avidity $Fc_{\gamma2a}$ receptor. In this regard, it is interesting that activation of macrophages by live bacillus Calmette-Guérin or lymphokine results in an increase in binding sites for IgG2a and a decrease in the binding sites for IgG2b (Ezekowitz et al 1983).

Another development of interest is the demonstration that in murine serum there is a soluble Fc receptor related antigenically to that on the cells. Khayat et al (1984) and Pure et al (1984) reported essentially similar results demonstrating protein reactive with MAb 2.4G2 in murine serum, and the removal of this material by passage over insoluble IgG columns. The size of the protein precipitated from murine serum by 2.4G2-Sepharose was $48\,000\,M_r$, significantly smaller than that found on the cell membrane. The concentration of soluble $Fc_{\gamma}R$ in murine serum was $\sim 10^{-9}$ M and increased with age. Levels of soluble $Fc_{\gamma}R$ in germ-free mice were less than those in neonatal mice, suggesting that release of the soluble $Fc_{\gamma}R$ is correlated with activation of the immune system. Further evidence for this thesis comes from the observation by Pure et al (1984) that the amount of soluble MAb 2.4G2-reactive $Fc_{\gamma}R$ released by both splenic B cells and the cloned B cell line BCL-1 CW 13.20-3B3 was increased dramatically by stimulation with lipopolysaccharide.

Analysis of human Fc_{γ} receptors has lagged somewhat behind analysis of the murine model. It is now clear, however, that human leucocytes have at least two Fc_{γ} receptors that differ in antigenicity and ligand-binding properties. The initial observation made by Kurlander & Batker (1982) was that the association constant for the binding of human IgG1 dimers and trimers to monocytes was 100–1000 times higher than that for binding to neutrophils. Confirming these results, Fleit et al (1982) also found a lack of binding of human IgG1 monomer to neutrophils. It is interesting that the dramatic difference in avidity between the neutrophil and monocyte had not been observed previously, despite extensive experimentation that led to the definition of high avidity binding sites on monocytes and relative affinities for binding to monocytes of the different human IgG subclasses (see Dickler 1976, for review).

Fleit et al (1982) then isolated an MAb, 3G8, that was directed against the low avidity Fc_{γ} receptor ($Fc_{\gamma}R_{lo}$). The hybridoma cell supernatants were screened for inhibition of rosetting on neutrophils of IgG-sensitized erythrocytes. Quantitative binding studies revealed that neutrophils bear 1.3×10^5 3G8 Fab binding sites per cell, and the 3G8 Fab fragment totally blocked the binding of both IgG-sensitized erythrocytes and soluble immune complexes to neutrophils, but had no effect whatsoever on binding of monomeric IgG1 to monocytes or the U937 human cell line, which bears a high avidity Fc$_\gamma$ receptor (Fc$_\gamma$R$_{hi}$). The epitope defined by MAb 3G8 was totally absent from blood monocytes, but was present on 60% of lung macrophages and was also present on monocytes after culture for one week *in vitro*, demonstrating the status of Fc$_\gamma$R$_{lo}$ as an induced or a differentiation antigen. Fleit et al (1984) also examined the ontogeny of Fc$_\gamma$R$_{lo}$ synthesis during myeloid differentiation, and concluded that it is a relatively late differentiation antigen, appearing during the metamyelocyte stage.

These results have been extended by Kurlander et al (1984), who examined the binding of IgG1 dimers to blood monocytes and resident peritoneal macrophages obtained at laparoscopy. Scatchard analysis of the binding data showed that blood monocytes had a high avidity site for IgG1 dimers with a K_a of $2.6 \times 10^9 \text{M}^{-1}$. Peritoneal macrophages, in addition to the high avidity site, had a more abundant low avidity site with a K_a of $1.1 \times 10^7 \text{M}^{-1}$. It is the low avidity site (Fc$_\gamma$R$_{lo}$) that we believe corresponds to the receptor identified by MAb 3G8.

A variety of anti-Fc$_\gamma$R$_{lo}$ MAbs have been isolated and their characteristics compared by Perussia et al (1984). These MAbs are directed against different epitopes on the same molecule, and thus might be expected to differ in their capacity to inhibit immune complex binding, which they do. More surprising, however, is the observation that MAb B73.1, originally isolated as a reagent specific for human NK cells, is directed against an epitope present on neutrophils of 50% of individuals tested. The basis for this cell and population polymorphism is not understood. Anderson et al (1985) produced a goat antiserum directed against the receptor, but no monoclonal reagents have been reported directed against the high avidity receptor.

In addition to Fc$_\gamma$ receptor heterogeneity deduced by analysis of the binding of ligand and MAbs, analysis of the proteins by affinity chromatography or immunoprecipitation reveals a wealth of complexity. All the immunoprecipitation experiments reported with the various anti-Fc$_\gamma$R$_{lo}$ MAbs discussed by Perussia et al (1984) identify a protein migrating with a diffuse M_r of 51–73 000. There is some controversy about eosinophil Fc$_\gamma$ receptors. Fleit et al (1982) report that the epitope recognized by MAb 3G8 is present on human eosinophils, but Kulczycki (1984) reported that IgG binding proteins isolated by affinity chromatography from labelled eosinophils and neutrophils were clearly different. The neutrophil had a 52–68 000 M_r receptor not capable of binding to IgG3-Sepharose and the eosinophil had a 43 000 M_r receptor that bound to both IgG1 and IgG3. In similar affinity chromatography studies on IgG-Sepharose Cohen et al (1983) found that different proteins were isolated from monocytes, B lymphocytes and non-B lymphocytes by affinity chromatography. The Fc$_\gamma$ receptor isolated from human monocytes by affinity chromatography was of 60–68 000 M_r; the goat anti-Fc$_\gamma$ receptor serum prepared by Anderson et al (1985) immunoprecipitated peptides of 72 000 and 40–43 000 M_r.

As with the murine Fc$_\gamma$ receptors discussed previously, the role that the high and low affinity Fc$_\gamma$ receptors play in macrophage and lymphocyte physiology is not clearly understood, but it would seem that the great difference in association constants for monomeric IgG would dictate the function. The Fc$_\gamma$R$_{hi}$ must be saturated with IgG, given that the concentration of IgG in serum is $\sim 10^{-5}$ M. The Fc$_\gamma$R$_{lo}$, by contrast, is probably more 'available' for ligand binding, and may play an important role in clearance of immune complexes. It is likely that the Fc$_\gamma$R$_{hi}$ is analogous in function to the murine Fc$_{\gamma2a}$R. Supporting this is the observation of Guyre et al (1983) that interferon-γ specifically induced Fc$_\gamma$R$_{hi}$ expression on monocytes and the U937 cell line. In addition to priming the cell for cytolytic function in release of activated oxygen metabolites (see Nathan & Tsunawaki, this volume), IFN-γ probably increases the sensitivity of the macrophage/monocyte recognition systems.

We have begun a series of experiments to study the *in vivo* role of Fc$_\gamma$R$_{lo}$, and first have examined its distribution, by MAb 3G8 immunoperoxidase staining of frozen sections, in human organs (M. Witmer & J. C. Unkeless, unpublished work). Intense 3G8 staining was found in those areas traditionally thought to be the loci of immune complex clearance—the Kupffer cells of the liver and the red pulp of the spleen. There was little or no immunoperoxidase product in splenic white pulp. The phylogenetic distribution of the epitope recognized by MAb 3G8 was restricted to the great apes; it was not found in any monkeys we examined. The distribution of MAb 3G8 reactivity on peripheral leucocytes of the chimpanzee and the inhibition of neutrophil Fc$_\gamma$ receptor function was identical to that found with human cells (S. B. Clarkson & J. C. Unkeless, unpublished work).

The chimpanzee was thus the only animal suitable for *in vivo* studies of the effect of MAb 3G8 on the kinetics of immune complex clearance. Preliminary experiments have shown that infusion of MAb 3G8 at a dose of 1 mg/kg body weight totally blocks clearance of IgG-sensitized chimpanzee erythrocytes for about two weeks, and the clearance kinetics return to normal by six weeks. Immediately after infusion of the MAb there was a transitory drop in monocyte, lymphocyte and neutrophil numbers. The monocyte and lymphocyte populations returned to normal by 24 h; the neutrophil count, which dropped to $\sim 1000/mm^3$ immediately after infusion of MAb 3G8, returned to normal levels more slowly, but was normal at two weeks (S. B. Clarkson & J. C. Unkeless, unpublished work). No other untoward side-effects were observed in the animals. These results demonstrate the feasibility of *in vivo* blockade of Fc-mediated clearance phenomena using monoclonal reagents. Further controls with which we can define the cause of the blockade more clearly are being prepared.

Acknowledgement

This work has been supported by grants AI-14603 and CA-30198. J. Unkeless is an American Cancer Society Research Scholar.

REFERENCES

Anderson CL, Spence JM, Edwards TS, Nusbacher J 1985 Characterization of a polyvalent antibody directed against the IgG Fc receptor of human mononuclear phagocytes. J Immunol 134:465-470

Cohen L, Sharp S, Kulczycki A Jr 1983 Human monocytes, B lymphocytes, and non-B lymphocytes each have structurally unique Fc$_\gamma$ receptors. J Immunol 131:378-383

Diamond B, Scharff MD 1980 IgG1 and IgG2b share the Fc receptor on mouse macrophages. J Immunol 125:631-633

Diamond B, Yelton DE 1981 A new Fc receptor on mouse macrophages binding IgG3. J Exp Med 153:514-519

Diamond B, Bloom BR, Scharff MD 1978 The Fc receptors of primary and cultured phagocytic cells studied with homogeneous antibodies. J Immunol 121:1329-1333

Dickler HB 1976 Lymphocyte receptors for immunoglobulin. Adv Immunol 24:167-214

Ezekowitz RAV, Bampton M, Gordon S 1983 Macrophage activation selectively enhances expression of Fc receptors for IgG2a. J Exp Med 157:807-812

Fleit HB, Wright SD, Unkeless JC 1982 Human neutrophil Fc$_\gamma$ receptor distribution and structure. Proc Natl Acad Sci USA 79:3275-3279

Fleit HB, Wright SD, Durie CJ, Valinsky JE, Unkeless JC 1984 Ontogeny of Fc receptors and complement receptor (CR3) during human myeloid differentiation. J Clin Invest 73:516-525

Guyre PM, Morganelli PM, Miller R 1983 Recombinant immune interferon increases IgG Fc receptors on cultured human mononuclear phagocytes. J Clin Invest 72:393-397

Herlyn D, Koprowski H 1982 IgG2a monoclonal antibodies inhibit tumor growth through interaction with effector cells. Proc Natl Acad Sci USA 79:4761-4765

Khayat D, Dux Z, Anavi R, Shlomo I, Witz P, Ran M 1984 Circulating cell-free Fc$_{\gamma2b/\gamma1}$R in normal mouse serum: its detection and specificity. J Immunol 132:2496-2501

Kulczycki A Jr 1984 Human neutrophils and eosinophils have structurally distinct Fc$_\gamma$ receptors. J Immunol 133:849-854

Kurlander RJ, Batker J 1982 The binding of human immunoglobulin G1 monomer and small, covalently cross-linked polymers of immunoglobulin G1 to human peripheral blood monocytes and polymorphonuclear leukocytes. J Clin Invest 69:1-8

Kurlander RJ, Ellison DM, Hall J 1984 The blockade of Fc receptor-mediated clearance of immune complexes *in vivo* by a monoclonal antibody (2.4G2) directed against Fc receptors on murine leukocytes. J Immunol 133:855-862

Kurlander, RJ, Haney AF, Gartrell J 1984 Human peritoneal macrophages possess two populations of IgG Fc receptors. Cell Immunol 86:479-490

Lane BC, Bricker MD, Cooper SM 1982 Fc receptors of mouse cell lines II. IgG binding specificity and identification of the Fc receptor on a lymphoid leukemia. J Immunol 128:1825-1831

Lane BC, Cooper SM 1982 Fc receptors on mouse cell lines I. Distinct proteins mediate the IgG subclass-specific Fc binding activities of macrophages. J Immunol 128:1819-1824

Matthews TJ, Collins JJ, Roloson GJ, Thiel HJ, Bolognesi DP 1981 Immunologic control of the ascites form of murine adenocarcinoma 755 IV. Characterization of the protective antibody in hyperimmune serum. J Immunol 126:2332-2336

Mellman IS, Unkeless JC 1980 Purification of a functional mouse Fc receptor through the use of a monoclonal antibody. J Exp Med 152:1048-1069

Nathan C, Tsunawaki S 1986 Secretion of toxic oxygen products by macrophages: regulatory cytokines and their effects on the oxidase. This volume, p 211-226

Perussia B, Trinchieri G, Jackson A et al 1984 The Fc receptor for IgG on human natural killer cells: phenotypic, functional and comparative studies with monoclonal antibodies. J Immunol 133:180-190

Pure E, Durie CJ, Summerill CK, Unkeless JC 1984 Identification of soluble Fc receptors in mouse serum and conditioned medium of stimulated B cells. J Exp Med 160:1836-1849

Ralph P, Nakoinz I, Diamond B, Yelton D 1980 All classes of murine IgG antibody mediate macrophage phagocytosis and lysis of erythrocytes. J Immunol 125:1885-1888

Teillaud J-L, Diamond B, Pollock RR, Fajtova V, Scharff MD 1985 Fc receptors on cultured myeloma and hybridoma cells. J Immunol 134:1774-1779

Unkeless JC 1979 Characterization of a monoclonal antibody directed against mouse macrophage and lymphocyte Fc receptors. J Exp Med 150:580-596

Unkeless JC, Eisen HN 1975 Binding of monomeric immunoglobulins to Fc receptors of mouse macrophages. J Exp Med 142:1520-1533

Unkeless JC, Kaplan G, Plutner H, Cohn ZA 1979 Fc-receptor variants of a mouse macrophage cell line. Proc Natl Acad Sci USA 76:1400-1404

Walker WS 1976 Separate Fc receptors for immunoglobulins IgG2a and IgG2b on an established cell line of mouse macrophages. J Immunol 116:911-914

DISCUSSION

Gordon: Have you looked at the effect of MAb 2.4G2 on clearance in the mouse?

Unkeless: Roger Kurlander found a fairly dramatic effect on immune complex clearance but no effect on the clearance rate of monomeric immunoglobulin (Kurlander et al 1984), which is what one would predict. In that paper Kurlander reported that there was no effect on the composition of the lymphocyte populations, which I found surprising in view of our results in chimpanzees infused with MAb 3G8.

Nathan: You showed all the other cells in the blood but what about the platelet count?

Unkeless: We didn't do platelet counts.

Singer: What function do you assign to the high avidity receptor?

Unkeless: I suspect it may be involved in antibody-dependent cytotoxicity. Matthews et al (1981), Herlyn & Koprowski (1982) and Herlyn et al (1985) have reported that murine IgG2a is effective in eradicating tumours by antibody-dependent cytotoxicity. In the mouse system the $Fc_\gamma 2a$ receptor is the high avidity receptor and it may be analogous to the high avidity receptor on human monocytes.

Singer: Are the two receptors physically independent in the membrane?

Unkeless: Yes; as I showed, they are regulated independently. We also used human monocytes that had been cultured *in vitro* for a week, at which time they begin to express the low avidity receptor. We plated *in vitro* matured monocytes on surfaces coated with Fab fragments of monoclonal antibody 3G8; this removes the low avidity receptor but the high avidity receptor is still there and it rosettes quite nicely.

Roos: Von dem Borne and colleagues in our institute have shown that the low avidity receptor you spoke about carries the neutrophil-specific antigen NA1 (Werner et al 1985). They have made a monoclonal against the Fc$_\gamma$ receptor that reacts only with neutrophils from NA1-positive donors and not with K lymphocytes. Inhibition of EA rosette formation, immunoprecipitation and blocking studies with anti-NA sera all point to the conclusion that the NA1 antigen is located on the Fc receptor. It also means that the Fc receptors on K lymphocytes and neutrophils are different, because the NA1 antigens are not present on lymphocytes.

Unkeless: I am not sure that the difference lies at the level of the genome. It could equally likely be due to different post-translational modification.

Roos: That is possible. There are different epitopes, but not necessarily different proteins.

Unkeless: Some recent work shows that the lymphocyte receptor in murine B cells may be different, at least in specificity, from the receptor on macrophages, even though both receptors bear the epitope for 2.4G2. We do not know unequivocally that these are different gene products.

Cole: Have you tried to accelerate the expression of Fc receptors on human monocytes during the first three to seven days by addition of IFN-γ or any other substances?

Unkeless: IFN-γ doesn't induce low avidity Fc$_\gamma$ receptor expression. We haven't studied other cytokines.

Moore: Is the Fc receptor a monomer, a dimer or a polymer?

Unkeless: We have no data bearing on that question.

Moore: Why do some cells such as large granulocytes tend to lose their Fc receptor expression quite rapidly on culture in interleukin 2, for example?

Unkeless: I don't really know. In the Langerhans cells, for example, the transient expression of 2.4G2 is lost during culture as the cells mature, as Drs Ralph Steinman and Gerald Schuler have found (Schuler & Steinman 1985). I don't know why expression is not maintained. There may be cytokines that drive the expression of those receptors in the site where they reside.

Gordon: What about shedding experiments where B lymphocytes release Fc$_\gamma$ receptor antigen?

Unkeless: Pure et al (1984) and Khayat et al (1985) have shown that a soluble form of receptor immunoreactive with MAb 2.4G2 is present in mouse serum at a low concentration, 10^{-9} or 10^{-8} M. Dr Pure's results suggest that this is B cell-derived because the amount of material is greatly increased by lipopolysac-charide stimulation. We don't know whether the release of soluble Fc_γ is due to proteolysis of the molecule on the surface of the B cells or to some other kind of processing of message, or even to an entirely different gene product which bears the epitope recognized by the monoclonal antibody.

Dean: Does the soluble release receptor have lipid associated with it in the same way as the *in situ* receptor does? Is the 'smear' of the immunoprecipitated material you showed due to the association with lipid? For instance, is it removed by delipidation or a high concentration of SDS? It looks very like what one gets with LDL-labelled protein.

Unkeless: We don't know whether any lipid is associated with the receptor. The smear collapses if Asn-linked carbohydrate synthesis is blocked by tuni-camycin. I suspect there is differential glycosylation.

Dean: But does it disappear if you positively put a high concentration of SDS in during sample preparation?

Unkeless: We haven't done that.

Roos: In human Fc_γ receptor preparations, you can get rid of carbohydrate chains by incubation with endoglycosidases.

van Furth: How do you explain the rapid disappearance of monoclonal antibodies in the chimpanzee? The usual half-life is 21 days so one would expect them to be there for much longer than two weeks. Did you find antibodies against the murine immunoglobulins?

Unkeless: Presumably the neutrophils that are maturing and being released from the bone marrow bear the epitope recognized by MAb 2.4G2. That is, there is a continuing 'sink' for that antibody which might explain why it is cleared more rapidly than might be expected. The chimpanzees developed anti-murine immunoglobulin antibody.

Schreiber: Macrophages treated with immune complexes or adherent to IgG-coated dishes are inhibited in their ability to express tumoricidal activity or express Ia antigens when exposed to IFN-γ. This raises the possibility that the low avidity of the Fc receptor might be important in the regulation of mac-rophage function. Can the monoclonals in either system regulate macrophage function directly?

Unkeless: We haven't looked at that. Plating macrophages on immune complexes is a fairly drastic thing to do to the cells because immune complexes trigger these cells to do almost everything they are capable of doing. I don't know how we are altering the physiology of the cell when we deliver what is really an optimal frustrated phagocytic stimulus.

Nathan: If you plate 2.4G2 on a dish and add activated mouse macrophages, this does not trigger substantial respiratory burst activity, although in soluble form even the Fab of 2.4G2 blocks antibody-dependent cell-mediated cytoto-xicity (Nathan et al 1980).

Cohn: Do you get ligand-dependent down-regulation of the 3G8 receptor?

Unkeless: That hasn't been looked at adequately.

Humphrey: Can you be sure that the autologous erythrocytes coated with chimpanzee IgG didn't activate complement?

Unkeless: We are injecting the cells back into the animal and the animal hasn't been decomplemented, so I can't rule that out. If complement is activated presumably it is only going to go as far as C4 in any case, because in a homologous system one rarely gets activation past that point.

Humphrey: The effect was clearly due to the monoclonals but what is the mechanism?

Unkeless: Clearance of sensitized erythrocytes in the animal infused with 3G8 was clearly faster than clearance of non-opsonized autologous erythrocytes would have been. Some clearance mechanism is operating there that is not blocked by 3G8.

Humphrey: Could you see where the erythrocytes are cleared to?

Unkeless: No. Radioisotope imaging is needed for that and it is difficult to do.

Humphrey: In the human spleen stained with monoclonals, if you had examined deeper into the white pulp would you see staining of follicular dendritic cells?

Unkeless: I can't say.

Springer: There could be some damage to Kupffer cells in your system. For example monocytes or neutrophils might bind to the antibody in Kupffer cells and damage the cells. You could also have a very high phagocytic load due to clearance of neutrophils. Have you tested whether any other mechanisms of clearance are affected by the MAb infusion? Have you looked at heat-treated red cells?

Unkeless: Those are all things that should be done. The animals survived quite happily but the problem is that these experiments are difficult to arrange.

Whaley: Do both the high and low avidity Fc receptors on the human macrophage cause membrane depolarization when they interact with a suitable ligand?

Unkeless: We are trying to make monoclonal antibodies now against the high avidity receptor on human monocytes, in an effort to get probes with which we can do those sorts of experiments.

Singer: Is there any indication of similar heterogeneity in IgE or other Fc receptors?

Unkeless: The classic high avidity IgE receptor is present on basophils and mast cells, as described by Dr Henry Metzger and many others. There is an IgE receptor on lymphocytes, and possibly monocytes as well, which has a much lower avidity and is apparently a different molecule. There seem to be receptors for every conceivable immunoglobulin ligand, with the exception of IgM.

Singer: How many of these receptors for immunoglobulins are present on neutrophils?

Unkeless: Neutrophils have only the low avidity receptor. Neutrophils also have an Fc receptor for IgA (Fanger et al 1983).

Singer: And the macrophages?

Unkeless: There are high avidity and low avidity immunoglobulin G receptors and there are reports of IgE receptors on U937 cells and monocytes (Anderson & Spiegelberg 1981, Melewicz et al 1982). I don't know about IgA.

Schreiber: You showed that HL60 presumably doesn't have the 3G8 epitope, although it has high avidity Fc receptors. If you use DMSO to induce HL60 to become neutrophils, are the original high avidity receptors lost?

Unkeless: We have tried to do that experiment. The overall number of IgG1 binding sites did not change much. We need to do that on a cell-by-cell basis because incubating HL60 with DMSO results in differentiation of the cells to the point where the low avidity Fc_γ receptor is expressed by only 20 or 30% of the population. We need to see whether the 20 or 30% of cells that express the epitope for MAb 3G8 lose the high avidity receptor. Since we were doing population binding studies, we can't answer the question.

Ezekowitz: Could you treat tissue macrophages, such as lung macrophages, with IFN-γ and induce a high avidity receptor, as we did in mice (Ezekowitz et al 1983)?

Unkeless: I would think so.

REFERENCES

Anderson CL, Spiegelberg HL 1981 Macrophage receptors for IgE: binding of IgE to specific IgE Fc receptors on a human macrophage cell line, U937. J Immunol 126:2470-2473

Ezekowitz RAB, Bampton M, Gordon S 1983 Macrophage activation selectively enhances expression of Fc receptors for IgG2a. J Exp Med 157:807-812

Fanger MW, Goldstine SN, Shen L 1983 The properties and role of receptors for IgA on human leukocytes. Ann NY Acad Sci 409:552-563

Herlyn D, Koprowski H 1982 IgG2a monoclonal antibodies inhibit human tumor growth through interaction with effector cells. Proc Natl Acad Sci USA 79:4761-4765

Herlyn D, Powe HJ, Ross AH, Herlyn M, Koprowski H 1985 Inhibition of human tumor growth by IgG2a monoclonal antibodies correlates with antibody density on tumor cells. J Immunol 134:1300-1304

Khayat D, Dux Z, Anavi R, Shlomo Y, Witz IP, Ran M 1984 Circulating cellfree Fcγ2b/γ1 receptor in normal mouse serum: its detection and specificity. J Immunol 132:2496-2501

Kurlander RJ, Ellison DM, Hall J 1984 The blockade of Fc receptor-mediated clearance of immune complexes in vivo by a monoclonal antibody (2.4G2) directed against Fc receptors on murine leukocytes. J Immunol 133:855-862

Matthews TJ, Collins JJ, Roloson GJ, Thiel HJ, Bolognesi DP 1981 Immunologic control of the ascites form of murine adenocarcinoma 755. IV. Characterization of the protective antibody in hyperimmune serum. J Immunol 126:2332-2336

Melewicz FM, Plummer JM, Spiegelberg HL 1982 Comparison of the Fc receptors for IgE on human lymphocytes and monocytes. J Immunol 129:563-569

Nathan C, Brukner L, Kaplan G, Unkeless J, Cohn A 1980 Role of activated macrophages in antibody dependent lysis of tumour cells. J Exp Med 152:183-197

Pure E, Durie CJ, Summerill CK, Unkeless JC 1984 Identification of soluble Fc receptors in mouse serum and the conditioned medium of stimulated B cells. J Exp Med 160:1836-1849

Schuler G, Steinman RM 1985 Murine epidermal Langerhans cells mature into potent immunostimulatory dendritic cells in vitro. J Exp Med 161:526-546

Werner G, von dem Borne AEG, Bos MJE et al 1985 Localization of the human NA1 alloantigen on neutrophil Fcγ receptors. In: Reinherz EL et al (eds) Leucocyte typing II. Springer-Verlag, Berlin, in press

The importance of the Mac-1, LFA-1 glycoprotein family in monocyte and granulocyte adherence, chemotaxis, and migration into inflammatory sites: insights from an experiment of nature

TIMOTHY A. SPRINGER* and DONALD C. ANDERSON†

*Dana-Farber Cancer Institute, Harvard Medical School, 44 Binney Street, Boston, Massachusetts 02115, and †Baylor College of Medicine and Texas Children's Hospital, 6621 Fannin, Houston, Texas 77030, USA

Abstract. The Mac-1, LFA-1 (lymphocyte function-associated 1), p150,95 family of glyco-proteins, which share a common β subunit of M_r 95 000, are of widespread importance in leucocyte adhesion reactions. This paper focuses on the role of this glycoprotein family in granulocyte and monocyte adhesion and chemotaxis *in vitro*, and in migration into inflammatory sites *in vivo*. Most findings have been made with granulocytes, but results with monocytes are similar. Some studies have used leucocytes from patients exhibiting a severe or moderate deficiency in expression of this glycoprotein family, which is secondary to a defect in the common β subunit. Patients are susceptible to bacterial infections and have defective pus formation and Rebuck skin-window tests, despite chronic granulocyto-sis. Granulocytes from such patients exhibit defective adherence to serum albumin and fibronectin-coated glass or plastic, defective orientation and directed migration in response to chemoattractants, and are defective in chemoattractant-stimulated aggregation and hyperadherence. Antibodies to the common β subunit, to the Mac-1 α subunit, and to a lesser extent to the LFA-1 and p150,95 α subunits, inhibit many of the same functional responses by normal cells. In normal granulocytes and monocytes chemoattractants stimu-late a five-fold increase in Mac-1 and p150,95 surface expression, by mobilization of a latent, presumably intracellular, pool. Cells from patients are deficient in up-regulation of these molecules but show normal up-regulation of other surface receptors, degranulation and oxidative burst. The hypothesis is presented that Mac-1 and p150,95 regulate or directly mediate the increase in granulocyte and monocyte adhesivity, which is essential for diapede-sis, chemotaxis and migration into inflammatory sites.

1986 Biochemistry of macrophages. Pitman, London (Ciba Foundation Symposium 118) p 102-126

Cell surface adherence reactions are of central importance in a wide spectrum of granulocyte, monocyte and lymphocyte functions which contribute to host defences against infection. Granulocyte and monocyte translocation *in vitro* and mobilization *in vivo* are influenced by the nature of cell–substrate adherence interactions. Studies using time-lapse photography have shown that granulocytes adhere preferentially to vascular endothelium adjacent to a site of inflammation before their diapedesis into tissues (Atherton & Born 1972). This 'directed' adherence is facilitated by by-products of inflammation such as C5a and *N*-formyl-methionyl peptides which bind to specific receptors on granulocytes and monocytes and initiate a sequence of events that enhance cellular adherence (reviewed in Snyderman & Pike 1984 and Tonnesen et al 1984). Much evidence exists that physical properties of endothelial cells or experimental substrates (glass, plastic, albumin, fibrinogen, fibronectin) influence adherence and, secondarily, the extent and direction of cell migration (Wilkinson 1982). Migration towards gradients of chemotactic factors *in vitro* appears to require intermittent adhesion which is sufficiently strong to allow attachment to a substrate but sufficiently localized temporally to allow selective detachment (Wilkinson 1982).

Adhesive interactions are fundamental to other granulocyte and monocyte functions. Specific recognition of opsonized microorganisms is facilitated by membrane receptors for immunoglobulin G (IgG) and for the third component of complement (C3), which mediate adhesion to opsonized microorganisms before the cytoskeletal events leading to endocytosis are triggered. Adhesion mediated by IgG (Fc) receptors can also trigger antibody-dependent killing of target cells, independently of endocytosis. In the absence of opsonins, some microorganisms may adhere to granulocytes and monocytes without undergoing ingestion, or may be phagocytosed inefficiently, depending on the physical properties of the microorganism (Dawson & Mandell 1980).

Many different cell surface proteins are important in these events. Among these, and of ubiquitous importance in the aforementioned granulocyte and monocyte adhesion reactions, and additionally in lymphoid adhesive interactions, are the Mac-1, LFA-1 (lymphocyte function-associated 1) family of glycoproteins (Table 1). These molecules appear to synergize with other receptors or act on their own to regulate or mediate a panoply of leucocyte functional interactions. The wide variety of these functions, and their common dependence on cell adhesion, suggests that the Mac-1, LFA-1 glycoproteins are of general importance in leucocyte adhesion reactions. In this sense, they may be analogous to the adhesion molecules of other tissues, such as the nervous system (N-CAM) or liver (L-CAM).

The thesis of this paper is that these glycoproteins regulate monocyte and granulocyte adherence and chemotaxis *in vitro*, and diapedesis and migration into inflammatory sites *in vivo*. Two types of studies are presented. The first uses monoclonal antibodies (MAb) to these glycoproteins (Sanchez-Madrid et al 1983). MAbs have been obtained which are specific for the αM, αL,

TABLE 1 The Mac-1, LFA-1 family[a]

	Mac-1 (OKM1, Mol)	LFA-1	p150,95
Subunits ($M_r \times 10^{-3}$)	αM β (170,95)	αL β (180,95)	αX β (150,95)
Cell distribution	Monocytes Macrophages Granulocytes Large granular lymphocytes	Lymphocytes Monocytes Granulocytes Large granular lymphocytes	Monocytes Macrophages Granulocytes
Stimulation increases surface expression	+	−	+
Functions inhibited by monoclonal antibodies	Complement receptor type three; Granulocyte adherence, stimulated adherence, spreading, aggregation and chemotaxis	Cytolytic T lymphocyte-mediated killing and T helper cell responses; Natural killing; Antibody-dependent cellular cytotoxicity; Phorbol ester-stimulated lymphocyte aggregation	?

Common features. The β subunits appear identical. The α subunits αM and αL are 35% homologous in sequence. The α and β subunits are non-covalently associated in $\alpha_1\beta_1$ complexes. Both α and β subunits are glycosylated and exposed on the cell surface. All functions shown require divalent cations.
[a] Reviewed in Springer et al (1982), Sanchez-Madrid et al (1983) and Springer & Anderson (1985a,b).

or αX subunits, and thus react only with Mac-1, LFA-1, or p150,95, respectively (Table 1). Another type of MAb reacts with the common β subunit, and hence with all three of these glycoproteins. The other type of study uses cells from patients with a recently discovered heritable deficiency of the entire glycoprotein family. This deficiency is detailed below. Before these studies, we describe a physiologically important property of the Mac-1 and p150,95 glycoproteins: their up-regulation by inflammatory stimuli.

Up-regulation of Mac-1 and p150,95 on granulocytes and monocytes

N-formyl-methionyl peptides such as f-Met-Leu-Phe, which are produced by bacteria, and the C5a anaphylatoxin, a product of complement activation, are chemoattractants for monocytes and granulocytes. These molecules bind with high affinity to specific receptors on these cells (Snyderman & Pike 1984).

In addition to chemotaxis, they trigger increased adherence to surfaces (termed 'hyperadherence'), granulocyte aggregation, the respiratory burst, and the secretion of about 20% of the lactoferrin and cobalamin-binding protein stored in granulocytes (Wilkinson 1982, Gallin 1982). These proteins are stored in the secondary or 'specific' granules of granulocytes. After granulocytes in suspension are stimulated with chemoattractants, electron microscope morphometric analysis demonstrates rapid bipolarization of the cell with the formation of lamellipodia at one end, the loss of about 30% of the secondary granules but no loss of primary granules, and an increase of about 25% in surface area. The increase in area can be accounted for by the fusion of the membrane bilayer surrounding secondary granules with the plasma membrane (Hoffstein et al 1982).

Importantly, the chemoattractant f-Met-Leu-Phe stimulates a marked increase in the amount of Mac-1 and p150,95 expressed on the surface of monocytes (Fig. 1) and granulocytes (Springer et al 1984). Mac-1 and p150,95 increase fivefold on both granulocytes and monocytes (Springer et al 1984 and unpublished). In contrast, the related LFA-1 glycoprotein is not increased. The increases are stimulated by 10^{-8}M f-Met-Leu-Phe, which is within the concentration range for chemotaxis (Wilkinson 1982). The chemoattractant C5a, and the secretagogues phorbol myristyl acetate (PMA) and calcium ionophore A23187 stimulate similar increases in surface expression (Anderson et al 1985). Up-regulation is maximal after 8 min at 37 °C, and is not impeded by inhibitors of protein synthesis (L. Miller et al, unpublished).

Thus, Mac-1 and p150,95 are stored in a latent pool in granulocytes and monocytes, and can be mobilized to the cell surface by chemoattractants (Fig. 2). The fivefold increase shows that the amount of Mac-1 and p150,95 is considerably higher than on the unstimulated cell surface. Furthermore, since the fivefold increase in Mac-1 and p150,95 is accompanied by an increase of only about 25% in granulocyte surface area (Hoffstein et al 1982), the density of Mac-1 and p150,95 in the membrane bilayer of the storage vesicle must be about 16-fold higher than on the cell surface. In granulocytes, the intracellular Mac-1 pool cosediments in sucrose gradients with secondary granules (Todd et al 1984), but further experiments are needed before it can be definitely established whether Mac-1 and p150,95 are stored in the membrane enclosing secondary granules or in some other secretory vesicle. The location of the latent pool in monocytes has not yet been examined.

Mac-1, LFA-1 deficiency disease

Recently, a disease has been recognized in which the Mac-1, LFA-1 and p150,95 glycoproteins are deficient (Springer et al 1984, Anderson et al 1985).

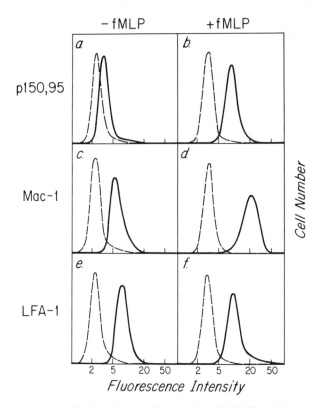

FIG. 1. Chemoattractant stimulates increased expression of p150,95 and Mac-1 but not LFA-1 on monocytes. Mononuclear cells were incubated for 30 min at 37 °C with 10^{-8}M-f-Met-Leu-Phe (fMLP), or held at 4 °C without fMLP as indicated. Cells were stained at 4 °C with specific (solid curves) or control (dashed curves) MAb, followed by fluorescein isothiocyanate anti-mouse IgG, and subjected to immunofluorescence flow cytometry. Both antibodies were used at saturating concentrations, so fluorescence is proportional to the number of antigen molecules per cell. Fluorescence of monocytes was determined by gating on 90° and forward angle light scatter to exclude lymphocytes.

Patients have recurrent, life-threatening bacterial infections, a lack of pus formation, and persistent granulocytosis (Table 2). The deficiency affects all cell lineages which normally express the Mac-1, LFA-1 glycoprotein family, i.e. monocytes, granulocytes and lymphocytes, and cell lines established from patients. Deficiency is inherited as an autosomal recessive mutation. Each of the three α subunits, and the common β subunit, is deficient on the surface of all patients' cells, as shown by immunofluorescent flow cytometry and immunoprecipitation with MAb specific for each subunit (Fig. 3). Two phenotypes

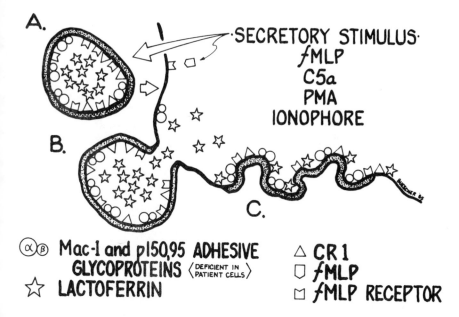

FIG. 2. Secretory vesicle mobilization in granulocytes. The components shown are all mobilized to the cell surface or secreted in response to the indicated stimuli. Deficient cells from patients lack an intracellular pool of Mac-1 and p150,95 and thus fail to mobilize them to the cell surface; the secretory response and mobilization of other surface components such as the CR1 and fMLP receptor is otherwise completely normal in cells from patients. Mac-1 and p150,95 the CR1 and fMLP receptor may be in storage sites distinct from one another and from that of lactoferrin in the secondary granule. They are shown in the same secretory vesicle only for ease of representation. (Drawing by Dr S. Buescher.)

have been defined, severe deficiency and moderate deficiency, with surface expression of <0.2% and 5%, respectively, of the normal amounts of Mac-1, LFA-1, and p150,95 (Fig. 3 and Anderson et al 1985). In both phenotypes, the underlying defect is in the common β subunit (Springer et al 1984), as summarized in Fig. 4. In normal cells, α and β subunit precursors (α' and β') are synthesized which become non-covalently associated, probably in the endoplasmic reticulum, and transported to the Golgi, where carbohydrate processing and a slight increase in relative molecular mass occurs. The mature molecules are then transported to the cell surface or to intracellular storage sites. Cells from patients, however, appear to lack β subunit synthesis or to make it in only small amounts. Normal α' precursors are made but do not undergo carbohydrate processing, suggesting that biosynthesis is blocked before transport to the Golgi apparatus. $\alpha\beta$ association appears to be required

TABLE 2 Clinical features of Mac-1, LFA-1 deficiency syndrome in patients in Texas[a]

Clinical features	Severe deficiency			Moderate deficiency				
	No. 1 F (6 yr)	No. 2 F (16 mths)[b]	No. 3 F (18 mths)[b]	No. 4 M (18 yr)	No. 5 M (15 yr)	No. 6 M (37 yr)	No. 7 M (8 yr)	No. 8 F (12 yr)
Delayed umbilical cord severance and infection	+	+	+	–	–	–	–	–
Persistent granulocytosis (15 000 – 161 000/mm³)	+++	+++	+++	+	+	+	+	+
Recurrent soft tissue infections: Necrotic/ulcerative cutaneous/subcutaneous abscess or cellulitis	+++	+++	+++	++	+	+++	+	+
Perirectal abscess/sepsis	+	+	+	–	–	–	–	–
Mucositis/stomatitis/pharyngitis/tracheitis	+++	+	++	+	+	+	–	
Gingivitis/peridontitis	+++	+	+	+++	+++	+++	+++	+++
Pneumonitis	+	+	+	–	–	+	+	–
Peritonitis/necrotizing enterocolitis	+	+	–	–	+	–	–	–
Impaired wound healing	+	+	+	+	+	++	±	±
Parental consanguinity	–	–		–	–	±	–	+
Ethnic background	Anglo-Saxon	Hispanic	Iranian	Hispanic	Hispanic	Hispanic	Hispanic	Hispanic

[a] Summarized from Anderson et al (1985).
[b] Deceased.

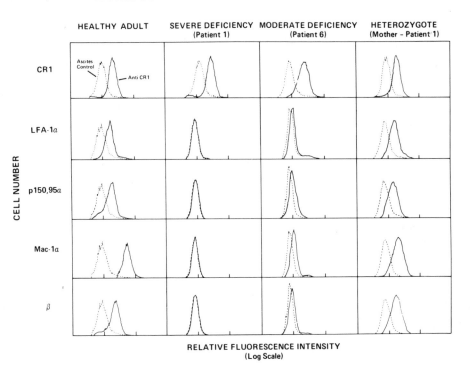

FIG. 3. Immunofluorescence flow cytometry of granulocytes of representative patients with severe and moderate deficiency, a heterozygote, and a healthy adult. Unstimulated granulocytes were indirectly stained with antibodies to the CR1 or the indicated α or β subunits (solid lines) or control MAb (dashed lines). Other methods as in legend to Fig. 1. A similar degree of deficiency was found if granulocytes from patients were stained after f-Met-Leu-Phe stimulation. (From Anderson et al 1985, with permission.)

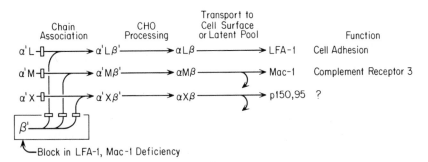

FIG. 4. Biosynthesis of the Mac-1, LFA-1 glycoprotein family (Sanchez-Madrid et al 1983, Springer et al 1984). The evidence for a primary block β subunit synthesis and a secondary block in α subunit processing in cells from patients is described in the text.

for processing and transport to the surface. The α chains are not expressed on the surface (severe deficiency) or are expressed in amounts which appear stoichiometrically limited by the small quantity of β produced (moderate deficiency). In addition to surface expression, granulocytes and monocytes from these patients lack the intracellular pool of Mac-1 and p150,95. After stimulation with f-Met-Leu-Phe or PMA there is little if any increase in Mac-1 and p150,95 surface expression (Springer et al 1984, Anderson et al 1985).

Mac-1, LFA-1 deficiency is a highly specific defect. Granulocytes from patients show normal surface expression of the Fc receptor, the complement receptor type 1 (CR1), and many other markers surveyed in an international monoclonal antibody workshop (Springer & Anderson 1985b). Up-regulation of CR1, secretion of granule constituents such as lactoferrin and lysozyme, the respiratory burst, and superoxide production in response to chemoattractants and PMA are completely normal in cells from patients. Thus, the granule mobilization response depicted in Fig. 2 and other biochemical changes appear normal in such cells, except that Mac-1 and p150,95 are absent from the intracellular compartment that is mobilized to the cell surface. This is in contrast to a distinct disorder involving specific granule deficiency (Gallin et al 1982).

The functional consequences of deficiency

The effects of this deficiency disease have taught us much about the importance of the Mac-1, LFA-1 glycoprotein family in leucocyte adhesion and migration (Anderson et al 1984, 1985). The first known function of Mac-1 was as the complement receptor type 3, which mediates binding and phagocytosis of particles opsonized with the iC3b ligand (Beller et al 1982, Wright et al 1983). Indeed, despite some initial controversy (Dana et al 1983), it is clear that patients are deficient in CR3 (Dana et al 1984, Anderson et al 1984). However, the functional defects are much broader than this.

The recurrent soft tissue infections in patients (Table 2) appear to be due to an inability of granulocytes and monocytes to migrate into inflammatory sites (Anderson et al 1984, 1985). There is no pus formation in the common necrotic, ulcerative skin lesions or in other less readily apparent infected sites. This is confirmed by biopsies, which show that granulocyte mobilization into infected tissues is profoundly impaired. Patients have severe gingivitis, yet a saline wash of the oral cavity reveals no polymorphonuclear leucocytes (PMN), as would be found in other types of gingivitis. Leucocyte mobilization was measured experimentally in patients by the Rebuck skin-window test. The skin was abraded, a coverslip was placed over the site, and granulocytes and monocytes present in the serous effusions were counted at two-hour intervals. Healthy controls showed immigrating neutrophils at 2 and 4 h followed by monocytes at 6 h. Severely deficient patients showed no mobilization of neutrophils or monocytes to the site even at the 24-hour time point, and leucocyte mobilization in moderately deficient patients was strikingly diminished and delayed. Thus, Mac-1, LFA-1 deficiency results in a profound defect in the ability of leucocytes to leave the circulation by migrating between endothelial cells and through the basement membrane into inflammatory sites, i.e. in diapedesis.

This dysfunction correlates with *in vitro* defects in chemotaxis and adhesion (Anderson et al 1984, 1985). Chemotaxis to f-Met-Leu-Phe and C5a was markedly depressed (Table 3). Patients' granulocytes exhibited a normal bipolar change in shape in suspension in response to chemoattractants, but failed to orient to gradients of f-Met-Leu-Phe or C5a when attached to surfaces (Anderson et al 1984). Granulocytes undergoing orientation to f-Met-Leu-Phe in Zigmond chambers were examined by scanning electron microscopy (Fig. 5). Healthy granulocytes oriented normally, with lamellipodia at their leading edge facing in the direction of the chemoattractant diffusing from the right (Fig. 5B,C). In contrast, patients' granulocytes failed to orient (Fig. 5E,F). Photographs taken in a plane perpendicular to the substrate and parallel to the gradient (Fig. 5C,F) showed that granulocytes from patients were clearly activated, since they were bipolar, but were in a plane perpendicular to the substrate rather than parallel to it (Fig. 5F). They were unable to initiate lateral or peripheral areas of attachment with the substrate.

The orientation and chemotaxis defects appear secondary to a defect in adherence. The percentage of granulocytes adhering to serum-coated glass under 'baseline' conditions was significantly ($P < 0.01$) diminished compared to adherence in healthy controls (Table 3). After stimulation with f-Met-Leu-Phe or PMA, there was little or no increase in adherence by severely deficient PMN and only a modest increase by moderately deficient PMN. In contrast, healthy control PMN demonstrated a normal hyperadherence response. The defect in adherence is also found for glass and plastic coated with other proteins, including fibronectin (Anderson et al 1984, Buchanan et al 1982). Those cells which adhere to protein-coated glass or to plastic demonstrate a profound defect in their ability to spread (Buchanan et al 1982, Anderson et al 1984). C5a, f-Met-Leu-Phe and PMA cause healthy granulocytes to aggregate into clumps, which can be measured in an aggregometer by changes in light transmittance. Deficient granulocytes failed to aggregate (Table 3). Although a change in surface charge on stimulation may contribute to granulocyte aggregation (Gallin 1982), there was no difference in charge between deficient and normal granulocytes (Anderson et al 1984). Phagocytosis of IgG and iC3b-opsonized Oil Red O particles and C3-opsonized zymosan was measured.

Phagocytosis of C3-opsonized particles by deficient granulocytes was diminished (Table 3), as would be expected from the CR3 defect. Deficient granulocytes phagocytosed IgG-opsonized particles normally (Table 3). PMNs demonstrate phagocytosis of many microorganisms in the absence of opsonization, although at a slower rate than after opsonization. Under these conditions, deficient granulocytes demonstrate diminished phagocytosis of some but not all microorganisms. Defects are found for *Staphylococcus aureus* and zymosan (Anderson et al 1984, Thompson et al 1984).

TABLE 3 Assessments of adherence-dependent granulocyte functions[a]

Functional assay	Severe[b] deficiency	Moderate[c] deficiency	Healthy adults
Chemotaxis			
f-Met-Leu-Phe (10^{-8}M)	43 ± 6^d	66 ± 7	105 ± 4
C5a	42 ± 5	68 ± 14	108 ± 7
Adherence			
Baseline (PBS)	12 ± 2^e	16 ± 9	38 ± 6
f-Met-Leu-Phe (10^{-8}M)	12 ± 3	28 ± 12	63 ± 6
PMA (5 µg/ml)	16 ± 4	31 ± 12	67 ± 9
Aggregation			
C5a	16 ± 11^f	15 ± 12	100 ± 0
f-Met-Leu-Phe (10^{-7}M)	16 ± 4	14 ± 13	40 ± 6
PMA (10 µg/ml)	15 ± 9	22 ± 3	105 ± 7
Phagocytosis			
Oil Red O-(IgG)	1.4 ± 0.6^g	1.4 ± 0.5	1.7 ± 0.4
Oil Red O(iC3b)	1.9 ± 1.2^g	2.4 ± 1.2	7.0 ± 3.1
C3-opsonized zymosan	4.6 ± 0.7^h	7.9 ± 3.2	17.4 ± 4.0

[a] Results with each functional assay are represented by mean $\pm$ 1 SD value for each patient category, derived from mean values for individual patients in two to six separate experiments. Summarized from Anderson et al (1985).
[b] Includes assessments on severe deficiency patients 1, 2 and 3.
[c] Includes assessments on moderate deficiency patients 4, 6, 7 and 8.
[d] Boyden assay values (mean $\pm$ 1 SD) for f-Met-Leu-Phe or C5a (10% zymosan-activated serum) expressed as µm migration/40 min incubation.
[e] Percentage of granulocytes adhering to serum (6%)-coated glass under baseline or stimulated conditions at 21 °C.
[f] Granulocyte aggregation responses to C5a (10% zymosan-activated plasma), f-Met-Leu-Phe or PMA, at 37 °C, measured by the increase in light transmittance and expressed as % of the response to C5a.
[g] Dionylphthalate uptake (µg/10^6 granulocytes in 15 min).
[h] Slope of chemiluminescence evolution (c.p.m.$^2 \times 10^{-5}$).
PBS, phosphate-buffered saline; PMA, phorbol myristate acetate.

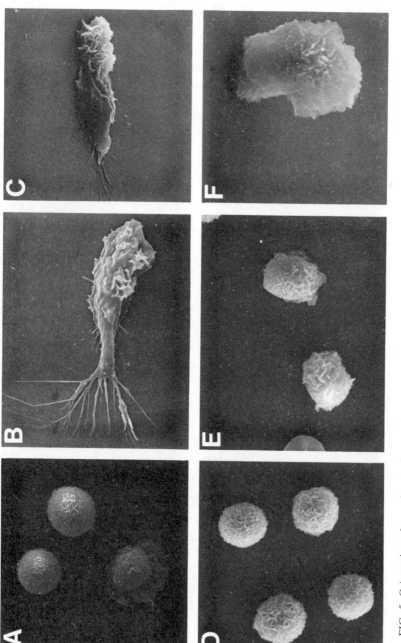

FIG. 5. Orientation of granulocytes from patients or controls in chemotactic gradients. Scanning electron micrographs show the sequence of cell ruffling and spreading on the substrate (A) and achievement of polarity and orientation by healthy adult PMNs (B,C), and parallel experiments on deficient PMNs (D–F). Cells adhere to the coverslip over the bridge in a Zigmond orientation chamber and respond to f-Met-Leu-Phe diffusing from the right. Cells in A, B, D, and E are photographed in a plane parallel to the coverslip, and in C and F perpendicular to the coverslip. (From Anderson et al 1984, with permission.)

Inhibition of adherence-dependent functions by MAb

Binding of monoclonal antibodies to normal granulocytes reproduced the defects found in Mac-1, LFA-1-deficient patients. Both baseline and f-Met-Leu-Phe-stimulated adherence were strikingly inhibited (Fig. 6). Spreading, chemotaxis and aggregation were also inhibited (sumarized in Table 4). The order of potency was anti-β > anti-Mac-1 α > anti-p150,95α > anti-LFA-1. This suggests that all members of the glycoprotein family may contribute to these reactions; the order of potency reflects their relative amounts on the granulocyte surface (Springer & Anderson 1985a). These effects are quite

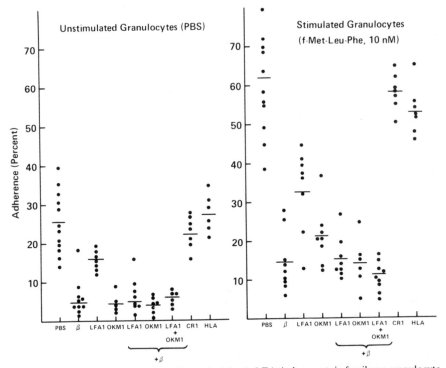

FIG. 6. Effects of monoclonal antibodies to the Mac-1, LFA-1 glycoprotein family on granulocyte adherence. Granulocytes were preincubated with MAbs, washed and then incorporated into Smith Hollers adherence chambers in which they were allowed to adhere to serum (6%)-coated glass substrates under unstimulated (PBS) or stimulated (f-Met-Leu-Phe, 10 nM) conditions at 21 °C. MAb preparations used for the studies shown included: the OKM1 MAb to Mac-1 α (5 µg/ml), F(ab')$_2$ fragments of the TS1/22 MAb to LFA-1 α (5 µg/ml), and F(ab')$_2$ fragments of the TS1/18 MAb to the common β subunit of Mac-1 and LFA-1 (5 µg/ml). Control MAbs included saturating concentrations of an F(ab')$_2$ fragment of rabbit IgG directed against the human C3b receptor (anti-CR1) and an MAb to HLA framework antigen (W6/32).

TABLE 4 Effects of subunit specific monoclonal antibodies to Mac-1 proteins on adherence-dependent and adherence-independent granulocyte functions

Granulocyte function[a]	Monoclonal antibody specificity					
	Mac-1 α		LFA-1 α	p150,95 α	β	HLA-A,B
	OKM1	LM2/1.6	TS1/22 F(ab')₂	SHCL-3	TS1/18 F(ab')₂	W6/32
Adherence (6% serum-coated glass)	+	+	±	+	+	–
Hyperadherence (6% serum-coated glass, 10 nm fMLP)	+*	+	±	+	+	–
Spreading, glass	+	+*	±	±*	+*	–
Aggregation, C5a	+	+	–	+*	+*	–
Chemotaxis, C5a	+*	±	±	±*	+*	–
Phagocytosis (iC3b-ORO)	+		–	–	+	–
Shape change (suspension)	–	–	–	–	–	–
f-Met-Leu-³H-Phe binding	–	–	–	–	–	–
Superoxide generation (PMA)	–	–	–	–	–	–
Secretion of β-glucuronidase, vitamin B₁₂ transport protein (PMA)	–	–	–	–	–	–
Phagocytosis (IgG-ORO)	–	–	–	–	–	–

[a] For most experiments, granulocytes were preincubated in saturating concentrations of MAbs or their F(ab')₂ fragments, washed and then assayed.
+ Consistently and significantly blocks function.
± Inconsistent or minimal blockage.
– No blockage.
*Requires presence of monoclonal antibody during assay for inhibitory effect.
ORO, Oil Red O.

specific. They are obtained with F(ab')$_2$ fragments (anti-β and anti-LFA-1) and are not given by IgG MAb bound to other surface molecules (CR1 and HLA-A,B). These MAbs did not inhibit functions that were not deficient in cells from patients, i.e. shape change in suspension, f-Met-Leu-Phe binding, superoxide generation, secondary granule secretion, and phagocytosis of Oil Red O (Table 4).

A dynamic model of chemotaxis and diapedesis

The specific molecular and functional deficits observed in cells from patients suggest that in normal cells adherence and chemotaxis are mediated by the Mac-1, LFA-1 glycoprotein family, and that chemoattractant-stimulated hyperadherence and aggregation are mediated by the increased surface expression of Mac-1 and p150,95. MAb blocking experiments confirm these findings. We believe chemotaxis is profoundly deficient in patients because of the underlying inability of cells to adhere properly to substrates. We propose that, *in vivo*, chemoattractants diffusing from sites of inflammation into the circulation induce Mac-1 and p150,95 up-regulation, leading to increased adherence of monocytes and granulocytes to blood vessels in the inflammatory site (Fig. 7). We further propose that, in analogy to the importance of the Mac-1, LFA-1, and p150,95 glycoproteins in chemotaxis *in vitro*, these glycoproteins mediate essential adherence functions during diapedesis and migration into the inflammatory site. The most important clinical manifestation of Mac-1, LFA-1 deficiency is the inability of granulocytes to migrate into inflammatory sites and form pus. We propose that this is due to a lack of up-regulation of adhesiveness, which is normally regulated by the increased surface expression of Mac-1 and p150,95.

The molecular mechanisms by which these glycoproteins mediate or regulate adhesivity are not known, and are an interesting area for further research. If adhesion is mediated by binding to specific ligands, the experiments with protein-coated glass and plastic substrates suggest that the ligand would first be secreted by the granulocytes or monocytes, then adhere to the substrate, thus allowing attachment of adhesion proteins. It has been demonstrated that the Mac-1 molecule binds at least one specific ligand, iC3b (Wright et al 1983); however, other adhesive interactions mediated by Mac-1 might involve different ligand binding sites or different adhesive mechanisms. It is possible that the Mac-1, LFA-1 glycoproteins each bind several different ligands, or have highly flexible conformations and act as molecular glues, binding to a wide range of molecules. Alternatively, the Mac-1, LFA-1 glycoproteins might not bind ligands directly, but might regulate adhesion through other surface molecules. It should be pointed out that all of the adhesive interactions in which these molecules participate require metabolic energy and temperatures higher than 4 °C, and thus are not dependent on simple receptor–ligand interactions alone. The Mac-1, LFA-1 glycoproteins may regulate active processes, such as energy-dependent modification of the activity of other molecules, or remodelling of the topography of the plasma membrane.

Whatever the mechanism, the delivery of adhesive proteins to the cell surface in discrete packages, by fusion of secretory vesicles with the plasma membrane, allows an interesting speculation about chemotaxis. Cells undergoing chemotaxis orient in the gradient with lamellipodia at their anterior end and the uropod with retraction fibres at their posterior end (Fig. 5). Sensing of the chemoattractant stimulates not only orientation and motility but also release of secondary granules or some other secretory vesicle containing the Mac-1 and p150,95 glycoproteins. As explained earlier, the concentration of these glycoproteins is much higher in the membrane bilayer of the storage compartment than in the plasma membrane of the unstimulated cell. We propose that during chemotaxis the secretory vesicles containing Mac-1 and p150,95 fuse with the plasma membrane at the leading edge of the cell. The site of fusion is hypothesized to be directed by the same chemoattractant-sensing machinery that guides the ruffling lamellipodia towards the chemoattractant.

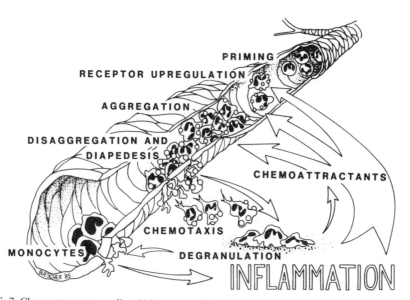

FIG. 7. Chemoattractant-mediated Mac-1 and p150,95 up-regulation, changes in leucocyte adherence, and diapedesis at inflammatory sites. (Drawing by Dr S. Buescher.)

A focal point of high Mac-1 and p150,95 concentration would thus be formed in the plasma membrane at the site of fusion. Adhesion would be initiated or strengthened at this focal point. After further cell translocation, this focal point of attachment would approach the cell uropod. By this time, diffusion of the adhesion proteins in the plane of the membrane, during moments when they are dissociated from ligand, would have lowered their concentration and the strength of adhesion. Alternatively, other time-dependent processes could regulate dissipation of the adhesive force. Detachment in the area of the uropod and its retraction fibres could thus occur, allowing further translocation. Because each granulocyte contains hundreds of specific granules, this cycle could be repeated many times. This process would allow intermittent adhesion sufficiently strong to allow attachment to a substrate but sufficiently localized temporally to allow selective detachment. This process would be superimposed on endocytic recycling of membrane, with endocytosis over the entire surface of the cell, and readdition at the leading edge of the cell. This allows bulk membrane flow from the leading edge to the uropod, and has been hypothesized to effect cell locomotion (Bretscher 1984).

Previous observations are consistent with this model. We found that granulocyte spreading and chemotaxis are inhibited in the continued presence of excess MAb to the Mac-1 α subunit or the common β subunit, but not if cells are pretreated with MAb (Table 4). This is consistent with the idea that these processes require mobilization of Mac-1 from the intracellular latent pool to the cell surface. A role for secondary granule secretion in adherence and chemotaxis has previously been proposed, although it was related to changes in surface charge rather than to Mac-1 and p150,95 up-regulation (Gallin 1982). Chemotaxis through micropore filters is accompanied by secondary granule release, and release is greatest from the granulocytes that migrate furthest. Degranulation occurs at the leading edge of the cell, and has been seen to occur from pseudopodia at points of close apposition to the filter matrix. Furthermore, spreading of neutrophils on glass beads or nylon fibres results in secondary but not primary granule release (Wright & Gallin 1979). Exudate granulocytes accumulating in sterile exudates from heat blisters, or in skin chambers, are selectively depleted in secondary granules, and secondary granule constituents are found in the exudate fluid (Wright & Gallin 1979). Circulating granulocytes from patients with burns are depleted in their stores of secondary granules and deficient in chemotaxis (Gallin 1982). Patients whose granulocyte developmental defect consists of having no secondary granules show a chemotactic defect (Gallin et al 1982). Exposure of granulocytes to step increases in the concentration of f-Met-Leu-Phe induces adhesion sites at the lamellipodia, followed by their redistribution to the uropod, as shown by binding of albumin-coated latex beads (Smith & Hollers 1980). These observations on chemotaxis, adherence and secondary granule release may all be related to chemoattractant-stimulated Mac-1 and p150,95 up-regulation.

More detailed studies of the intracellular location of Mac-1 and p150,95, the coordination of their up-regulation with cell adhesion, orientation and chemotaxis, the formation and dissipation of the adhesive foci, and the structural basis for the adhesion functions of these proteins, promise to provide important insights into the molecular mechanisms of leucocyte chemotaxis and diapedesis.

REFERENCES

Anderson DC, Schmalstieg FC, Arnaout MA et al 1984 Abnormalities of polymorphonuclear leukocyte function associated with a heritable deficiency of high molecular weight surface glycoproteins (GP138): Common relationship to diminished cell adherence. J Clin Invest 74:536-551

Anderson DC, Schmalstieg FC, Finegold MJ et al 1985 The severe and moderate phenotypes of heritable Mac-1, LFA-1, p150,95 deficiency: Their quantitative definition and relation to leukocyte dysfunction and clinical features. J Infect Dis, in press

Atherton A, Born GVR 1972 Quantitative investigations of the adhesiveness of circulating polymorphonuclear leucocytes to blood vessel walls. J Physiol (Lond) 222:447-474

Beller DI, Springer TA, Schreiber RD 1982 Anti-Mac-1 selectively inhibits the mouse and human type three complement receptor. J Exp Med 156:1000-1009

Bretscher MS 1984 Endocytosis: Relation to capping and cell locomotion. Science (Wash DC) 224:681-686

Buchanan MR, Crowley CA, Rosin RE, Gimbrone MA, Babior BM 1982 Studies on the interaction between GP-180-deficient neutrophils and vascular endothelium. Blood 60:160-165

Dana N, Todd, R, Pitt J, Colten HR, Arnaout MA 1983 Evidence that Mo1 (a surface glycoprotein involved in phagocytosis) is distinct from the C3bi receptor. Immunobiology 164:205-206

Dana N, Todd RF, Pitt J, Springer TA, Arnaout MA 1984 Deficiency of a surface membrane glycoprotein (Mo1) in man. J Clin Invest 73:153-159

Dawson P, Mandell O 1980 Phagocyte strategy vs. microbial tactics. Rev Infect Dis 2:817-836

Gallin JI 1982 Role of neutrophil lysosomal granules in the evolution of the inflammatory response. In: Karnovsky ML, Bolis L (eds) Phagocytosis: past and future. Academic Press, New York, p 519-541

Gallin JI, Fletcher MP, Seligmann BE, Hoffstein S, Cehrs K, Mounessa N 1982 Human neutrophil-specific granule deficiency: A model to assess the role of neutrophil-specific granules in the evolution of the inflammatory response. Blood 59:1317-1329

Hoffstein ST, Friedman RS, Weissmann G 1982 Degranulation, membrane addition, and shape change during chemotactic factor-induced aggregation of human neutrophils. J Cell Biol 95:234-241

Sanchez-Madrid F, Nagy J, Robbins E, Simon P, Springer TA 1983 A human leukocyte differentiation antigen family with distinct alpha subunits and a common beta subunit: The lymphocyte-function associated antigen (LFA-1), the C3bi complement receptor (OKM1/Mac-1), and the p150,95 molecule. J Exp Med 158:1785-1803

Smith CW, Hollers JC 1980 Motility and adhesiveness in human neutrophils: Redistribution of chemotactic factor-induced adhesion sites. J Clin Invest 65:804-812

Snyderman R, Pike MC 1984 Chemoattractant receptors on phagocytic cells. Annu Rev Immunol 2:257-281

Springer TA, Anderson DC 1985a Functional and structural interrelationships among the Mac-1, LFA-1 family of leukocyte adhesion glycoproteins, and their deficiency in a novel, heritable disease. In: Springer TA (ed) Hybridoma technology in the biosciences and medicine. Plenum, New York, p 191-206

Springer TA, Anderson DC 1985b Antibodies specific for the Mac-1, LFA-1, p150,95 glycoproteins or their family, or for other granulocyte proteins. In: Reinherz EL et al (eds) Leucocyte typing II. Springer-Verlag, Berlin, in press

Springer TA, Davignon D, Ho MK, Kürzinger K, Martz E, Sanchez-Madrid F 1982 LFA-1 and Lyt-2,3, molecules associated with T lymphocyte-mediated killing; and Mac-1, an LFA-1 homologue associated with complement receptor function. Immunol Rev 68:111-135

Springer TA, Thompson WS, Miller LJ, Schmalstieg FC, Anderson DC 1984 Inherited deficiency of the Mac-1, LFA-1, p150,95 glycoprotein family and its molecular basis. J Exp Med 160:1901-1918

Thompson RA, Candy DCA, McNeish AS 1984 Familial defect of polymorph neutrophil phagocytosis associated with absence of a surface glycoprotein antigen (OKM1). Clin Exp Immunol 58:229-236

Todd RFI, Arnaout MA, Rosin RE, Crowley CA, Peters WA, Babior BM 1984 Subcellular localization of the large subunit of Mo1 (Mo1 alpha; formerly gp 110), a surface glycoprotein associated with neutrophil adhesion. J Clin Invest 74:1280-1290

Tonnesen MG, Smedly LA, Henson PM 1984 Neutrophil-endothelial cell interactions: modulation of neutrophil adhesiveness induced by complement fragments C5a and C5a des arg and formyl-methionyl-leucyl-phenylalanine in vitro. J Clin Invest 74:1581-1592

Wilkinson PC 1982 Chemotaxis and inflammation, 2nd edn. Churchill Livingstone, London

Wright DG, Gallin JI 1979 Secretory responses of human neutrophils: Exocytosis of specific (secondary) granules by human neutrophils during adherence in vitro and during exudation in vivo. J Immunol 123:285-294

Wright SD, Rao PE, Van Voorhis WC et al 1983 Identification of the C3bi receptor of human monocytes and macrophages with monoclonal antibodies. Proc Natl Acad Sci USA 80:5699-5703

DISCUSSION

Singer: Are you suggesting that LFA-1 is in a different granule from Mac-1, as they are not simultaneously expressed?

Springer: Mac-1 and p150,95 are up-regulated and LFA-1 is not. LFA-1 is not stored inside the cell but is expressed only on the cell surface. There are two possible mechanisms for this compartmentalization. One is that the α subunit controls storing, so the LFA-1 α subunit directs its αβ complex only to the cell surface and the other subunits direct their αβ complexes to both the cell surface and the secondary granule. The other possibility concerns the fact that secondary granules form at a very late stage in granulocyte differentiation. The primary granules are formed at the promyelocyte stage and the secondary granules bud off from the Golgi at the myelocyte stage. We know that there is differential regulation of α subunit expression during granulocyte or myeloid differentiation. The LFA-1 on the cell surface may be synthesized at the promyelocyte stage but at the myelocyte stage no LFA-1 may be made, which would explain why it is not in secondary granules.

Hogg: Götze & Sundsmo (1981) demonstrated that complement components can cause spreading and adhesion of macrophages. Could the complement receptor function of the CR3 molecule therefore be involved in adhesion? Does adhesion perhaps occur via the complement component?

Springer: Götze & Sundsmo (1981) reported that factor B causes spreading of the cells, but factor B does not interact with CR3 so I haven't been able to make any connection between those studies and this work.

Schreiber: Those studies showed that B was ineffective. They reported that activated factor B and C5a were antagonists of one another. Since you are now proposing that chemoattractants increase the expression of this family of proteins it might be worth seeing whether activated factor B decreases the expression of these proteins, as it antagonizes the chemotactic action of complement.

Stanley: What about the role of these antigens in monocyte and macrophage adhesion?

Springer: I think the results with monocytes would be similar to those for granulocytes, because Rebuck skin-window tests show that in both monocytes and granulocytes diapedesis is deficient.

Unkeless: D.T. Fearon (personal communication) looked at Fc receptors on neutrophils and didn't find that the low avidity Fc$_\gamma$ receptor was mobilized.

Springer: We found the same thing with your 3G8 antibody.

Unkeless: Is there any kind of up-regulation of the Mac-1 and LFA-1 family of monocytes?

Springer: Yes. We see a fivefold up-regulation on blood monocytes of Mac-1 and p150,95.

Nathan: Zanvil Cohn alluded in his opening remarks to the role of monocyte adherence and emigration under the endothelium of large arteries in initiating the fatty streak. Have any of your teenage or older patients shown unexpected absence of fatty streaks in the large vessels at autopsy?

Springer: We haven't had any who died in their teens. One person of 20 died here in England but the family didn't give permission for an autopsy.

Nathan: Do cells in these patients who get granulocyte transfusions mobilize normally? Could a factor other than that expressed in the patients' leucocytes produce this profound deficiency?

Springer: Granulocyte transfusions have only been stop-gap measures in preventing infectious diseases and weren't given to any of the patients I have studied directly. However, on finding that the parents of a patient deceased in 1981 have amounts of Mac-1 α and β on the surface of their granulocytes which are 68% and 58% of normal, we have typed them as heterozygote carriers of Mac-1, LFA-1 deficiency. Thus in retrospect, their son appears to have had Mac-1, LFA-1 deficiency. The case history is strongly suggestive of this diagnosis. This patient, studied by Drs T. Holbrook, F. Southwick, and T. Stossel, was given leucocyte transfusions. In answer to your question, this patient was converted from negative to positive in the Rebuck skin window by leucocyte transfusion. The failure of diapedesis in his own granulocytes was thus inherent, rather than due to extrinsic factors. Drs A. Fischer and C. Griscelli in Paris have treated the disease successfully by bone marrow transplantation (Fischer et al 1983). The chimeras are healthy.

Singer: Up-regulation may happen very rapidly but chemotaxis has to go on for a very long time. Up-regulation may be of great interest in adhesion and it could be important at the onset of chemotaxis. But if it is involved in adhesion and chemotaxis, these components must be continually appearing at the leading edge of the cell. The burst may have less to do with the ultimate chemotaxis than with its initial onset and with the initial adhesion.

Springer: In up-regulation experiments, we are inducing an artificial situation when we give 10^{-8} M f-Met-Leu-Phe and see a large, immediate response. In contrast, in chemotaxis assays *in vitro* the ligand diffuses very slowly towards the granulocyte. The granulocyte probably meets a very low concentration of ligand and one would expect a small proportion of the secondary granules to be released at a time. I imagine that this cycle recurs continually and there is some evidence for that. If you put two filters in a Boyden chamber and allow chemotaxis to occur, you can separate those two filters and look at the amount of degranulation in the filter where the cells have moved the furthest. The cells that have moved the furthest have released more secondary granular constituents than the other cells (Wright & Gallin 1979).

Singer: Does your monoclonal antibody for LFA-1 inhibit chemotaxis?

Springer: No.

Cohn: Were your studies done in the presence of cytochalasin?

Springer: No.

Gordon: Are there any patients who lack only the Mac-1 and not the whole family? How do you distinguish between the effects of the lack of one molecule versus the lack of all three molecules in relation to these functions? Could you resolve this with antibody-blocking experiments?

Springer: All 20 patients who have been looked at by a number of different groups appear to lack the entire family of glycoproteins. All these molecules are expressed on monocytes and granulocytes, so the only way to sort out the contribution by individual molecules is by antibody blocking experiments on normal cells. The adherence experiments indicate that all the antibodies have inhibited to a certain extent but there is a definite order of inhibition. The anti-Mac-1 and anti-β are strongest, followed by anti-p150, 95. Anti-LFA-1 is the weakest. This order of inhibition is in rough proportion to the concentration of these molecules on the granulocyte surface. So they may all contribute to adherence. There is quite good evidence that CR3 is inhibited by anti-Mac-1 antibodies and not by anti-LFA-1 antibodies or anti-p150, 95 antibodies.

Werb: Are any of these molecules expressed on either HL60 or U937?

Springer: On uninduced U937 and HL60 we see LFA-1. If we induce with phorbol ester on U937 we see a very dramatic increase in Mac-1 and p150, 95, while LFA-1 remains level. On HL60 there is some induction of Mac-1.

Werb: What is the evidence that Mac-1 or p150, 95 is really a specific granule membrane constituent of the neutrophil?

Springer: Todd et al (1984) showed that when granule fractions are prepared by sucrose density sedimentation, Mac-1 antigen co-sediments in the secondary granule fraction. Gallin and co-workers have obtained similar results and have also shown that patients who have a genetic defect in which they lack secondary granules appear to lack up-regulation of Mac-1 (O'Shea et al 1985).

Werb: HL60 doesn't have secondary granules so I wondered in what form they express Mac-1.

Springer: They do express it on the cell surface.

Cole: Are the patients and the individuals with moderate to low LFA expression heterozygotes?

Springer: No, they are clearly homozygotes. Their parents have 50% of normal surface expression. The moderately deficient patients have only 5% surface expression.

Cole: Are the β subunits identical by criteria other than immunological cross-reactivity?

Springer: Yes, in the mouse we demonstrated identity by peptide mapping. In humans they are also identical by isoelectric focusing.

Cole: Are you certain that there is one α subunit and one β subunit per unit of LFA or Mac-1?

Springer: Yes. We use a bifunctional cross-linking reagent and we wind up with a cross-linked heterodimer of M_r about 260 000. When we break the cross-links we get the α and β subunits. If we had an $\alpha_2\beta_2$ complex we would get something of twice that M_r. We see absolutely no species at the 520 000 position or at any other position greater than 260 000 M_r.

Cole: Can defects of these kinds of proteins be acquired or are they always due to a genetic defect?

Springer: There is no evidence that they are acquired.

Nathan: There are reports that ethanol and aspirin ingestion decrease neutrophil adherence (MacGregor et al 1974). Would these have any effect on the function of LFA *in vitro*?

Springer: We haven't tested that.

Cohn: Does that happen by acetylation?

Nathan: I don't know. There are clear-cut effects *in vitro* after *in vivo* or *in vitro* treatment.

Springer: Ethanol inhibits the up-regulation. We learnt that as a result of doing the proper control for adding cytochalasin dissolved in ethanol.

Sorg: Did you test adherence in endothelial cell cultures? In other words, what is the natural substrate of adherence of protein coating?

Springer: The Seattle group have similar patients and looked directly at adherence to endothelial cells, which was deficient (Beatty et al 1984).

Cohn: Are there substrates to which these cells attach normally?

Springer: Yes, they adhere well to uncoated glass or plastic. That is a kind of irreversible adhesion which is not dependent on divalent cations and which does not allow chemotaxis. Cells also spread normally on IgG-coated substrates.

Cohn: Presumably via the Fc receptor. Is there specificity in terms of types of protein that you use to coat the glass?

Springer: No, you can use serum albumin, which is not glycosylated, ruling out lectin-like activity. You can also use whole serum, fibrinogen and fibronectin and get equivalent results.

Cohn: Have you used defatted albumin or just fatty acid-containing albumin?

Springer: We used fatty acid-containing albumin.

Singer: You say that calcium is required for adhesion. Is it required for neutrophil motility in a chemotactic gradient?

Springer: We haven't looked at that but it is well documented by Gallin & Rosenthal (1974) and others that magnesium is required for both adhesion and chemotaxis.

Nicola: In the same time course the same chemotactic peptide, f-Met-Leu-Phe, down-regulates granulocyte colony-stimulating factor receptors on human blood neutrophils. That occurs within 15–20 minutes over the range 10^{-9}–10^{-7} M. The amount of down-regulation is about 50% and then the response reaches a plateau (N.A. Nicola et al, unpublished). At the same time as this chemotactic peptide is up-regulating some receptors, it is also down-regulating at least one other, and other more complicated interactions may be going on.

Springer: Fearon and co-workers (Changelian et al 1985) have shown for complement receptor type 1 that after an initial up-regulation, phorbol esters can stimulate down-regulation. That may be due to increased endocytosis.

Whaley: Do patients with a moderate deficiency of CR3 show the same biosynthetic defects as those with severe deficiency?

Springer: Yes, we have seen the same β subunit defect in moderately deficient and severely deficient patients. Both have normal α subunits, which were also normal by isoelectric focusing. We don't have any direct evidence for this but our model for the difference between moderately and severely deficient patients is that the moderates synthesize about 5% of the normal amount of the β subunit, which stoichiometrically limits the amount that appears on the cell surface.

Cohn: Are both molecules on the cell surface?

Springer: In moderately deficient patients both subunits are expressed on the cell surface. If you immunoprecipitate with anti-LFA antibody, for example, you pull down the β chain as well, so moderately deficient patients have αβ complexes.

Cohn: What do you think the non-covalent linkage is?

Springer: Typical hydrophobic bonds, etc.

Singer: Do the macrophages of these patients show normal chemotaxis? It would be interesting to know to what extent macrophage motility and neutrophil motility are related in their mechanisms.

Springer: We haven't looked at macrophages. Don Anderson may have looked at monocytes.

Nathan: The absence of monocytes in the Rebuck window doesn't necessarily establish an intrinsic monocyte defect. Monocytes may depend on the prior accumulation of neutrophils to respond. One of John Gallin's patients with absent neutrophil specific granules had defective neutrophil and monocyte accumulation in Rebuck windows but the monocytes showed normal chemotaxis *in vitro* while the neutrophils did not (Gallin et al 1982).

Springer: I have seen reports that in the absence of neutrophils there is still an influx of monocytes, i.e. monocyte emigration is normal in patients with neutropenia (Dale & Wolff 1971).

Nathan: This may be due to a quantitative versus a qualitative difference.

Roos: We have a patient with a few per cent of the normal amount of LFA-1 in the lymphocytes. We find normal K and NK function, but this can be inhibited with very small quantities of antibody against the LFA-1 antigen. The amount of LFA-1 on the patient's T cells is apparently enough to give normal function, but it is on the borderline of what is necessary.

Springer: We have similar observations. We have been using target cells which are LFA-1 positive and in moderately deficient patients part of the inhibitory effect is due to binding of LFA-1 antibody to target cell LFA-1. For one of the severely deficient patients we see inhibition which is due to binding to target cell LFA-1. So it appears that LFA-1 can mediate bidirectional interactions between effector and target cells (Krensky et al 1985).

REFERENCES

Beatty PG, Harlan JM, Rosen H et al 1984 Absence of monoclonal-antibody-defined protein complex in boy with abnormal leucocyte function. Lancet 1:535-537

Changelian PS, Jack RM, Collins LA, Fearon DT 1985 PMA induces the ligand-independent internalization of CR1 on human neutrophils. J Immunol 134:1851-1858

Dale DC, Wolff SM 1971 Skin window studies of the acute inflammatory responses of neutropenic patients. Blood 38:138

Fischer A, Descamps-Latscha B, Gerota I et al 1983 Bone-marrow transplantation for inborn error of phagocytic cells associated with defective adherence, chemotaxis, and oxidative response during opsonised particle phagocytosis. Lancet 2:473-476

Gallin JI, Rosenthal AS 1974 The regulatory role of divalent cations in human granulocyte chemotaxis. Evidence for an association between calcium exchanges and microtubule assembly. J Cell Biol 62:594-609

Gallin JI, Fletcher MP, Seligmann BE, Hoffstein S, Cehrs K, Mounessa N 1982 Human neutrophil-specific granule deficiency: a model to assess the role of neutrophil-specific granules in the evolution of the inflammatory response. Blood 59:1317-1329

Götze O, Sundsmo JS 1981 A role for membrane associated complement proteins in the spreading of human mononuclear phagocytes. In: Forster O, Landy M (eds) Heterogeneity of mononuclear phagocytes. Academic Press, London, p 115-121

Krensky AM, Mentzer SJ, Greenstein JL et al 1985 Human cytolytic T lymphocyte clones and their function-associated cell surface molecules. In: Springer TA (ed) Hybridoma technology in the biosciences and medicine. Plenum, New York

MacGregor RR, Spagnuolo PJ, Lentnek AL 1974 Inhibition of granulocyte adherence by ethanol, prednisone, and aspirin, measured with an assay system. N Engl J Med 291:642-646

O'Shea JJ, Brown EJ, Seligmann BE, Metcalf JA, Frank MM, Gallin JI 1985 Evidence for distinct intracellular pools of receptors for C3b and C3bi in human neutrophils. J Immunol 134:2580-2587

Todd RFI, Arnaout MA, Rosin RE, Crowley CA, Peters WA, Babior BM 1984 Subcellular localization of the large subunit of Mol (Mol alpha; formerly gp 110), a surface glycoprotein associated with neutrophil adhesion. J Clin Invest 74:1280-1290

Wright DG, Gallin JI 1979 Secretory responses of human neutrophils: exocytosis of specific (secondary) granules by human neutrophils during adherence in vitro and during exudation in vivo. J Immunol 123:285-294

Interaction and regulation of macrophage receptors

R. A. B. EZEKOWITZ* & S. GORDON†

*Division of Hematology/Oncology, Harvard Department of Pediatrics, 320 Longwood Avenue, Boston, MA 02115, USA, and †Sir William Dunn School of Pathology, South Parks Road, Oxford, OX1 3RE, UK

Abstract. Macrophages express distinct plasma membrane receptors for different isotypes of immunoglobulin, bear at least two receptors for cleaved third complement component (CR1 and CR3) and have a lectin-like receptor that mediates endocytosis of glycoproteins or glycoconjugates with terminal mannose or fucose residues (MFR). Interferon-γ, a macrophage-activating factor, induces effects common to other interferons as well as having unique effects on cell function. The down-regulation of MFR, induction of IgG2a Fc receptors and Class II antigens and enhanced production of superoxide and hydrogen peroxide can be considered interferon-γ-specific effects on macrophages.

   Previous reports described synergism of various interferon preparations in anticellular and antiviral effects. However, interferon-α/β can selectively antagonize the down-regulation of macrophage MFR by interferon-γ. The macrophage MFR and CR3 also play a synergistic role in the uptake of zymosan and *Leishmania donovani* in the absence of serum. The receptors may act independently or in concert. Cleaved third complement components can be specifically eluted from zymosan particles in the absence of exogenous complement and are derived from the macrophages themselves. These studies indicate a role for macrophage complement in local opsonization of pathogens at extravascular sites and focus on the role of the tissue macrophage in first-line host defence.

1986 Biochemistry of macrophages. Pitman, London (Ciba Foundation Symposium 118) p 127-136

All cells involved in antigen recognition are required to recognize a wide variety of different antigens. For lymphocytes, this challenge is met by clonal proliferation of T and B cells which possess disulphide-linked heterodimers which confer antigen specificity. By contrast, the repertoire of antigens recognized by mononuclear phagocytes is dependent on exogenous opsonins such as antibody and complement or on the presence of ubiquitous molecules on antigens, for example carbohydrates, specifically mannose. Macrophages are unique in that they express distinct Fc receptors for different isotypes of immunoglobulin (Unkeless et al 1981), bear at least two distinct receptors for fragments of activated third complement component (C3) (Ross et al 1982), and express a lectin-like receptor for mannosyl- or fucosyl-terminated ligands (MFR) (Stahl et al 1980). They also possess receptors for fibronectin (Bevilacqua et al 1981), laminin (Bohnsack et al 1985) and various pinocytosed ligands, including different hormones and substrates required for cellular homeostasis (reviewed by Steinman et al 1983).

The functional state of the macrophages can be selectively altered by soluble factors from antigen- or mitogen-stimulated lymphocytes termed lymphokines. Recently, it has been shown that interferon-γ (IFN-γ), a product of T lymphocytes, has macrophage-activating activity (Celada et al 1984). IFN-γ and IFN-α/β induce common effects on macrophages, including induction of class I major histocompatibility antigens (Lindahl et al 1976) and secretion of plasminogen activator (Jones et al 1982). However, induction of Ia antigens, transient cytolytic activity and enhanced production of superoxide/hydrogen peroxide, which appears to mediate much (though not all) antimicrobial activity, are IFN-γ-specific effects (Nathan et al 1983). We have found that lymphokines and IFN-γ selectively increase the level of IgG2a FcR but decrease expression of MFR activity. The regulation of macrophage receptor function by cytokines contributes to their adaptability in phagocytic and cytolytic recognition.

Effects of lymphokines and interferons on receptor expression

Treatment of adherent mouse macrophages for one to three days with lymphokine derived from antigen-stimulated spleen cells or recombinant IFN-γ results in a selective twofold increase in IgG2a Fc receptor and a threefold decrease in expression of MFR, but little change in the third complement receptor (CR3), antigen Mac-1 (Table 1). Both lymphokine and IFN-γ effects are specifically inhibited by anti-IFN-γ antisera. This suggests that, for the effects studied, IFN-γ can account for all the activity in the crude lymphokine. IgG2aFcR are more effective triggers of the respiratory burst in activated macrophages (Ezekowitz & Gordon 1984). The selective enhancement of IgG2aFcR by macrophage activation could account for the efficacy of homologous antibody in mediating cytotoxicity in some systems (Mathews et al 1981), although a role for natural killer cells should not be discounted (Kipps et al 1985). The down-regulation of MFR activity is a highly reproducible indicator of macrophages activated to secrete enhanced levels of O_2^-/H_2O_2 in humans (Mokoena & Gordon 1985) and mice (Ezekowitz et al 1981). Although the levels of expression are decreased, all macrophages express the receptor, which effectively triggers a respiratory burst on interaction with unopsonized zymosan particles (Berton & Gordon 1983).

TABLE 1 Effect of lymphokines and interferons on receptor expression

	Receptor expression (molecules of macrophages $\times$ 10^{-4})			
Treatment[a]	CR3(Mac I)	IgG2aFcR	IgG2bFcR	MFR
0	55 ± 3	7.2 ± 2	9.0 ± 5	12 ± 3
Lymphokine	53 ± 4	12.5 ± 1.5	7.6 ± 2	4 ± 0.5
+anti-IFN-γ antisera	50 ± 3	ND	ND	11 ± 3
+anti-IFN-α/β antisera	ND	ND	ND	4 ± 1
Interferon-γ	52 ± 5	ND	ND	5 ± 1
+anti-IFN-γ antisera	52 ± 5	ND	ND	12 ± 3
+anti-IFN-α/β antisera	ND	ND	ND	5 ± 1

[a] Macrophages were cultivated for 48–72 h in the presence of 10% immune lymphokine, 1–10 units of recombinant murine IFN-γ or 100–1000 U of IFN-α/β from a murine cellular source. Erythrocytes opsonized with IgG2a and IgG2b mouse antibodies bound to IFN-γ-treated cells as follows: 665 and 360/100 macrophages respectively; values for untreated controls were 380 and 490/100 macrophages. Results show the mean $\pm$ SD of at least eight independent experiments. ND, not done.

Selective antagonism by IFN-α/β of IFN-γ-induced down-regulation of MFR

Addition of IFN-α/β results in a dose-dependent antagonism of reduction of mouse macrophage MFR activity by recombinant murine IFN-γ, provided that IFN-α/β is present during the first 4 h of exposure to IFN-γ (R. A. B. Ezekowitz et al, unpublished). Celada et al (1984) have noted a similar 4-h requirement for exposure to IFN-γ and induction of cytolytic activity. Antagonism between IFN-α/β and IFN-γ is selective for MFR activity. The linked association between a decrease in MFR activity and enhanced O_2^-/H_2O_2 secretion is strengthened by observations that human recombinant IFN-α or β decreases the capacity of recombinant IFN-γ-activated human monocytes to secrete reactive reduced oxygen metabolites (C. Nathan, personal communication). Interactions of different interferons may therefore be antagonistic (MFR, H_2O_2 activity), additive as in secretion of plasminogen activator, antiviral and antiproliferative activity, or neutral, as in expression of Ia antigens.

The mechanism of antagonism between different interferons is not known. Plasma membrane receptors for these interferons are distinct, although binding of one cytokine could decrease expression of the other ligand, as described (Hanigen et al 1984). However, since other effects of both interferons are observed, it is likely that the antagonism depends on a post-receptor mechanism. We do not know if this interaction is specific for macrophages. The restriction of antagonism to markers of macrophage activation (decreased

MFR, enhanced respiratory burst) implies that the phenotype associated with immune activation of macrophages is distinct from marker changes (e.g. plasminogen activator secretion) mediated by non-activating cytokines such as colony-stimulating factors, perhaps at the level of gene regulation.

Interactions between phagocyte receptors

Opsonins, as first defined by Wright & Douglas (1904), promote phagocytosis, and this process involves both attachment and ingestion. The consequences of ligand–receptor interactions are different for IgG and C3. While Fc receptors constitutively promote phagocytosis and trigger the release of powerful oxidants, the ability of C3 receptors to promote phagocytosis is regulated and ligation of these receptors does not appear to stimulate oxidant release (Wright & Silverstein 1983). Fibronectin-coated ligands (Bevilacqua et al 1981) and laminin (Bohnsack et al 1985) bind to distinct receptors on macrophages which appear to modulate phagocytic activity. Fibronectin and laminin promote both Fc- and C3-mediated phagocytosis, possibly by increasing contact between the cell and the phagocytic target, but indirect mechanisms may also contribute to enhanced ingestion. Wright et al (1984) have reported that substratum-bound fibronectin can activate CR3 on the upper surface of monocytes. It is not known whether cooperative interactions between receptors are mediated within the plane of the plasma membrane, via the cytoskeleton or soluble signals.

A cooperative interaction between CR3 and MFR may also be involved in other instances of phagocytic recognition, especially in the absence of exogenous opsonin. Earlier studies showed that under serum-free conditions macrophage ingestion of zymosan, a mannose-rich yeast and excellent activator of the alternative complement pathway, could be mediated by MFR (Berton & Gordon 1983, Sung et al 1983). However, macrophage populations that lack MFR activity, e.g. human monocytes and J774 cells, nevertheless bind or ingest unopsonized zymosan. We showed that uptake of 'unopsonized' zymosan by mononuclear phagocytes can be mediated by receptors for complement as well as MFR and that these receptors may act independently or in concert (Ezekowitz et al 1984). We demonstrated that C3-derived components are present even in the absence of exogenous complement, and we have shown that macrophages themselves can generate all the alternative pathway components required for local opsonization (Ezekowitz et al 1985). The covalently bound CR3 ligand iC3b has been eluted from zymosan particles after co-cultivation with human monocytes under serum-free conditions. Recent studies by Blackwell et al (1985) have provided evidence that a similar mechanism can contribute to the initial macrophage-specific binding of *Leish-*

mania donovani promastigotes, which also activate the alternate complement pathway of complement. Amastigotes do not activate the alternative pathway and their uptake by macrophages appears to be mediated by a process which does not involve MFR and CR3.

The mechanism by which these two receptors cooperate in phagocytic recognition is not clear. Selective modulation of macrophage receptors onto anti-complement receptor antibody or onto mannose-rich yeast mannan confirmed that the complement and lectin receptors are distinct (Blackwell et al 1985). In addition, soluble mannan did not inhibit rosette formation with iC3b-coated erythrocytes, nor did anti-CR3 antibody inhibit MFR activity. Together, these results exclude a role for mannose in iC3b–CR3 interaction. We do not know whether the two receptors recognize distinct ligands on the zymosan or parasite surface, or whether a complex ligand such as mannose-rich glycoproteins or peptidoglycan found in yeast cells, parasites and some bacteria, can act as an acceptor surface for initial complement deposition as well as a source of exposed mannose residues. Further deposition of complement could mask free mannosyl residues so that uptake in the presence of excess complement (presence of serum) proceeds almost exclusively via the CR3. The latter mechanism would apply to phagocytes circulating in serum, to monocytes and to polymorphonuclear leucocytes which lack MFR but express high levels of CR3. However, at extravascular sites local secretion of complement by macrophages could contribute significantly to opsonization. Exposed mannose residues on target organisms or cells could also provide ligands for the relatively high levels of MFR expressed by tissue macrophages. Interestingly, zymosan uptake greatly stimulated C3 secretion by macrophages (R. A. B. Ezekowitz & H. S. Auerbach, unpublished). A possible explanation may be that extracellular fluid-phase C3 regulates a feedback mechanism as found with C4 (Auerbach et al 1984), in which deposition of macrophage C3 on the surface of zymosan would lower extracellular C3 and thereby stimulate C3 secretion. Serum complement may also inhibit monocyte C3 secretion by a similar mechanism.

Conclusion

The mechanisms by which cells of the immune system interact with one another or with particulate targets are more complex than was once thought. Even phagocytic recognition, in which plasma membrane receptors appear to act within a local segment of membrane and to a large extent independently, may involve multiple receptor functions in certain circumstances, e.g. in the absence of high levels of an exogenous opsonin. Control of binding, ingestion and extracellular lysis at the surface of macrophages is precise and selective and involves interaction of plasma membrane receptors with one another and with elements in the cytoskeleton and extracellular matrix. These interactions are modulated further by secretory products and surface molecules of participant cells and targets. The identification of the molecules involved and their functions will be facilitated by the development of new monoclonal antibodies and suitable *in vitro* assays.

Acknowledgements

Supported by grants from the Medical Research Council (UK). We would like to thank Ms Maxine Hill for excellent technical assistance, Dr H. Auerbach for useful discussion, especially in regard to the C3 feedback mechanism, and Ms J. Reynolds and E. Gregory for preparation of the manuscript.

REFERENCES

Auerbach HS, Baker RD, Matthews WI, Colten HR 1984 Molecular mechanism for feedback regulation of C4 biosynthesis in guinea pig peritoneal macrophages. J Exp Med 159: 1750-1761
Berton G, Gordon S 1983 Modulation of macrophage mannose-specific receptors by cultivation on immobilised zymosan. Effects on superoxide-anion release and phagocytosis. Immunology 49:705-715
Bevilacqua M, Amrani D, Mosesson M, Bianco C 1981 Receptors for cold-insoluble globulin (plasma fibronectin) on human monocytes. J Exp Med 153:42-60
Bohnsack JF, Kleinman HK, Takahashi T, O'Shea JJ, Brown EJ 1985 Connective tissue proteins and phagocytic cell function. Laminin enhances complement and Fc-mediated phagocytosis by cultured human macrophages. J Exp Med 16:912-923
Blackwell JM, Ezekowitz RAB, Roberts MB, Channon JY, Sim RB, Gordon S 1985 Macrophage complement and lectin-like receptors bind Leishmania in the absence of serum. J Exp Med 162:324-331
Celada A, Gray PA, Rinderknecht E, Schreiber RD 1984 Evidence for a gamma-interferon receptor that regulates macrophage tumoricidal activity. J Exp Med 160:55-74
Ezekowitz RAB, Gordon S 1984 Alterations of surface properties by macrophage activation: Expression of receptors for Fc and mannose-terminal glycoproteins and differentiation antigens. Contemp Top Immunobiol 13:33-56
Ezekowitz RAB, Austyn JA, Stahl P, Gordon S 1981 Surface properties of Bacillus Calmette-Guerin-activated mouse macrophages. Reduced expression of mannose specific endocytosis, Fc receptors and Ag F4/80 accompanies Ia induction. J Exp Med 154:60-76
Ezekowitz RAB, Sim R, Hill M, Gordon S 1984 Local opsonisation by secreted macrophage complement components. Role of receptors for complement in uptake of zymosan. J Exp Med 159:244-260
Ezekowitz RAB, Sim RB, MacPherson GG, Gordon S 1985 Interaction of human blood monocytes, macrophages and polymorphonuclear leukocytes with zymosan. Role of CR3 and macrophage derived complement. J Clin Invest, in press

Hanigen GE, Fish EN, Williams BRE 1984 Modulation of human interferon-α receptor expression by human interferon-β. J Biol Chem 259:8084-8086

Jones CM, Varesio L, Herberman R, Pestka R 1982 Interferon activates macrophages to produce plasminogen activator. J Interferon Res 2:377-81

Kipps TJ, Parham P, Purt J, Herzenberg LA 1985 Importance of immunoglobulin isotype in human antibody dependent cell mediated cytotoxicity directed by murine monoclonal antibodies. J Exp Med 161:1-15

Lindahl P, Gressor IM, Leary P, Tovey M 1976 Interferon treatment of mice: enhanced expression of histocompatibility antigens on lymphoid cells. Proc Natl Acad Sci USA 73:1984-1987

Mathews IJ, Collins JJ, Roloson CJ, Thick HJ, Bolognosi DP 1981 Immunological control of the ascites form of adenocarcinoma. J Immunol 126:2332-2336

Mokoena T, Gordon S 1985 Human macrophage activation. Modulation of mannose, fucosyl receptor activity in vitro by lymphokines, gamma and alpha interferons and dexamethasone. J Clin Invest 75:624-631

Nathan CF, Murray HW, Wiebe M, Rubin BY 1983 Identification of interferon-γ as the lymphokine that activates human macrophage oxidative metabolism and antimicrobial activity. J Exp Med 158:670-689

Ross GD, Lambris JD, Cain JA, Newman SL 1982 Generation of three different fragments of bound C3 with purified factor I or serum. Requirements for factor H vs CR cofactor activity. J Immunol 129:2051-2058

Stahl P, Schlesinger PH, Sigardson E, Rodman JS, Lee YS 1980 Receptor-mediated pinocytosis of mannose glycoconjugates by macrophages. Characterization and evidence for membrane recycling. Cell 19:207-214

Steinman R, Mellman IS, Muller WA, Cohn ZA 1983 Endocytosis and recycling of plasma membrane, J Cell Biol 96:1-18

Sung SI, Nelson RS, Silverstein SC 1983 Yeast mannose inhibits binding and phagocytosis of zymosan by mouse peritoneal macrophages. J Cell Biol 96:160-168

Unkeless J, Fleit H, Mellman IS 1981 Structural aspects and heterogeneity of immunoglobulin Fc receptors. Adv Immunol 31:247-268

Wright AE, Douglas SR 1904 Role of blood fluids in phagocytosis. Proc R Soc Lond B Biol Sci 72:357

Wright S, Silverstein S 1983 Receptors for C3b abd C3bi promote phagocytosis but not the release of toxic oxygen from human phagocytes. J Exp Med 158:2016-2023

Wright SD, Licht MR, Craigmyle LS, Silverstein SC 1984 Communication between receptors for different ligands on a single cell: ligation of fibronectin receptors induces a reversible alteration in the function of complement receptors on cultured human monocytes. J Cell Biol 99:336-339

DISCUSSION

Roos: Did you try to block the macrophage response by monoclonal antibody or other inhibitors?

Ezekowitz: Yes. We found we could block the response of zymosan in BCG-activated cells. If we added Mac-1 to BCG-activated cells we could at least partially block the respiratory burst activity.

Roos: Did you preincubate the neutrophils with anti-CR3 monoclonal antibody and then add it to the interactive system referred to (p 130)?

Ezekowitz: No. It would also be useful to look at patients who were defective in these molecules to see whether that was a mechanism of mediation. I am now trying to work out what is involved in this complex interaction.

Dean: In the oxidative experiments you had a monolayer of macrophages and pulsed them with neutrophils. Have you compared the two conditions where on the one hand the zymosan is completely internal and no longer exposed on the macrophage surface and on the other hand there is some remaining on the surface?

Ezekowitz: No. Scanning electron micrographs of these clusters show that some zymosan is still on the cell surface and that the polymorph is adhering to the zymosan in a 'cup' of membrane which is the beginnings of the phagosome. But that is just extrapolation from looking at those clusters.

Hogg: You said that zymosan caused a fivefold or sixfold increase in factor B. Does antibody to CR3 or CR1 or binding of the ligands cause a similar increase?

Ezekowitz: We haven't looked at that.

Hogg: It would also be interesting to know whether Fc receptor occupation causes an increase in factor B.

Whaley: If you put an Fc receptor ligand on the Fc receptor you get an increase in synthesis of C2, B, C3 and C1 inhibitor. If you put a C3b ligand on CR1, synthesis is reduced.

Werb: There are two issues to this question. One is whether there is a burst of secretion related to things that are already synthesized and may be stored, and the second is whether there is an increase in the total biosynthesis. In some systems one occurs, in other systems both occur. Reiko Takemura in my laboratory gets a burst of secretion related to ligation of a number of receptors, including the Fc receptor, over a period of a few minutes to an hour after adding a particular ligand. At 6 h or more some of these things also affect secretion.

Springer: In the adherence of monocytes and granulocytes to unopsonized zymosan, both direct interaction with the particle and interaction with the particle after opsonization such as you described have been reported to play a role. To further distinguish between these two mechanisms, it would be interesting to look at patients with C3b inactivator deficiency, since they would be unable to convert C3b to iC3b. Have granulocytes or monocyte from these patients been looked at?

Ezekowitz: No. We thought about looking at C3-deficient patients. There is the question of whether the macrophage C3 is also deficient. The two are not necessarily causally related. In fact the reason why these patients do so well may be that the macrophage C3 is not totally deficient.

Cole: In people who are congenitally C3-deficient, monocytes and macrophages synthesize about 25% of the normal amount of C3. I haven't specifically looked at C3b inactivator-deficient monocytes and macrophages.

Ezekowitz: Initially we discounted a role for CR1 in this mechanism because we used the monoclonal antibody which we assumed was inhibiting rosetting of C3b-coated ligands. Then we found that was not so. The role of the CR1 mechanism is therefore still open.

Cole: In the experiments where you rosetted with C3-coated erythrocytes, was any ^{125}I-labelled ligand taken up when the cells were coated with sheep red cells?

Ezekowitz: We didn't do it like that. We plated the cells on a Fab fragment of monoclonal antibody so that all the complement receptors were modulated to the under-surface of the cell. To test that they had all moved laterally within the membrane we then looked at iC3b-coated rosetting and showed that to be absent. We then took those cells and looked for ^{125}I-labelled mannose–BSA uptake.

Bellavite: It has recently been demonstrated that low doses of chemotactic peptides and complement factor prime neutrophils to respond to other stimuli (Bender et al 1983). We have confirmed these observations. If stimulated macrophages produce complement factors, as you observed, this may be a priming phenomenon carried out by the macrophages to the neutrophils. The molecular basis of this finding is not well understood but perhaps the target of the priming is the same as the respiratory burst enzyme.

Whaley: I think Ross and his colleagues have shown that iC3b binding to CR3 can be inhibited by a sugar. Is that correct?

Ezekowitz: I am not sure.

Whaley: Can zymosan bind to CR3?

Ezekowitz: Ross et al (1985) have claimed that it can. They claim that something on the cell surface of zymosan is very similar to complement. They therefore postulate that the binding is carbohydrate-mediated and that CR3 is a lectin-like receptor. The concentrations of *N*-acetylglucosamine they need to add would make the affinity about 10^{-2}M, which is a very high concentration. We showed that the well-characterized lectin receptor on macrophages, the mannose receptor, is distinct from the complement receptor. Other adhesion molecules may be involved in the direct recognition of ligands, so enhancing the contact and making the ligand available for phagocytic receptors.

Whaley: Your inhibition studies using Fab anti-C3 show that C3 on the *Leishmania donovani* promastigote is an important ligand. Did you do the same sort of experiment with zymosan?

Ezekowitz: Yes, but with zymosan we got only about 38 or 40% inhibition with the Fab fragment of C3. The inhibition effect of both monoclonal antibody and mannan can be overcome in time. That suggests that there must be another mechanism of entry into the cell. After 40–60 minutes you can get entry by another mechanism, even if you leave the monoclonal antibodies in the culture. We usually leave them in for between 15 and 20 minutes and then wash them out. Certainly for the *Leishmania donovani* promastigote another mechanism doesn't seem necessary.

Schreiber: Gordon Ross has reported that, using monoclonal antibodies with different epitope specificities to the Mac-1 α chain he can selectively inhibit binding to C3bi with OKM10 and inhibit binding to zymosan with OKM1, while Mac-1 inhibits both types of interaction. Have you confirmed those findings?

Ezekowitz: Yes. OKM10 was as good as Mac-1 or MO-1 in the inhibition of ligands. A monoclonal made by Sam Wright (Wright et al 1983), 1B4, didn't inhibit in that system, while Tim Springer's β chain antibodies enhanced uptake. I think Tim has found the same in other systems. I have no idea why that happens.

Gordon: It is going to be very important in the long run to distinguish monocyte/macrophages and granulocytes. Granulocytes do not secrete complement components and don't take zymosan well without opsonization, but they can perform other adhesion-related functions, apparently in the absence of an exogenous source of complement.

Ezekowitz: Polymorphs live in a sea of complement, as do monocytes, so physiologically they have been in complement before they encounter ligands that could activate the alternative pathway. Outside the tissues, if you could get selective migration of polymorphs without serum proteins, perhaps local secretion of complement would be sufficient, again leading to the idea that polymorphs would never see a ligand without complement being around.

Schreiber: Have you looked at whether IFN-α and IFN-β antagonize IFN-γ by inducing prostaglandin production? PGE_2 can be an IFN-γ antagonist for some functional activities.

Ezekowitz: We haven't looked at that. What are the kinetics of prostaglandin secretion in response to IFN-α or IFN-β?

Aderem: In our hands IFN-α and IFN-β do not cause the release of any prostaglandins. In fact at high concentrations they down-regulate the release of prostaglandins in response to other stimuli.

REFERENCES

Bender JG, McPhail L, Van Epps DE 1983 Exposure of human neutrophils to chemotactic factors potentiates activation of the respiratory burst enzyme. J Immunol 130:2316-2323

Ross GD, Cain JA, Lachmann PJ 1985 Membrane complement receptor type three (CR_3) has lectin-like properties analogous to bovine conglutinin and functions as a receptor for zymosan and rabbit erythrocytes as well as a receptor for iC3b. J Immunol 134:3307-3315

Wright SD, Rao PE, Van Voorhis WC et al 1983 Identification of the C3bi receptor of human monocytes and macrophages by using monoclonal antibodies. Proc Natl Acad Sci USA 80:5699-5703

General discussion 2

Chemotaxis

Singer: We have been doing some experiments on cell motility, in particular on the motility of fibroblasts and on what happens inside the cells when fibroblasts receive a stimulus to move. We don't know whether a chemotactic factor is involved. When we wound a confluent monolayer with a rubber policeman, the cells at the edge of the wound migrate into the empty space created by the wounding. They do this in a synchronous fashion and in a particular direction. Immunofluorescent labelling of these cells for microtubules reveals the so-called microtubule organizing centre from which microtubules grow out. In an interphase cell the microtubule organizing centre (MTOC) contains the pair of centrioles. In addition we use another antibody that specifically recognizes the Golgi in double immunofluorescence experiments. The MTOC and the Golgi are found to be superimposed in a perinuclear position in all the cells. In the confluent portion of the monolayer this superposition is always seen but the organelles are randomly oriented with respect to the ultimate direction of motion. In cells placed at the edge of a wound, however, the MTOC and the Golgi are coordinately positioned in the direction of subsequent migration. This reorientation occurs within minutes after wounding (Kupfer et al 1982).

We think that the function served by this reorientation, in accordance with what Michael Abercrombie and his colleagues (1970) suggested many years ago for motile cells, is to direct the insertion of new membrane mass into the leading edge of the cell. New membrane mass is derived from the Golgi apparatus and is directed by the reorientation of the Golgi to that part of the cell surface which becomes the leading edge.

In a model system containing cells infected with a virus, we demonstrated that the first surface expression of a viral membrane protein was indeed at the leading edge, which supports the notion that this is where new membrane insertion occurs (Bergmann et al 1983). Along with new membrane insertion one would also expect secretory components derived from the Golgi to be directed to the leading edge.

We observed the same kind of reorientation phenomenon in mouse peritoneal macrophages subjected to a chemotactic gradient of activated mouse serum. The MTOCs were always oriented in one direction whereas in normal mouse serum there was no directional orientation. Likewise the Golgi was oriented preferentially in the direction forward of the nucleus, along with the

MTOC, whereas in unstimulated cells there is no directionality to the position of the Golgi (Nemere et al 1985).

Cell motility is a very complicated multifactorial process. I think John Hartwig has emphasized the role of the cytoskeleton, particularly the actin filament system, in generating an internal force against the leading edge. We think that in addition the insertion of new membrane mass into the leading edge, and perhaps also the secretion of adhesive components at the leading edge, play important roles. Inserting new membrane mass into the leading edge of the cell doesn't of itself guarantee that the cell will move in that direction. The new membrane mass has to be fastened down to the substratum by adhesion. Insertion of new membrane mass and the deposition of adhesive components are probably happening simultaneously at the leading edge as a result of this Golgi reorientation phenomenon.

The motility characteristics of neutrophils may be quite different from those of macrophages. The multifactorial kind of motility mechanism we have been discussing may occur in cells that show long-term chemotaxis or directed migration. Cells that have only to migrate for a relatively short period of time, with a burst of motility, may not need the full panoply of mechanisms involved in long-term migration.

On the other hand, Malech et al (1977) showed some time ago in a Boyden chamber type of experiment that very soon after a chemotactic gradient was applied to neutrophils on a filter, the pair of centrioles in each cell was seen to orient within minutes in the direction of the gradient. I think they were observing the same reorientation of the Golgi and MTOC (containing the centriole pair) in a neutrophil that we have described in a macrophage. It is not clear, however, if such reorientation plays an important role in very short-term migration of the neutrophil.

Cohn: Does this also relate to the directionality of new microtubules?

Singer: The microtubules are distributed throughout but they emanate from the MTOC. They may help to direct the vesicular traffic to the leading edge.

Cohn: Could there be other sources of membrane, such as focusing endocytic vesicles in a unidirectional manner during recycling or from the Golgi?

Singer: There is substantial evidence that at least some endocytic vesicles go through the Golgi. The mechanism we have been discussing in effect polarizes membrane recycling that goes through the Golgi. In an unstimulated immobile cell membrane recycling is presumably going on at random all over the cell surface, but by focusing the Golgi in a particular direction you polarize that recycling process.

Hartwig: In polymorphonuclear leucocytes and macrophages treated with colchicine, the microtubules can be completely dissolved and cells still retain the ability to move directionally toward particles, although not very fast, as untreated cells.

Singer: You have to be careful how you do that experiment. If you incompletely depolymerize microtubules you do not disrupt the Golgi apparatus. If we treat a fibroblast with 30μM-nocodazole for 90 minutes, the MTOC appears to be completely disrupted and the Golgi is dispersed into the cell periphery. The Golgi is still functional—membrane proteins still get to the cell surface, fully glycosylated and at the same rate as in the untreated cells. But the membrane proteins arrive at the cell surface in a uniform distribution. As a result membrane insertion cannot be polarized if you completely depolymerize the microtubules.

This mechanism of reorientation of the Golgi and MTOC in response to a polar signal apparently occurs not only with motile cells after some kind of chemotactic or other stimulus, but also with cytotoxic lymphocytes bound to a susceptible target cell (Kupfer et al 1983, 1985). Presumably the secretion of some cytotoxic component, derived from the Golgi, from the effector to the target cell is involved in this killing. In the natural killer (NK) cell or cytotoxic T lymphocyte, the Golgi and MTOC reorientate very rapidly to face the target cell. No such reorientation occurs in the target cell. This reorientation in the effector cell appears to be a prerequisite for cell killing. For example, killing by cytotoxic T lymphocytes requires calcium, but binding of the cytotoxic T lymphocyte to its target cell occurs in the absence of calcium. When the binding phenomenon occurs in the absence of calcium and in the presence of magnesium this Golgi reorientation in the killer cell does not occur. The addition of calcium results in an immediate Golgi reorientation in the killer cells. It looks as if a similar kind of signalling mechanism operates in both cell motility and cytoxicity.

Unkeless: Our attempts to clone the Fc receptor led to a serendipitous by-product. Andrew Luster, Jeff Ravetch and I have cloned an IFN-γ-induced protein that we called IP10. This protein is homologous with two other proteins, platelet factor 4 (PF4) and β-thromboglobulin. These small proteins, which are located in the α-granules of platelets, are used widely in clinical work as a measure of platelet degranulation.

There are areas of γIP10 where there is rigid conservation of the amino acid sequence of γIP10 in comparison to PF4 and β-thromboglobulin. In particular there are four cysteines in the molecule which form interchain disulphide bridges in PF4 and β-thromboglobulin; these bridges are rigidly conserved in the protein we are discussing. The N terminus of the protein has a classic leader sequence with a hydrophobic core and is in all probability cleaved. PF4 and β-thromboglobulin are chemotactic for neutrophils and monocytes, with an optimal concentration in the nanomolar range. PF4 has heparin-anticoagulant activity and there is a report that both these proteins inhibit collagenase and elastase and stimulate mast cell granule release. Senior et al (1983) have shown that β-thromboglobulin is chemotactic for fibroblasts at exceedingly low concentrations. This also binds to heparin but does not inhibit anticoagulant activity.

We (Luster et al 1985) have shown that the mRNA coding for γIP10 is produced rapidly, with a detectable response to IFN-γ at 30 minutes. Induction of γIP10 mRNA is not inhibited by cycloheximide, and it is probably a primary gene activation event. γIP10 is induced in a variety of cells, including monocytes, fibroblasts and endothelial cells. We have shown by nuclear run-off that synthesis of the message is transcriptionally controlled.

γIP10 may play an important role in inflammation, in that it may constitute a major signal for the emigration of inflammatory cells, monocytes and macrophages into a site where IFN-γ is being synthesized. Preliminary experiments show that conditioned media from IFN-γ-pulsed U937 cells have chemotactic activity for monocytes. This can be removed by passage of the conditioned medium over heparin–Sepharose and the chemotactic activity can be recovered by elution with 0.5 M-NaCl.

Gordon: Is there good evidence that the platelets themselves synthesize the other two products, or could they be taking them up from monocytes? Some platelet granule contents are taken up from outside.

Unkeless: There is no evidence that monocytes and macrophages synthesize PF4. We tried to immunoprecipitate PF4 from U937 cells using anti-PF4 serum supplied by Dr Deuel, with no success.

REFERENCES

Abercrombie M, Heaysman JEM, Pegrum SM 1970 The locomotion of fibroblasts in culture. III. Movements of particles on the dorsal surface of the leading lamella. Exp Cell Res 62:389-398

Bergmann JE, Kupfer A, Singer SJ 1983 Membrane insertion at the leading edge of motile fibroblasts. Proc Natl Acad Sci USA 80:1367-1371

Kupfer A, Louvard D, Singer SJ 1982 The polarization of the Golgi apparatus and the microtubule organizing center in cultured fibroblasts at the edge of an experimental wound. Proc Natl Acad Sci USA 79:2603-2607

Kupfer A, Dennert G, Singer SJ 1983 Polarization of the Golgi apparatus and the microtubule organizing center within cloned natural killer cells bound to their targets. Proc Natl Acad Sci USA 80:7224-7228

Kupfer A, Dennert G, Singer SJ 1985 The reorientation of the Golgi apparatus and the microtubule organizing center in the cytotoxic effector cell is a prerequisite in the lysis of bound target cells. J Mol Cell Immunol 2:37-49

Luster AD, Unkeless JC, Ravetch JV 1985 γ-Interferon transcriptionally regulates an early-response gene containing homology to platelet proteins. Nature (Lond), in press

Malech HL, Root RK, Gallin JI 1977 Structural analysis of human neutrophil migration. Centriole, microtubule, and microfilament orientation and function during chemotaxis. J Cell Biol 75:667-693

Nemere I, Kupfer A, Singer SJ 1985 Reorientation of the Golgi apparatus and the microtubule organizing center inside macrophages subjected to a chemotactic gradient. Cell Motil 5:17-29

Senior RM, Griffin GL, Huang JS, Walz DA, Deuel TF 1983 Chemotactic activity of platelet alpha granule proteins for fibroblasts. J Cell Biol 96:382-385

Regulation of complement protein biosynthesis in mononuclear phagocytes

HARVEY R. COLTEN, ROBERT C. STRUNK, DAVID H. PERLMUTTER and F. SESSIONS COLE

Harvard Medical School, and the Children's Hospital, 300 Longwood Avenue, Boston, MA 02115, USA

Abstract. Proteins of the complement system (with the exception of the terminal components C6–9) are synthesized in mononuclear phagocytes. The extrahepatic macrophage is therefore an important local source of the complement proteins which may serve as a first-line host defence mechanism. Net synthesis and secretion of complement by these cells is a function of maturation of the mononuclear phagocytic series, the tissue from which the cells are isolated, and the state of macrophage activation.

To define some of the mechanisms for regulation of complement gene expression in mononuclear phagocytes, the major histocompatibility complex class III genes and C3 have been investigated. These genes are expressed constitutively in hepatocytes and mono-cytes/macrophages. In the mononuclear phagocyte, interferon-γ, at physiological concentrations, effects a dose- and time-dependent increase in factor B and C2 mRNA and a corresponding increase in factor B and C2 biosynthesis. This effect is specific inasmuch as the expression of other genes (e.g. C3) is decreased by interferon-γ, and interferon-α and β at concentrations one to two logs greater have only a minimal effect on C2 and factor B gene expression. Endotoxin acting directly on monocytes has qualitatively different effects on expression of the complement genes. These complex regulatory mechanisms are being investigated with the use of murine fibroblasts transfected with human DNA bearing the relevant complement genes.

1986 Biochemistry of macrophages. Pitman, London (Ciba Foundation Symposium 118) p 141-154

The many important biological functions served by macrophages may be divided into three broad categories: (a) the uptake and degradation of infectious agents, immune aggregates and endogenous biological substances; (b) a focal point for delivery of antigens to cells that mediate specific immune responses; (c) the source of many secreted products which act locally or at remote sites on soluble and cellular elements of several homeostatic systems. Among the large number of proteins secreted by the macrophage are components of the complement system (reviewed in Bentley et al 1981). The recent isolation of cDNA probes corresponding to several of these complement components, together with methods for the analysis of the biosynthesis and post-synthetic processing of complement proteins in cell culture and under cell-free conditions, has provided insight into the molecular changes that accompany maturation of mononuclear phagocytes and the biochemical regulation of macrophage-mediated inflammation.

The complement system consists of 20 proteins that function as effectors of host defences against microbial infection and as mediators of immunopathological events. During the past two decades, many aspects of the functional and structural features of this complex system have been elucidated. Each of the complement proteins and proteins that control complement activation has been isolated to homogeneity, and partial amino acid sequence data are available for many.

The first complement component (C1) is a macromolecular complex of three proteins designated C1q, C1r and C1s. C1q ($M_r \sim 410\,000$) consists of six subunits each composed of three polypeptide chains (M_r 21 000–24 000). C1r and C1s are single-chain proteins in their zymogen forms which are activated when they are cleaved. Both are serine proteinases, as are the classical pathway protein C2 ($M_r \sim 110\,000$) and alternative pathway proteins factor B (M_r 95 000) and factor D ($M_r \sim 24\,000$). The third (C3), fourth (C4) and fifth (C5) components are structurally related multichain glycoproteins which are the mediators of many complement-dependent biological effects. The mechanisms of activation of the classical and alternative pathways of the complement system and the biological activities of complement peptides have also been intensively investigated. This work has been reviewed by Reid & Porter (1981) and will not be discussed further.

Early studies suggested that the liver was the principal site of synthesis of serum complement proteins. This was to a great extent confirmed when it was shown that for several components (C3, C6, C8 and factor B) orthotopic liver transplantation from a donor with a distinct genetic variant of the relevant protein resulted in complete conversion from the recipient to the donor allotype (Alper et al 1980). Moreover cDNA clones for C1q, C2, C4, C3, C5, C8, C9 and factor B have been isolated from human cDNA liver libraries, demonstrating the presence of mRNA for each. These findings, and studies of complement synthesis in hepatoma cell lines, suggest that the hepatocyte synthesizes most, if not all, of the complement proteins. On the other hand, extrahepatic synthesis of complement components of the classical and alternative pathways through C5 has been demonstrated in cells of the monocyte-/macrophage series (Colten et al 1979). Except for the membrane lesions induced by assembly of the terminal complement proteins, the biological effects of this system can be generated by macrophage-derived complement. Thus, local production of complement proteins by the macrophage may provide the initial response to tissue injury or microbial invasion plus a mechanism for recruiting intravascular humoral and cellular mediators of host defences. That is, the components necessary for generation of the activated complement peptides that alter vascular permeability and induce directed movement of leucocytes are produced locally by mononuclear phagocytes.

Complement gene structure and biosynthesis of complement proteins

Among the macrophage-derived complement proteins, the major histocompatibility complex class III gene products C2, factor B and C4 have been the focus of considerable interest, but data pertaining to synthesis of C3 and other components will be discussed as well.

A single copy of the C2 gene is found within the human (Fu et al 1974, Carroll et al 1984) and murine (D. H. Perlmutter et al, unpublished) major histocompatibility complex (MHC) less than 1.0 kilobase (kb) 5' to the factor B gene. Three distinct C2 primary translation products are generated from human mRNA (Perlmutter et al 1984), the most abundant of which is an 84 kilodalton (kDa) product. This protein is glycosylated and secreted within 1–2 hours. Two forms of lower molecular mass (79 kDa and 70 kDa) remain cell-associated for many hours; the function of these proteins is unknown.

Synthesis of the factor B primary translation product (83 kDa) is directed by an mRNA of ~2.5 kb. Single loci for the human (Carroll et al 1984) factor B gene of ~6 kb and the murine (Chaplin et al 1983) factor B gene have been identified 3' to the C2 gene. The human factor B gene is divided into 18 exons separated by introns of variable length. Analysis of the structure of this gene (Campbell et al 1984) has provided insights into the evolution of factor B and its relationship to other serine proteinases.

Synthesis of the 185 kDa single-chain precursor of the fourth component (pro-C4) (Hall & Colten 1977) is directed by a 5 kb mRNA in which the subunits of the native C4 proteins (β, α, γ) are separated by arginine-rich linking peptides (Ogata et al 1983, Carroll & Porter 1983) similar to the interchain peptides of pro-C3 (Domdey et al 1982) and pro-C5 (Lundwall et al 1985). Postsynthetic processing of pro-C4 involves glycosylation (Roos et al 1980), limited proteolysis, modification within the thiol ester site (Karp 1983) and sulphation. The two human C4 loci (Carroll et al 1984) and the corresponding murine genes, Slp and C4 (Chaplin et al 1983), are 3' to the factor B gene within the MHC.

The third component is synthesized as a single-chain precursor, prepro-C3 (Wiebauer et al 1982), which is cleaved by a signal peptidase and a plasmin-like enzyme to generate native C3 (Goldberger et al 1981). The central role of the C3 protein in the biological effects of complement and the presence of

C3 receptors on mononuclear phagocytes emphasizes the importance of studies designed to elucidate the mechanisms regulating C3 gene expression.

Regulation of C2 and factor B synthesis

Evidence has been obtained that factors B and D of the alternative pathway are synthesized by guinea-pig peritoneal macrophages (Bentley et al 1981). The same authors demonstrated a lack of D synthesis (in its active form) by either stimulated or resident murine macrophages. The lack of active D synthesis allowed detection of functional factor B in the culture media from the mouse macrophage preparations (reviewed in Colten et al 1979). Similar studies established that factor I (Whaley 1980) and factor D are synthesized in human monocytes and macrophages.

C2 is also synthesized in cells of the monocyte/macrophage series. Studies of extrahepatic synthesis of C2 in guinea-pig and human mononuclear phago-cytes (Alpert et al 1983, Cole et al 1985) revealed changes in the proportion of complement-producing cells and in rates of synthesis as a function of cell maturation. For instance, no C2-producing cells are detected in guinea-pig bone marrow but 10% of the blood monocyte population are C2 plaque-forming cells. In different tissues, the proportion of macrophages producing C2 varies from about 45% in spleen and peritoneum to 2.5% in lung. The subpopulation of cells producing C2 characteristic of each tissue remains quite constant for several days in culture. Complement-producing macrophages from guinea-pig lung synthesize C2 at a rate 5–10 times greater than the rate of synthesis in complement-producing peritoneal macrophages. This com-pensates for the 20-fold difference in the proportion of C2-producing cells, so the absolute amount of C2 generated from equal numbers of unfractionated peritoneal and lung macrophages is comparable. An unresolved question raised by these observations is whether specific subpopulations of monocytes migrate to different tissues or whether regulatory signals characteristic of a given tissue provide local control of C2 gene expression.

Induction of an inflammatory response leads to increased local C2 produc-tion by two mechanisms: (a) an increase in macrophage cell number and (b) a twofold to threefold increased rate of synthesis per cell. This increased rate of C2 synthesis per cell is the result of an increase in C2 mRNA but probably reflects a general effect on transcription and translation since both total cellular RNA and protein secreted are increased in the inflammatory cells. The proportion of C2-producing cells in such an inflammatory exudate is similar to that in a resting cell population, i.e. there is no evidence for selective recruitment of complement-producing cells.

Human mononuclear phagocytes also display characteristic differences in

C2 and factor B synthesis as a function of maturation, tissue site and response to specific stimuli that elicit an inflammatory exudate. Haemolytically active C2 is secreted by monocytes in tissue culture for several months and the rate of C2 synthesis per cell varies as a function of the length of time the cells are maintained *in vitro*; i.e. the rate of C2 synthesis at two months is about three times the rate during the second week of culture. Moreover, little or no C2 is secreted during the first three to six days. Similar kinetics of factor B biosynthesis have also been observed (Whaley 1980).

Manipulation of the culture conditions alters baseline rates of C2 secretion by human monocytes. For example, the initial lag in C2 biosynthesis can be abolished by the addition of a soluble product of antigen-stimulated lymphocytes to the medium (Littman & Ruddy 1977). This observation prompted our recent studies (unpublished) on the effect of defined cytokines on C2 and factor B gene expression in mononuclear phagocytes. Recombinant-generated human interferon-γ (IFN-γ) at concentrations of 1 to 1000 units/ml induces a dose-dependent increase in C2 and factor B-specific mRNA in human monocyte cultures. This increase is accompanied by increased synthesis of the corresponding proteins without a significant effect on secretion or stability of C2 or factor B proteins. The effect of IFN-γ on factor B synthesis is detected earlier (<6 h) than its effect on C2 (~24 h after exposure to the lymphokine). Two observations established the specificity of this effect of IFN-γ on C2 and factor B gene expression: (a) Recombinant-generated IFN-α and IFN-β had only minimal effects on C2 and B synthesis at concentrations one to two logs greater than the concentration of IFN-γ required to effect a comparable increase. (b) IFN-γ decreased expression of the C3 gene as judged by a decrease in the steady-state C3 mRNA content and pro-C3 synthesis. It is difficult to understand how this effect on C3 gene expression is of biological advantage. This problem will be addressed when the direct effect on macrophages of a bacterial product (endotoxin) is considered (see below). Other stimuli result in decreased C2 biosynthesis by monocytes, e.g. Fc fragment of IgG, concanavalin A or serum-treated immune complexes. Certain lipids also inhibit C2 biosynthesis in human monocytes and guinea-pig macrophages. Although it is clear that the effect of lipid is independent of the type of free fatty acid, the mechanism accounting for this mode of regulation of C2 biosynthesis and its physiological importance is as yet unknown.

Synthesis of C2 and factor B is initiated without lag, and rates of synthesis are several times greater than in monocytes harvested from the peripheral blood of the same individuals. In addition, the ratio of C2 to factor B secreted by the macrophage differs from the relative rates of secretion in monocytes even after prolonged culture. That is, secretion of haemolytically active C2 exceeds factor B by 3.5- to 7-fold in milk and bronchoalveolar macrophages respectively, whereas the ratio of C2 to factor B secreted by the monocytes is constant $(C2/B = 1)$ for several weeks *in vitro*. In addition, variation in the proportion of C2-producing cells among human macrophage populations, similar to those observed in the guinea-pig, have been recognized. Changes in rates of post-translational modification, secretion, or stability of the extracellular products have been excluded as significant factors accounting for these differences between human monocyte and macrophage C2 and factor B biosynthesis. Finally, studies utilizing specific cDNA probes for factor B and C2 suggest that this regulation is exerted at a pretranslational level, i.e. is either the result of transcriptional control or post-transcriptional processing (Cole et al 1985). The signals that mediate this change, however, are not yet understood.

Regulation of C3 gene expression

Thorbecke et al (1965) first demonstrated that many tissues, including lymph nodes, spleen, liver, lung, bone marrow, etc., synthesize C3. However, other evidence indicated that the liver is the primary source of serum C3. Interest in extrahepatic synthesis of C3 was renewed by the observation that short-term cultures of synovial tissue from patients with rheumatoid arthritis synthesized and secreted biologically active C3, though similar cultures from patients with degenerative joint disease did not (Ruddy & Colten 1974). These studies suggested an important role for locally produced C3 in immunopathological events.

The molecular details of C3 biosynthesis were first examined by Brade et al (1977) in short-term cultures of guinea-pig liver and peritoneal macrophages. This work showed that radiolabelled C3 protein immunoprecipitated from cell lysates or from an endogenous cell-free translation mixture is a single-chain peptide of approximately 180 kDa (pro-C3) which undergoes intracellular proteolytic cleavage before secretion as the native two-chain protein. Similar work established that mouse (Domdey et al 1982) and human (Morris et al 1982) C3 are also synthesized as single-chain precursors.

More recently Strunk et al (1985) have shown that the lipid A portion of endotoxin induces a 5–30-fold increase in C3 biosynthesis by human mononuclear phagocytes without a significant effect on C2, factor B or lysozyme synthesis. The increase in C3 synthesis is associated with an increase in C3 mRNA, suggesting a pretranslational regulatory mechanism. Significant increases in C2 and factor B mRNA were also observed, although these were not reflected in an increased rate of synthesis of the corresponding proteins. The possibility must be considered that a second signal is required for an increase in synthesis of these two proteins. That is, although endotoxin effects an increase in specific mRNA, another signal may be required for alteration in specific translation rates.

Regulation of C4 biosynthesis

Murine C4 is synthesized in short-term cultures of peritoneal macrophages (Newell et al 1982). The rate of C4 secretion falls rather rapidly within the first few hours in culture, although total protein synthesis remains approximately constant. In addition, there is an increase in factor B synthesis during the first two days in culture. Both feedback inhibition and instability of secreted C4 were ruled out as possible explanations for the striking decrease in C4 production as a function of time in culture. More recently it has been possible to exclude changes in secretion rate or postsynthetic processing of the precursor protein as mechanisms accounting for this phenomenon, and to demonstrate that the change in synthetic rate is a function of the concentration of specific C4 mRNA per cell (Sackstein & Colten 1984). In addition, there is a reciprocal increase in steady-state levels of factor B mRNA, indicating that the change in cellular C4 mRNA levels is not simply the result of a limitation of the culture conditions. The most likely explanation for these findings is a change in rate of transcription of C4 and factor B RNA during the time the macrophages are in culture, but the signal(s) for this change is (are) not known. Alternative explanations include changes in post-transcriptional processing or stability of the specific C4 and factor B mRNA.

Elicited or activated murine peritoneal macrophages generated by injection with oil, casein, thioglycollate, concanavalin A or lipopolysaccharide produce markedly less C4, even in the initial few hours in culture, than resident macrophages produce (Newell & Atkinson 1983). About 3–10 times more C4 is synthesized and secreted in the resident cells than in the elicited cell populations. This is also the result of control of transcription, post-transcriptional processing or (less likely) stability of the specific C4 mRNA, because the steady-state C4 mRNA levels correlate with the pro-C4 synthesis rates in the resident and elicited cells (Sackstein & Colten 1984).

Serum levels of C4 differ in strains of mice designated high Ss and low Ss by about 10–20-fold as assessed functionally and immunochemically. Only recently has any insight into the basis for this difference been obtained. Initial studies showed that peritoneal macrophages obtained from high and low C4 strains synthesized C4 at comparable rates during the initial period in culture or at later time periods when the amount of C4 synthesized in both cell types decreased (Newell et al 1982). These results suggested either (a) that the mechanisms regulating serum levels of C4 in the various strains are present only in liver, not in macrophages, or (b) that catabolism of C4 in the strains with low serum levels is markedly greater than in strains with high levels. Evidence for the former hypothesis was obtained from two lines of investigation. Primary hepatocyte cultures produce C4 at rates that correspond to the strains from which the liver is obtained (Rosa & Shreffler 1983). A parallel difference in content of liver C4-specific mRNA from high and low C4 strains has been noted (Ogata et al 1983, Chaplin et al 1983) but C4 mRNA content is not significantly different in macrophages from high and low Ss strains (Sackstein & Colten 1984), indicating that the regulation of C4 mRNA levels in the hepatocyte differs from that in the macrophage.

Important differences in regulation of C4 synthesis by murine and guinea-pig macrophages have been observed. The sensitivity and specificity of the haemolytic assay for guinea-pig C4 has allowed studies of C4 biosynthesis on a single-cell level. These studies indicate that differences in tissue-specific regulation may even be more complicated than was appreciated from investigations of murine C4 biosynthesis. Alpert et al (1983) showed that approximately 10% of bone marrow-derived adherent mononuclear phagocytes and a comparable proportion of the circulating monocytes produce C4 haemolytic plaques but about 40–50% of the macrophages derived from bronchoalveolar wash, peritoneal cavity and spleen generate C4 plaque-forming cells.

About 20–25% of peritoneal macrophages bear surface C4 antigen but the surface C4-bearing cell population is not stable, since incubation of the cells in medium containing or lacking preformed fluid-phase C4 alters the proportion of C4 surface-positive cells (Auerbach et al 1984). The ability to separate cells displaying surface C4 from those lacking surface C4 permitted the presence of surface C4 antigen to be correlated with functional characteristics of the cells, namely the secretion of C2 and C4. The C4-bearing cells constitute the majority of peritoneal macrophages that secrete haemolytically active C4. However, within 6–12 hours secretion of C4 decreases. The C4 surface-negative cell population initially contains relatively few C4-secreting cells but this proportion increases when the macrophages are cultured in fresh medium or in C4-deficient conditioned medium. In contrast, when C4 purified from plasma, or conditioned medium containing C4, is added to the culture, the cells fail to produce C4. These and other experiments suggested a relationship between the binding of C4 (derived from the medium) to the cell surface and secretion of C4. This effect is specific, since the presence of fluid-phase or surface-cell-bound C4 antigen does not affect the rate of C2 secretion per cell or the proportion of C2-producing cells. Most of the cell-surface-bound C4 is native C4, although trace amounts of smaller C4 peptides are detected. Further work will be required to define the precise ligand and the specificity of its interaction with cell-surface-acceptor sites.

Although the specific signal remains obscure, it is clear that binding of C4 protein to the cell surface results in selective inhibition of C4 biosynthesis and this correlates with a decrease in the steady-state level of C4 mRNA (Auerbach et al 1984). Inhibition of C4 synthesis (a) is accomplished with both serum-derived and macrophage-derived C4 (the former probably of hepatocyte origin), (b) is independent of haemolytic activity of the C4, and (c) is reversible. The specific decrease of C4 mRNA in cells incubated in the presence of extracellular C4 is not accompanied by a change in factor B-specific mRNA or total RNA content. These observations suggest that the selective feedback inhibition of C4 biosynthesis is regulated at the level of transcription or post-transcriptional processing. It is unlikely that specific mRNA stability has been altered, but this possibility has not been excluded.

The direct regulation by extracellular C4 of C4 production by macrophages would have important consequences for regulation of an inflammatory response. That is, it would provide a mechanism for controlling constitutive secretion of C4 in resting macrophages as well as a basis for repletion of C4 after complement consumption or diffusion from the site of inflammation. The direct control of C4 synthesis would thus not depend on or necessarily correlate with plasma concentrations of C4, but would reflect the local concentration of extracellular C4 in the tissue environment. Notwithstanding the aforementioned differences between the guinea-pig and murine systems, this observation is consistent with the demonstration that macrophages from high and low C4 strains produce comparable amounts of C4.

Conclusion

It should be clear from this brief summary of the studies undertaken in the past few years that progress has been made towards understanding the molecular regulation of complement biosynthesis by mononuclear phagocytes. This has resulted from isolation of the relevant cDNA probes and use of new methods for studies of biosynthesis and postsynthetic processing. In the near future, direct studies of transcription *in vitro*, and further knowledge of the structure of the complement genes and the relevant monocyte/macrophage cell surface receptors, should make it possible to elucidate the network of biochemical mechanisms that control macrophage-mediated inflammation.

REFERENCES

Alper CA, Raum D, Awdeh Z, Petersen BH, Taylor PD, Starzl TE 1980 Studies of hepatic synthesis in vivo of plasma proteins including orosomucoid, transferrin, α_1-antitrypsin, C8 and factor B. Clin Immunol Immunopathol 16:84-89

Alpert SE, Auerbach HS, Cole FS, Colten HR 1983 Macrophage maturation: differences in complement secretion by marrow, monocyte, and tissue macrophages detected with an improved hemolytic plaque assay. J Immunol 130:102-107

Auerbach HS, Baker RD, Matthews WJ, Colten HR 1984 Molecular mechanism for feedback regulation of C4 biosynthesis in guinea pig peritoneal macrophages. J Exp Med 159:1750-1761

Bentley C, Zimmer B, Hadding U 1981 The macrophage as a source of complement components. Lymphokines 4:197-203

Brade V, Hall RE, Colten HR 1977 Biosynthesis of pro-C3, a precursor of the third component of complement. J Exp Med 146:759-765

Campbell RD, Bentley DR, Morley BJ 1984 The factor B and C2 genes. Phil Trans R Soc Lond B Biol Sci 306:379-388

Carroll MC, Porter RR 1983 Cloning of a human complement component C4 gene. Proc Natl Acad Sci USA 80:264-267

Carroll MC, Campbell DR, Bentley DR, Porter RR 1984 A molecular map of the human major histocompatibility complex class III region linking complement genes C4, C2 and factor B. Nature (Lond) 307:237-241

Chaplin DD, Woods DW, Whitehead AS, Goldberger G, Colten HR, Seidman JG 1983 Molecular map of the murine S region. Proc Natl Acad Sci USA 80:6947-6951

Cole FS, Auerbach HS, Goldberger G, Colten HR 1985 Tissue specific pretranslational regulation of complement production in human mononuclear phagocytes. J Immunol 134:2610-2616

Colten HR, Ooi, YM, Edelson PJ 1979 Synthesis and secretion of complement proteins by macrophages. Ann NY Acad Sci 332:482-490

Domdey H, Wiebauer K, Kazmaier M, Muller V, Odink K, Fey G 1982 Characterization of the mRNA and cloned cDNA specifying the third component of mouse complement. Proc Natl Acad Sci USA 79:7619-7623

Fu SM, Kunkel HG, Brusman HP, Allen FH, Fotino M 1974 Evidence for linkage between HLA histocompatibility genes and those involved in the synthesis of the second component of complement. J Exp Med 140:1108-1111

Goldberger G, Thomas ML, Tack BF, Williams J, Colten HR, Abraham GN 1981 NH_2-terminal structure and cleavage of guinea pig pro-C3, the precursor of the third complement component. J Biol Chem 256:12617-12619

Hall RE, Colten HR 1977 Cell free synthesis of the fourth component of guinea pig complement (C4): identification of a precursor of serum C4 (pro-C4). Proc Natl Acad Sci USA 74:1707-1710

Karp DR 1983 Post translational modification of the fourth component of complement. Effect of tunicamycin and amino acid analogs on the formation of the internal thiolester and disulfide bonds. J Biol Chem 258:14490-14495

Littman BH, Ruddy S 1977 Production of the second component of complement by human monocytes: stimulation by antigen activated lymphocytes or lymphokines. J Exp Med 145:1344-1352

Lundwall AB, Wetsel RA, Kristensen T et al 1985 Isolation of a cDNA clone encoding the fifth component of human complement. J Biol Chem 260:2108-2112

Morris KM, Aden DP, Knowles BB, Colten HR 1982 Complement biosynthesis by the human hepatoma-derived cell line, Hep-G2. J Clin Invest 70:906-913

Newell SL, Atkinson JP 1983 Biosynthesis of C4 by mouse peritoneal macrophages. II. Comparison of C4 synthesis by resident and elicited cell populations. J Immunol 130:834-838

Newell SL, Shreffler DC, Atkinson JP 1982 Biosynthesis of C4 by mouse peritoneal macrophages. I. Characterization of an in vitro culture system and comparison of C4 synthesis of 'low' vs 'high' C4 strains. J Immunol 129:653-659

Ogata RT, Shreffler DC, Sepich DS, Lilly SP 1983 cDNA clone spanning the alpha-gamma subunit junction in the precursor of the murine fourth complement component (C4). Proc Natl Acad Sci USA 80:5061-5065

Perlmutter D, Cole FS, Goldberger G, Colten HR 1984 Distinct primary translation products from human liver mRNA give rise to secreted and cell-associated forms of complement (C2). J Biol Chem 259:10380-10385

Reid KBM, Porter RR 1981 The proteolytic activation system of complement. Annu Rev Biochem 50:433-464

Roos MH, Kornfeld S, Shreffler DC 1980 Characterization of the oligosaccharide units of the fourth component of complement (Ss protein) synthesized by murine macrophages. J Immunol 124:2860-2863
Rosa PA, Shreffler DC 1983 Cultured hepatocytes from mouse strains expressing high and low levels of the fourth component of complement differ in rate of synthesis of the protein. Proc Natl Acad Sci USA 80:2332-2336
Ruddy S, Colten HR 1974 Rheumatoid arthritis: biosynthesis of complement proteins by synovial tissues. N Engl J Med 290:1284-1288
Sackstein R, Colten HR 1984 Molecular regulation of MHC class III (C4 and factor B) gene expression in mouse peritoneal macrophages. J Immunol 133:1618-1626
Strunk RC, Whitehead AS, Cole FS 1985 Pretranslational regulation of the synthesis of the third component of complement in human mononuclear phagocytes by the lipid A portion of lipopolysaccharide. J Clin Invest, in press
Thorbecke GJ, Hochwald GM, van Furth R, Muller-Eberhard HJ, Jacobson EB 1965 Problems in determining the sites of synthesis of complement components. In: Complement. J. & A. Churchill, London (Ciba Found Symp) p 99-119
Whaley K 1980 Biosynthesis of the complement components and the regulatory proteins of the alternative complement pathway by human peripheral blood monocytes. J Exp Med 151:501-516
Wiebauer K, Domdey H, Diggelman H, Fey G 1982 Isolation and analysis of genomic DNA clones encoding the third component of mouse complement. Proc Natl Acad Sci USA 79:7077-7081

DISCUSSION

Whaley: There is a lot of controversy about the importance of macrophages in making complement proteins. Leaving aside the fact that people who receive orthotopic liver transplants make complement proteins of donor origin, there are two observations indicating that macrophages are important sources of complement. First, in catabolic studies of patients with arthritis, radiolabelled C3 within a joint never equilibrates with what is in the plasma pool (Ruddy & Colten 1974). It looks as though at least half the complement in inflamed joints, and presumably therefore in other inflamed areas, is made locally, probably by macrophages. The second piece of evidence is the elegant work of Alan Ezekowitz, which was presented earlier.

Our interest is in the regulation of complement synthesis by macrophages at the cell membrane level. We use human monocytes and compare these with synovial fluid macrophages as a source of human tissue macrophages. We accept that these are probably activated macrophages rather than resident macrophages. Complement proteins are inducible products. The synthetic rates are much higher in macrophages than in monocytes. Monocytes make C3, D and I on day 0, but they require two to three days before they begin to synthesize C2, B and C1-inhibitor.

Whether the D and I activities in culture supernatant are really due to the presence of these two proteins or whether other enzymes are responsible for this effect has not been determined.

Lysozyme synthesis continues at a fairly constant secretory rate in macrophage and monocyte cultures. In these cultures we get 250–300 ng lysozyme/ μg DNA in 24 h (4×10^6 molecules/cell every hour), which is a fairly large quantity of protein. In monocyte cultures the secretion rate of C3 is about 0.07% that of lysozyme, C1 inhibitor is about 0.03%, C2 about 0.07% and B about 0.02%. In macrophage cultures these rates increase to 0.25% for C3, 0.2% for C2, 0.1% for B and 0.2% for C$\bar{1}$-inhibitor. Thus even in macrophage cultures complement components account for only a very small proportion of the secreted protein mass (<1.0% of lysozyme). If we compare the increase in the secretion rates of complement components in activated macrophages such as rheumatoid synovial fluid macrophages we find that there is some selectivity in the stimulation of synthesis of complement components. Synthesis of B and C$\bar{1}$ inhibitor synthesis are increased by fivefold to sixfold on average, whereas the synthesis rates of C3 and C2 increase by only about twofold to threefold.

We are also interested in the nature of the transmembrane signal. The agents which stimulate complement synthesis by macrophages include antigen–antibody complexes which activate Fcγ-receptors, acetylcholine which acts on nicotinic cholinergic receptors and adrenergic ligands acting on α_1 receptors. This stimulatory response can be blocked with calcium channel blockers and also with sodium channel blockers, which implies that influx of both sodium and calcium is needed to increase synthesis.

Histamine, PGE$_2$, C3b receptor ligands acting on CR1 and anaphylatoxins acting on specific receptors all activate adenylate cyclase and turn off synthesis of all complement proteins, but do not alter lysozyme synthesis. The kinetics of cyclic AMP accumulation shows a pattern with a fairly rapid rise which peaks after 15 minutes and then returns to baseline after 2 h. We think that a general switch-off signal in mononuclear phagocytes is adenylate cyclase activation, but there must be more specific signals.

Nathan: Interferon experts have made catalogues of two-dimensional gels for polypeptide synthesis in cells responding to interferons. They find 8 or 12 spots that are induced. People with specific interests and powerful probes are able to identify individual products. Can you bring these areas together? Are the complement components among those polypeptides that are abundant enough to be seen on gels without screening with specific probes?

Cole: We have not performed experiments to examine that question. The functions of interferon-induced proteins are not defined. Some may be involved in repressing or derepressing specific gene products, while others may be involved in signal transduction.

Nathan: Did you say that IFN-γ induces the secretion of C2 and factor B?

Cole: No. IFN-γ induces an increase in the synthetic rate of C2 and factor B but no change in the secretion rate that we have been able to detect.

Unkeless: In the effect of LPS, you showed that there was a dramatic increase in C3 but none in C2.

Cole: There was no increase in newly synthesized C2 protein, but we showed an increase in C2 mRNA. I assume that there is transcriptional regulation of C3 and translational regulation of C2 after exposure to LPS.

Aderem: Could you comment on your work with protein synthesis inhibitors?

Cole: They are dangerous experiments. We did them primarily to decide whether to direct our work at examining regulatory nucleotide sequences or induced regulatory proteins. For IFN-γ we were motivated to look at sequences, while for LPS we were motivated to look at proteins.

Dean: Have you looked at the effects of inhibiting mitochondrial protein synthesis?

Cole: No. Those would be interesting experiments to do.

Springer: You have shown that the species-specificity in IFN-γ induction resides at the level of the L cell that the gene is in, rather than in the species of the gene inside the cell. Is that controlled at the level of the L cell receptor for IFN-γ on the cell surface?

Cole: My understanding is that human IFN-γ has not had any effect in any mouse systems.

Schreiber: That is true. Competition experiments indicate that human interferon does not bind to the interferon receptor on murine cells.

Cohn: Can a macrophage assemble the entire attack complex? Could that play a role in cytolysis?

Cole: At present it appears that terminal complement components are not synthesized by monocytes or macrophages from humans or several animal species. The entire membrane complex cannot therefore be assembled by macrophage-derived components alone. We hypothesize that activation of macrophage-derived early-acting complement proteins liberates chemotactic peptides (C3a, C4a and C5a) which alter vascular permeability and permit transudation of plasma-derived late-acting components into the tissue or site of inflammation.

Humphrey: Is there a basal level of IFN-γ in humans? And does a rise in interferon detectably alter the rate of synthesis of the complement components? After total body irradiation there aren't many circulating macrophages left. What is happening at that stage?

Cole: We have not yet attempted to re-create an inflammatory environment by putting T cells that are secreting interferon back together with monocytes and macrophages. Human alveolar macrophages obtained by bronchial lavage from patients with high-intensity alveolitis from pulmonary sarcoidosis synthesize more C2 and factor B than macrophages from normal volunteers. They also have a lot of T cells in the alveolar lavage. Whether there is any causal relationship there is purely speculation. That is the closest we have come to seeing what the *in vivo* result of this kind of interaction might be.

Nathan: Anna Fels and I have been looking at peroxide release by alveolar macrophages from patients with sarcoidosis and find that these cells secrete about threefold more than normal bronchoalveolar lavage macrophages. The latter population can be induced to become like the sarcoid population with exogenous interferon-γ (Fels et al 1985). Crystal's group has shown that the T cells in the sarcoid lung are in fact secreting IFN-γ (Robinson et al 1985). But the connection has not been proved.

Ezekowitz: I was interested in the kinetics of factor B induction and its relationship to IFN-γ-induced spreading, which seems to be quite an early event. Is factor B important in that mechanism?

Whaley: We used cobra venom factor in some of our monocyte cultures. After a few days they had spread remarkably compared with normal monocytes. We were able to inhibit spreading with Fab fragments of B. It is possible that endogenous C3b could complex with B and produce a similar effect.

Werb: Although mouse macrophages produce large quantities of factor B, much more than in the human, it takes a long time, at least 4 hours and, more likely, 24 hours before any breakdown components such as B_b are seen. There is a high M_r early on and then one slowly sees generation of factor B_b-like fragments when one induces with IFN-γ. So something other than what is present in the serum-free condition may be needed for factor B to be able to be functionally active.

Schreiber: How did factor B production by interferon-treated monocytes compare to factor B production by tissue macrophages? Does interferon function by inducing monocyte differentiation into macrophages?

Cole: Interferon certainly causes other changes in cell functions. The advantages of these proteins are (1) they are discrete gene products whose regulation can be quantitatively and specifically studied and (2) they serve both as markers of monocyte response to migration from the bloodstream into the tissue and as markers for the response to various inflammatory stimuli.

REFERENCES

Fels AOS, Nathan CF, Cohn ZA 1985 Generation of H_2O_2 by alveolar macrophages from sarcoidosis patients and normals. Am Rev Respir Dis, in press (abstr)

Robinson BWS, McLemore TL, Crystal RG 1985 Gamma interferon is spontaneously released by alveolar macrophages and lung T lymphocytes in patients with pulmonary sarcoidosis. J Clin Invest 75:1488-1495

Ruddy S, Colten HR 1974 Rheumatoid arthritis: biosynthesis of complement proteins by synovial tissues. N Engl J Med 290:1284-1288

The cell and molecular biology of apolipoprotein E synthesis by macrophages

ZENA WERB*†, JENNIE R. CHIN*, REIKO TAKEMURA*, ROSA LAURA OROPEZA*, DOROTHY F. BAINTON‡, PAULA STENBERG‡, JOHN M. TAYLOR§¶, and CATHERINE REARDON¶

*Laboratory of Radiobiology and Environmental Health, Departments of †Anatomy, ‡Pathology, and §Physiology, and ¶Gladstone Foundation Laboratories for Cardiovascular Disease, University of California, San Francisco, California 94143, USA

Abstract. Mononuclear phagocytes secrete over 50 different proteins that are regulated during differentiation and that are under the influence of various materials and factors in their extracellular milieu as part of the inflammatory response. The complex nature of the regulation of the expression of these molecules is displayed by apolipoprotein E (ApoE). ApoE mRNA first appears as monocytes differentiate into macrophages, and this expression is paralleled by the secretion of ApoE by the cells. In mature macrophages ApoE synthesis and secretion are decreased by activation of macrophages with endotoxin and interferon-γ. Although these macrophages contain abundant translatable ApoE mRNA, little ApoE is synthesized, suggesting that this decrease occurs largely at the translational level. ApoE is also controlled at the level of secretion. ApoE is concentrated in the Golgi complex of macrophages and is also found in endoplasmic reticulum, secretion vesicles and coated vesicles. When macrophages come in contact with immune complexes the intracellular ApoE compartment degranulates rapidly. Therefore, ApoE is regulated at the levels of secretion, translation and transcription.

1986 Biochemistry of macrophages. Pitman, London (Ciba Foundation Symposium 118) p 155-171

Mononuclear phagocytes secrete into their extracellular milieu at least 50 different proteins and peptides (Table 1). These products are not secreted coordinately by all mononuclear phagocytes, but vary with the functional states of the cells. Because the secretion products of macrophages are particularly sensitive to alteration in response to inflammation and other changes in the macrophage environment (Takemura & Werb 1984a), the secretory profile of a macrophage is particularly useful in defining its phenotype (Werb 1983). Apolipoprotein E (ApoE) is used here as an example to demonstrate the multiple pathways for regulating macrophage secretion.

TABLE 1 Secreted proteins of macrophages

Enzymes

Plasminogen activator (urokinase)	Lysozyme
Metal-dependent elastase	Transglutaminase
Collagenase types I-, II-, III-, VIII-specific	Lipoprotein lipase
Collagenase type V-specific (gelatinase)	Arginase
Stromelysin	Acid hydrolases
Cytolytic proteinase	Phosphatases

Plasma proteins

α_2-Macroglobulin	Apolipoprotein E
Coagulation factors	Complement components 1,2,3,4,5,
Fibronectin	properdin, factors, B,D,H,I
Thrombospondin	

Factors

Interleukin 1	Fibroblast mitogen
Angiogenesis factor	Endothelial cell mitogen
Erythropoietin	Inhibitory factor for tumour
Colony-stimulating factors	cells
Interferon	Inhibitory factor for
	Listeria monocytogenes

Modified from Takemura & Werb (1984a).

Characterization of macrophage-derived ApoE

ApoE, the M_r 33 000 major secretory product of resident peritoneal macrophages in mice (Werb & Chin 1983a, Basu et al 1981, Basu et al 1982), constitutes 7–25% of the total protein secreted by these cells and is produced at a rate of 1–10 µg per 10^6 cells per 24 h (Werb & Chin 1983a, Takemura & Werb 1984b). ApoE, a constituent of plasma lipoproteins used in receptor-mediated clearance of lipids from the circulation (Brown & Goldstein 1983, Brown et al 1981) and in immune regulation (Avila et al 1982, Curtiss & Edgington 1981), is synthesized and secreted by resident and thioglycollate-elicited macrophages, but not by endotoxin-treated, immunologically activated or immature macrophages (Werb & Chin 1983a,b,c). ApoE secretion may be regulated both positively (Basu et al 1981, Takemura & Werb 1984b, Werb & Chin 1983c) and negatively (Takemura & Werb 1984b) by receptor-mediated endocytosis.

Onset of ApoE secretion during differentiation of bone marrow-derived mononuclear phagocytes

Human monocyte-derived macrophages do not secrete ApoE until they have been cultured for at least five days (Basu et al 1981), suggesting that there may be stage-specific expression of this protein. Bone marrow proliferation in culture in response to colony-stimulating factor-1 (CSF-1) makes the various stages in the differentiation of mononuclear phagocytes accessible, so the developmental regulation of genes expressed by macrophages can be defined. In the mouse the onset of secretion of ApoE, a major gene product of mature macrophages in culture, occurs relatively late during differentiation, with expression beginning in most cells at nine days (Fig. 1) (Werb & Chin 1983c). Because the onset of ApoE synthesis and secretion is paralleled by the appearance of ApoE mRNA, detected with a cDNA probe to rat ApoE (McLean et al 1983), this favours transcriptional control during differentiation. In bone marrow cultured without CSF-1, only the few cells with characteristics of mature macrophages express ApoE, and there is no clonal heterogeneity for ApoE. Thus, diversity of macrophages in tissues probably arises either from the modulation of expression of ApoE by the interaction of these cells with their extracellular milieu, or from the recruitment of less mature cells from the bone marrow, particularly under conditions of stress. ApoE regulation

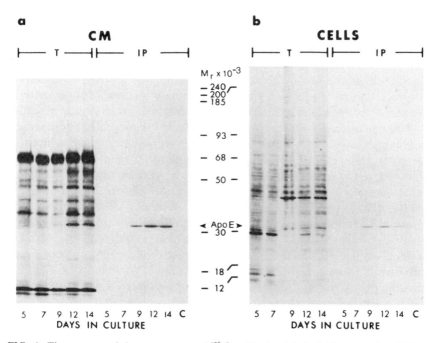

FIG. 1. Time course of the appearance of [^{35}S]methionine-labelled (a) secreted and (b) cell-associated ApoE in BMM cultured in the presence of CSF-1. CM, conditioned medium; T, total acid-precipitable proteins; IP, proteins immunoprecipitated with anti-ApoE IgG. Molecular weight markers and migration of ApoE are indicated. Reproduced from Werb & Chin (1983c), by permission of The Rockefeller University Press.

in bone marrow-derived macrophages (BMM) is different from that in tissue macrophages. Whether or not peritoneal macrophages secrete ApoE immediately after being explanted into culture, secretion is initiated by two to three days of culture in medium containing serum, and by seven days ApoE is secreted in large quantities (Werb & Chin 1983a). In contrast, BMM begin ApoE secretion only after nine days, and then at relatively modest rates (Werb & Chin 1983c). Withdrawal of the source of proliferation–differentiation factor (CSF-1) from BMM does not prompt premature initiation of ApoE secretion, and CSF-1 does not suppress secretion of ApoE by mature peritoneal macrophages.

Initiation of ApoE secretion is correlated with a decrease in plasminogen activator secretion in both peritoneal macrophages (Werb & Chin 1983a) and BMM. However, the relationship of elastase secretion to ApoE secretion is different in mature macrophages and BMM. BCG-activated macrophages, which do not secrete ApoE, usually have very low elastase secretion (Werb & Chin 1983a), whereas BMM secrete elastase at high rates until the onset of ApoE secretion (Werb & Chin 1983c).

Distinct phenotypes of macrophages in secretion of ApoE

Immediately after they are explanted in culture, the macrophages derived from mice that have received various inflammatory stimuli display patterns of secreted proteins that are markedly different from each other (Fig. 2a,b). Resident macrophages and macrophages elicited by thioglycollate both secrete ApoE at high rates, and $NaIO_4$-elicited macrophages secrete ApoE at intermediate rates. However, macrophages obtained from animals infected with bacille Calmette-Guérin (BCG) or treated with pyran copolymer or lipopolysaccharide endotoxin (LPS) have lower total rates of protein secretion and low rates of secreted ApoE (Fig. 2, Table 2). Within 24–48 h in culture, both the rate of secretion and the pattern of secreted proteins from inflammatory macrophages change markedly (Werb & Chin 1983a). Although the resident and thioglycollate-elicited macrophages continue to secrete ApoE in the same relative proportions, the total secretion of proteins is stimulated considerably, increasing up to fivefold by seven days in culture (Werb & Chin 1983a). By 24–72 h, activated macrophages from animals treated with BCG or LPS initiate ApoE secretion (Werb & Chin 1983a).

Suppression of ApoE secretion correlates with activation of macrophages, as measured by the development of the capacity to secrete H_2O_2 in response to triggering stimuli (Werb & Chin 1983a,b). All macrophages with little or no ApoE secretion have enhanced rates of H_2O_2 production (Table 2). When BCG- or pyran-elicited macrophages are cultured for 48–72 h, they regain

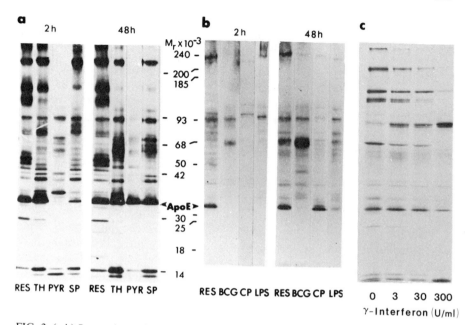

FIG. 2. (a,b) Secreted proteins of resident macrophages and macrophages elicited by inflammatory agents radiolabelled with [^{35}S]methionine for 2 h, at 2 or 48 h after being explanted into culture. Results are from two different experiments. RES, resident; TH, thioglycollate-elicited; PYR, pyran copolymer-elicited; SP, NaIO$_4$-elicited; LPS, endotoxin-elicited; CP, whole *Corynebacterium parvum*-elicited; BCG, BCG-elicited. Reproduced from Werb & Chin (1983a), by permission of The Rockefeller University Press. (c) Secreted proteins of resident macrophages treated with interferon-γ for 24 h. Molecular weight markers and migration of ApoE are indicated.

TABLE 2 Comparison of ApoE secretion and H$_2$O$_2$ production

Stimulus	ApoE secreted after 2 h in culture (% of total)	H$_2$O$_2$ secreted after 2 h in culture[a] (nmol min-1)/10^6 cells)
None	8.8	<0.04
Thioglycollate	13.4	0.11
LPS	0.2	0.58
Pyran copolymer	1.9	0.74
BCG	0.2	0.96

Modified from Werb & Chin (1983a).
[a] H$_2$O$_2$ secretion was triggered by 12-O-tetradecanoylphorbol-13-acetate.

the ability to secrete ApoE, whereas their rates of secretion of H_2O_2 decrease to those for resident and thioglycollate-elicited macrophages.

Macrophages also modulate their secretion of ApoE in culture. Resident and thioglycollate-elicited peritoneal macrophages and BMM all decrease their ApoE secretion in response to 10 μg LPS/ml after 20 h of treatment, although secretion of other proteins, such as fibronectin (the major protein of M_r 220 000), is affected minimally. As little as 0.01 ng LPS/ml produces a detectable decrease in ApoE secretion, with a decrease of >70% at 1 ng/ml (Werb & Chin 1983b).

The response of macrophages depends on their state of activation. Basu et al (1981, 1982) showed that resident and thioglycollate-elicited macrophages increase ApoE and total protein secretion in response to acetylated low density lipoproteins (LDL) and that this is due to the increased cholesterol content in macrophages. However, dextran sulphate, which is recognized by the same receptor as acetylated LDL but does not contain cholesterol, does not increase ApoE and total protein secretion (Takemura & Werb 1984b). BCG- activated macrophages, which secrete little ApoE, do not respond to acetylated LDL, and $NaIO_4$-elicited macrophages, which secrete an intermediate level of ApoE, respond to acetylated LDL by decreasing ApoE secretion (Takemura & Werb 1984b); however, these macrophages take up acetylated LDL to a similar extent, as judged by the accumulation of lipid droplets in the cells. These observations suggest that whether macrophages secrete ApoE after ingestion of cholesterol is regulated by their functional state. Ingestion of antibody-coated erythrocytes reduces ApoE secretion by resident and $NaIO_4$- elicited macrophages (Takemura & Werb 1984b).

Interferon-γ has been shown to be the lymphokine that activates macrophage oxidative metabolism (Nathan et al 1983). Interferon-γ alone (Fig. 2c), or synergistically with very low concentrations of LPS, also decreases ApoE secretion by resident and $NaIO_4$-elicited macrophages (Oropeza et al 1985). Because decreased secretion of ApoE is a phenotype associated with activation of macrophages, these findings suggest that many stimuli activate macrophages *in vitro*.

The intracellular secretory pathway for ApoE

Macrophages that secrete biochemically measurable amounts of ApoE have intracellular ApoE throughout the secretory pathway of the macrophage concentrated in two to three stacks of the Golgi complex, as determined by electron microscopic immunocytochemistry (Fig. 3). In the resident and thioglycollate-elicited populations, virtually every macrophage is positive for ApoE antigen, whereas the occasional fibroblasts are negative. In contrast,

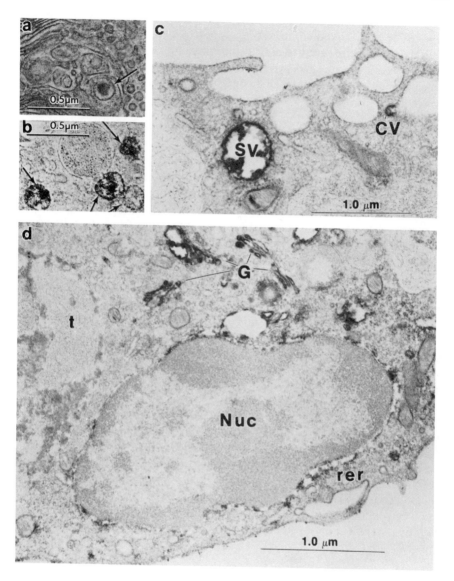

FIG. 3. Electron microscopic localization of ApoE in macrophages *in vivo*. (a) Golgi region of a tannic acid-stained resident macrophage. Note the granule containing a dense core (arrow) that (b) stains with immunoperoxidase anti-ApoE. (c,d) ApoE immunoperoxidase-stained thioglycollate-elicited macrophage. Note the ApoE in Golgi stacks (G), rough endoplasmic reticulum (rer), secretory vesicles (SV), and coated vesicles (CV). Nuc, nucleus; t, vacuoles containing thioglycollate broth component.

few of the macrophages elicited with pyran copolymer, *Corynebacterium parvum*, BCG or LPS show intracellular ApoE, whereas macrophages elicited with $NaIO_4$, which secrete ApoE at intermediate rates, have populations of macrophages negative and positive for ApoE. After 48 h in culture, when the cells elicited with $NaIO_4$, BCG and pyran copolymer have been induced to secrete ApoE, the proportion of cells containing ApoE increases to >90% (Werb & Chin 1983a).

There are two distinct pathways for secretory proteins in cells: a constitutive pathway through which proteins are secreted as fast as they are synthesized, and a regulated pathway in which proteins are stored in secretory granules and then secreted in response to specific stimuli (Gumbiner & Kelly 1982). Although some ApoE appears in the medium of macrophages within 30 min of pulse-labelling, the intracellular pool of ApoE corresponds to 2–4 h of synthesis (Werb & Chin 1983a), suggesting that some ApoE may be stored in the cells. Two sets of experiments have elucidated the nature of the intracellular ApoE pool.

When resident macrophages are plated on immobilized immune complexes, the cells spread within 20 min (Takemura & Werb 1983). When the spreading macrophages are stained with anti-ApoE, ApoE stain starts to disappear within the first 8 min and by 20 min most of the cells have lost their stain (Fig. 4). When the ultrastructural distribution of ApoE is examined in greater detail it becomes clear that small vacuoles containing a dense core and corresponding to storage granules are found in the Golgi region (Fig. 3), and these disappear after spreading. Therefore, the macrophage appears to secrete ApoE in response to ligation of Fc receptors.

A second source of intracellular ApoE could be through uptake of secreted ApoE. Macrophages have a variety of receptors for lipoproteins that could mediate this process (Brown & Goldstein 1983). When macrophages are cultured with radiolabelled ApoE in the form secreted by these cells, about 10% is taken up selectively in 1 h. Interestingly, in subsequent culture about half of the ApoE reappears in intact form in the medium, suggesting that active retroendocytosis operates for this protein in macrophages, as it does in other systems for lipoproteins (Greenspan & St Clair 1984).

ApoE synthesis is regulated both translationally and pretranslationally

The mechanism by which activating substances suppress ApoE synthesis in macrophages *in vivo* and in culture is not known. Although RNA synthesis is decreased in cytolytically activated macrophages (Varesio 1985), the activating stimuli affect overall protein synthesis relatively little when the decreased size of the activated cells is taken into consideration. Our findings indicate

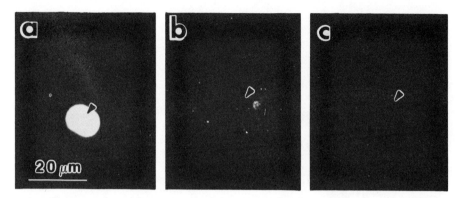

FIG. 4. Immunofluorescent localization of ApoE in resident macrophages plated for 60 min at 4 °C on immobilized BSA–anti-BSA immune complexes and then warmed to 37 °C for (a) 0, (b) 20 or (c) 120 min. Arrows indicate the position of the nucleus.

that *in vivo*-activated and non-activated macrophages contain similar amounts of total translatable mRNA for ApoE, but newly harvested pyran copolymer-activated macrophages contain no detectable translatable mRNA for ApoE, whereas ApoE mRNA is a major translatable species (~2%) in thioglycollate-elicited macrophages (Fig. 5).

When macrophages are placed in culture, ApoE mRNA increases. With pyran copolymer-elicited macrophages, ApoE mRNA appearance during culture reflects ApoE synthesis and secretion. These experiments favour transcriptional control of ApoE expression during transition of these activated immature macrophages to mature but unactivated macrophages.

The mechanism of suppression of ApoE synthesis and secretion in macrophages by LPS and interferon-γ in culture differs markedly. Although synthesis of ApoE is suppressed by these agents (Fig. 5), the amount of mRNA detected by a cDNA probe or by *in vitro* translation of protein-free mRNA is unchanged (Fig. 5). These data suggest that ApoE expression is controlled translationally in this system. The mechanism of the translational control has not been determined but may be due to competition for ribosomes, to alteration in specific tRNA, or to a specific protein complexing with ApoE mRNA.

Relation of ApoE secretion to cholesterol metabolism and immunoregulation by macrophages

Macrophage-derived ApoE may play a crucial role in controlling lipid metabolism and the immune response, because ApoE has functions both in the transport of lipoproteins (Brown et al 1981) and in immunoregulation (Curtiss

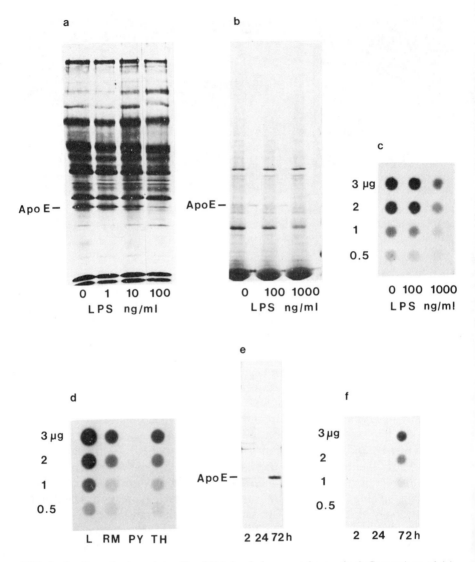

FIG. 5. ApoE synthesis and ApoE mRNA levels in macrophages. (a-c) Comparison of (a) [^{35}S]methionine-labelled secretion products, (b) *in vitro* translations and anti-ApoE immunoprecipitations of translation products of mRNA, and (c) dot blots of cytoplasmic RNA with ApoE cDNA from NaIO$_4$-elicited macrophages treated with 0–1000 ng/ml LPS for 24 h; (d) cytoplasmic dot blots of mRNA from liver (L) and from resident (RM), pyran copolymer (PY)-elicited, and thioglycollate (TH)-elicited macrophages cultured for 2 h with ApoE cDNA; (e) cytoplasmic mRNA dot blots and (f) immunoprecipitates with anti-ApoE of *in vitro* translation products of mRNA from pyran copolymer-elicited macrophages cultured for 2, 24 or 72 h. ApoE migration is indicated. Total RNA applied to the dot blots (μg) is indicated in (c), (d), and (f).

& Edgington 1981, Avila et al 1982). The immature BMM and immunologically activated macrophages (Werb & Chin 1983a,b,c) are the physiological
counterparts of the monensin-treated macrophages that have inhibited secretion of ApoE (Basu et al 1983). Because macrophages that do not secrete
ApoE still secrete cholesterol (Basu et al 1983), the 'reverse' cholesterol transport mechanisms involving ApoE may be disrupted in sites of inflammation
where immature or activated macrophages may be recruited. The decreased
local production of ApoE under these conditions may also serve to stimulate
the immune functions that are suppressed by ApoE. Macrophages have receptors that recognize ApoE-containing lipoproteins (Brown & Goldstein 1983)
and it is likely that macrophages take up their own newly secreted ApoE.
The receptors on macrophages for β-migrating very low density lipoproteins
(VLDL), chylomicron remnants and, in humans, LDL appear to recognize
both ApoE and apolipoprotein B, which is not produced by macrophages.

Thus, the LPS-induced decrease in ApoE synthesis may increase the concentration of circulating lipoproteins (Werb & Chin 1983b). The observed
increases in triglycerides and β-migrating VLDL after infection with Gram-
negative organisms and after injection of LPS may result from the reduced
clearance of these and other lipoproteins by receptors on other cells requiring
ApoE for recognition. In dyslipoproteinaemia, a disease in which ApoE has
an amino acid substitution that makes it poorly recognizable by the hepatic
lipoprotein receptors, there is a similar increase in circulating β-VLDL.
Because increased circulating lipids and lipoproteins may give rise to athero-
sclerotic-like syndromes and xanthomas in animals and humans, it is possible
that the LPS-induced modulation of macrophage ApoE secretion is a critical
initiating event in the pathogenesis of arterial wall disease. However, because
the genetic variability in susceptibility of macrophages to the suppressive
effects of LPS on ApoE secretion may alter the potentiation of host immune
responses or of increases in circulating lipoproteins, it is difficult to determine
the risks or benefits from modulation of ApoE secretion by macrophages
in vivo. Our ability to determine the ApoE secretory status of macrophages
by the immunocytochemical localization of intracellular ApoE makes it possible to carry out direct studies of ApoE secretion by macrophages in sites
of inflammation and lipid deposition.

Conclusions

There is a potential regulation of secretion of ApoE by four distinct regulatory
systems, one related to differentiation of mononuclear phagocytes (Werb &
Chin 1983c), a second to immunological regulation (Werb & Chin 1983a,b),

a third to cholesterol metabolism (Werb 1983, Basu et al 1982), and a fourth to receptor-mediated endocytosis (Takemura & Werb 1984b) (Table 3). ApoE secretion may also be regulated pharmacologically by inhibitors such as monensin (Basu et al 1983), colchicine and RNA synthesis inhibitors. ApoE secretion provides an interesting and accessible system for the investigation of a gene regulated developmentally and environmentally in macrophages at the levels of endocytosis, secretion, translation and transcription.

TABLE 3 Factors regulating macrophage ApoE secretion

Factor	Effect on secretion
Differentiation from monocyte to macrophage	Induction of ApoE mRNA
Non-specific inflammatory stimuli (thioglycollate, concanavalin A, NaIO$_4$)	Enhanced total protein and ApoE synthesis
Activating stimuli (BCG, *Trypanosoma cruzi*, pyran copolymer, *C. parvum*, interferon-γ, LPS)	Decreased total protein secretion, reduced synthesis of ApoE
Endocytosis of acetylated LDL	Increased total protein and ApoE synthesis
Endocytosis of zymosan, and immune complexes	Transient enhanced secretion of ApoE from regulated pathway; delayed decreased synthesis of ApoE
Monensin, colchicine	Inhibited secretion of ApoE

Acknowledgements

We thank Drs Thomas Innerarity and Steven Frisch for helpful discussions of many aspects of this work. This work was supported by the US Department of Energy (DE-AC03-76-SF01012) and the National Institutes of Health (AM10486 and AM31615).

REFERENCES

Avila EM, Holdsworth G, Sasaki N, Jackson RL, Harmony JAK 1982 Apoprotein E suppresses phytohemagglutinin-activated phospholipid turnover in peripheral blood mononuclear cells. J Biol Chem 257:5900-5909
Basu SK, Brown MS, Ho YK, Havel RJ, Goldstein JL 1981 Mouse macrophages synthesize and secrete a protein resembling apolipoprotein E. Proc Natl Acad Sci USA 78:7545-7549
Basu SK, Ho YK, Brown MS, Bilheimer DW, Anderson RGW, Goldstein JL 1982 Biochemical and genetic studies of the apoprotein E secreted by mouse macrophages and human monocytes. J Biol Chem 257:9788-9795

Basu SK, Goldstein JL, Brown MS 1983 Independent pathways for secretion of cholesterol and apolipoprotein E by macrophages. Science (Wash DC) 219:871-873

Brown MS, Goldstein JL 1983 Lipoprotein metabolism in the macrophage: implications for cholesterol deposition in atherosclerosis. Annu Rev Biochem 52:223-261

Brown MS, Kovanen PT, Goldstein JL 1981 Regulation of plasma cholesterol by lipoprotein receptors. Science (Wash DC) 212:628-635

Curtiss LK, Edgington TS 1981 Immunoregulatory plasma low density lipoprotein: the biologic activity and receptor-binding specificity is independent of neutral lipids. J Immunol 126:1008-1012

Greenspan P, St Clair RW 1984 Retroendocytosis of low density lipoprotein. Effect of lysosomal inhibitors on the release of undegraded ^{125}I-low density lipoprotein of altered composition from skin fibroblasts in culture. J Biol Chem 259:1703-1713

Gumbiner B, Kelly RB 1982 Two distinct intracellular pathways transport secretory and membrane glycoproteins to the surface of pituitary tumor cells. Cell 28:51-59

McLean JW, Fukazawa C, Taylor JM 1983 Rat apolipoprotein E mRNA. Cloning and sequencing of double-stranded cDNA. J Biol Chem 258:8993-9000

Nathan CF, Murray HW, Wiebe ME, Rubin BY 1983 Identification of interferon-γ as the lymphokine that activates human macrophage oxidative metabolism and antimicrobial activity. J Exp Med 158:670-689

Oropeza RL, Schreiber R, Werb Z 1985 Regulation of apolipoprotein E expression in macrophages by γ-interferon. In: Sorg C, Schimpl A (eds) Cellular and molecular biology of lymphokines. Academic Press, Orlando, FL, in press

Takemura R, Werb Z 1983 Redistribution of clathrin during spreading of mouse macrophages on immobilized immune complexes. J Cell Biol 97:174a

Takemura R, Werb Z 1984a Secretory products of macrophages and their physiological functions. Am J Physiol 246:C1-C9

Takemura R, Werb Z 1984b Modulation of apoprotein E secretion in response to receptor-mediated endocytosis in resident and inflammatory macrophages. J Exp Med 159:167-178

Varesio L 1985 Imbalanced accumulation of ribosomal RNA in macrophages activated in vivo or in vitro to a cytolytic stage. J Immunol 134:1262-1267

Werb Z 1983 How the macrophage regulates its extracellular environment. Am J Anat 166:237-256

Werb Z, Chin JR 1983a Apoprotein E is synthesized and secreted by resident and thioglycollate-elicited macrophages but not by pyran copolymer- or bacillus Calmette-Guerin-activated macrophages. J Exp Med 158:1272-1293

Werb Z, Chin JR 1983b Endotoxin suppresses expression of apoprotein E by mouse macrophages in vivo and in culture. A biochemical and genetic study. J Biol Chem 258:10642-10648

Werb Z, Chin JR 1983c Onset of apoprotein E secretion during differentiation of mouse bone marrow-derived mononuclear phagocytes. J Cell Biol 97:1113-1118

DISCUSSION

Cohn: Are there receptors for apolipoprotein E?

Werb: Several classes of receptors recognize ApoE. In humans a small number of LDL receptors recognize both ApoE and ApoB. There is a class of receptor that recognizes the very low density lipoprotein, β-VLDL, which requires ApoE for recognition. The acetylated VLDL receptor probably doesn't require ApoE. I don't think anyone has looked to see if there is an ApoE-specific receptor that doesn't involve a complex lipoprotein. In lymphocytes there may be such a receptor that will recognize delipidated ApoE.

Cohn: Secreted ApoE may complex with lipid and then be taken up with the complex.

Werb: Yes. The experiments I was talking about were done in serum-free medium so it would have to be lipid derived from the macrophage.

Cohn: Do these cells accumulate lipid under those conditions?

Werb: Not under serum-free conditions. If macrophages are loaded with cholesterol, say with acetylated LDL, the rate of secretion of ApoE goes up about fivefold while the message levels go up perhaps threefold, but the percentage of ApoE among the secreted proteins doesn't change. It is an overall trophic effect, in which most secreted proteins increase. So, even if there is no differential effect, there is still an enormous increase in ApoE secretion related to lipids. If the same experiment is done with macrophages elicited by periodate or BCG, protein synthesis and secretion go up but ApoE secretion does not. In fact the small amount of ApoE that is secreted in these elicited macrophages disappears.

Cole: Robert Sackstein and Harvey Colten (1984) have looked at C4 and factor B synthesis in elicited and resident murine macrophages, using thioglycollate-elicited macrophages; factor B synthesis increases and C4 decreases during the first 12 to 24 hours of culture.

Werb: We have done a few limited studies of C3. It is not regulated at all like factor B but we don't know any more details of the regulation.

Singer: In liver ApoE comes out as part of the VLDL particle. Is this true for macrophages as well?

Werb: Yes, mostly. Some 60% of the ApoB made in the liver gets taken back up by the liver. Re-uptake isn't unique to the macrophage but I don't know what it means.

Singer: So ApoB is not made in the macrophage?

Werb: No, absolutely not.

Singer: How does the ApoE come out?

Werb: Basu et al (1981) showed that it comes out as part of lenticular phospholipid protein complexes which may include a couple of other proteins but are certainly ApoE-rich. They did those experiments in the presence of serum. We tried to isolate the complexes by spinning them in the classic lipoprotein isolation schemes but we haven't found them. Other proteins may be needed to get that kind of structure. The dense core structures seen in the macrophages are similar to those seen in lipoprotein-rich vesicles in the Golgi region in the liver, although the macrophage vesicles are smaller.

Stanley: When you culture these cells in the presence of CSF-1 are they actively proliferating at day 12?

Werb: No, but in those kinds of experiments proliferation isn't related to whether the cells are making ApoE or not. It may affect how much they are making.

Stanley: All the CSF-1 in the medium may have been utilized by the cells.

Werb: We did those experiments using earlier stages of mononuclear phagocytes, removing the CSF-1, or adding it. We don't get premature onset. If we add CSF-1 at day 12 we see no difference. The rate of protein synthesis and secretion is affected by CSF-1 so if we add it back, all the protein synthesis goes up again and the cells start proliferating again.

Nicola: Macrophages elicited by these different compounds have different secretion properties. Is that because the inducing compounds alter the properties of a common set of macrophages or because they elicit different types of macrophages?

Werb: I don't know. We tried to get at that by using some of these proliferative stimuli under conditions where there is no influx. That is not so easy to do. One way we did it was to irradiate the mice, use an eliciting stimulus and show that no cells come in. The other way was to treat the mice with glucocorticoids and show that no new cells come in. In both cases if we use thioglycollate or pyran copolymer as the stimulus we get a macrophage which is at least 90% the phenotype it would have been *in vivo*. I don't know whether message levels and so on are reflected. When we change the phenotype but get no new influx of cells, these cells are never able to proliferate. But I wouldn't push that kind of experiment too far.

Gordon: When you look at bone marrow-cultured macrophages as colonies rather than as a mass culture you could say whether modulation of ApoE secretion is clonally heterogeneous.

Werb: Every colony turns on at more or less the same time for ApoE. At any given time there is heterogeneity within the colony, because the cells are approaching the critical stage of maturation at different times. It would be nice to do more of immunolocalization or *in situ* hybridization experiments on these populations. We can get populations that are heterogeneous in intracellular localization of ApoE from *in vivo* populations. In populations from some eliciting stimuli there are cells which are positive and cells which are negative. It would be interesting to re-evaluate these populations now we have shown that cells can be actively forced to secrete what they have inside, and that they don't regain appreciable intracellular ApoE for a few hours, so that immunolocalization at the light microscope level may not be the best way of determining population heterogeneity.

Gordon: Can you distinguish hepatocytes from Kupffer cells in the intact liver?

Werb: The Kupffer cells seem to have more ApoE inside than the hepatocytes, but I haven't done any detailed studies.

Cohn: What is known about the construction of the mature lipoprotein from ApoE? Can this occur extracellularly?

Werb: It can go on extracellularly. If you look at what the macrophages are secreting, the ApoE can be assembled onto human lipoproteins in a perfectly normal way. Those are hard experiments to do. Purified lipoproteins are always abnormal because of the way people purify them. Putting them through potassium bromide gradients is not normal for proteins.

Sorg: You said that IFN-γ has no effect on ApoE production whereas the recombinant IFN-γ does, and LPS does as well. Do other lymphokines have a regulatory influence?

Werb: That is very possible, especially as cells activated *in vivo* are really turned off in terms of their message. The only difference between the recombinant and the T-cell-derived IFN-γ is the effective amount of endotoxin. The amount of endotoxin needed to reconstitute the effect of rIFN-γ isn't enough to produce an effect of endotoxin itself. Many people have postulated that two signals are necessary. In our first few experiments with T-cell-derived IFN-γ we never saw an effect on the resident cells, then suddenly we did when we used rIFN-γ, and we wondered what we had done differently.

Dean: Do you get a burst of ApoE secretion even in response to ligands which themselves don't cause an influx of membranes? In other words, might it be due to a coupled membrane flux?

Werb: Endocytosis is not needed for that burst of secretion, nor is endocytosis by the Fc receptor needed for it to affect the down-regulation of synthesis that occurs later on, but we don't know the mechanism.

Gowans: Does the presence of ApoE in astrocytes mean that they play some special role in lipid metabolism in the central nervous system? Has anyone looked at astrocytes under conditions where lipid metabolism might normally be either very rapid, for example in the developing nervous system, or where membrane turnover would be very rapid in either demyelination or neuronal loss?

Werb: No one has looked yet. Fontana and his colleagues (1984) think that astrocytes are the major antigen-presenting cells in the brain in their models of demyelination. I thought that if that was true and if ApoE was involved in regulating the immune function, these cells should be making it. So I did the experiment and found they were making it. Neither endotoxin nor IFN-γ down-regulates synthesis by the astrocytes at all, so I don't know what is going on.

Gowans: I was thinking of a possible metabolic rather than immunological role.

Werb: There are lots of old reports of lipoproteins in cerebral spinal fluid, but I don't know of anything about lipid metabolism in the brain.

Gordon: Is the evidence based on *in situ* cytochemistry or have you isolated cells from the nervous system?

Werb: ApoE is there *in situ*. Not all astrocytes express it in culture. About 30% of the glial acidic fibrillary protein-positive cells show intracellular ApoE.

Gordon: What about other cells?

Werb: No other cells that we see in those populations are making ApoE.

Gordon: If your resident macrophages are negative, that doesn't fit in with other resident macrophages.

Werb: We were looking at cells that were quite far down in culture. They proliferate in the population. It looks as if the astrocytes are putting out a growth factor for the microglia.

REFERENCES

Basu SK, Brown MS, Ho YK, Havel RJ, Goldstein JL 1981 Mouse macrophages synthesize and secrete a protein resembling apolipoprotein E. Proc Natl Acad Sci USA 78:7545-7549
Fontana A, Fierz W, Wekerle H 1984 Astrocytes present myelin basic protein to encephalitogenic T-cell lines. Nature (Lond) 307:273-276
Sackstein R, Colten HR 1984 Molecular regulation of MHC class III (C4 and factor B) gene expression in mouse peritoneal macrophages. J Immunol 133:1618-1626

Respiratory response of phagocytes: terminal NADPH oxidase and the mechanisms of its activation

FILIPPO ROSSI, PAOLO BELLAVITE & EMANUELE PAPINI

Istituto di Patologia Generale, Università di Verona, Strada Le Grazie, 37134 Verona, Italy

Abstract. The chemical composition, properties and activation mechanism of the O_2^--forming NADPH oxidase of phagocytes were investigated, using partially purified enzyme preparations. Highly active NADPH oxidase was extracted as an aggregate of high M_r from the membranes of neutrophils and macrophages. The enzyme complex contained phospholipids and cytochrome b_{-245}, very little FAD and almost no quinones or NAD(P)H-dye reductase activity. The purification of a polypeptide with a relative molecular mass of 31 500 strictly paralleled the purification of NADPH oxidase, suggesting that this polypeptide is a component of the enzyme. This protein was identified as cytochrome b_{-245} after dissociation of the proteolipid complex and purification of the cytochrome moiety. The 31 500 M_r protein was phosphorylated in enzyme preparations from activated but not from resting cells. The results indicate that: (1) cytochrome b_{-245} is a major component of NADPH oxidase; (2) the involvement of NAD(P)H dye reductases in the O_2^--forming activity is questionable; (3) the cytochrome b_{-245}: FAD ratio in the enzyme complex is much higher than that indicated in crude preparations; (4) the M_r of pig neutrophil cytochrome b_{-245} is 31 500; (5) the activation of the O_2^--forming system involves a process of phosphorylation of cytochrome b_{-245}.

1986 Biochemistry of macrophages. Pitman, London (Ciba Foundation Symposium 118) p 172-195

The activation of respiration and production of toxic oxygen metabolites that is usually called the respiratory burst is one of the main functional responses by which phagocytes kill invading organisms and tumour cells. This response is induced by phagocytosis and by the interaction of the phagocytes with a number of soluble factors such as complement components, lectins, chemotactic peptides, phorbol esters, calcium ionophores, leukotrienes and platelet-activating factors (Babior 1978, Rossi et al 1982).

It is now generally agreed that the respiratory burst is due to the activation of an NADPH oxidase which we described about 20 years ago (Rossi & Zatti 1964). The active enzyme is located in the plasma membrane and it catalyses the one-electron reduction of oxygen to superoxide (O_2^-), using the reducing equivalents provided by NADPH, which in turn is formed by the dehydrogenases of the hexose monophosphate shunt for glucose oxidation. The reaction stoichiometry is the following: $NADPH + H^+ + 2O_2 \rightarrow NADP^+ + 2H^+ + 2O_2^-$. Two molecules of superoxide can then dismutate to hydrogen peroxide (H_2O_2) according to the reaction $2O_2^- + 2H^+ \rightarrow H_2O_2 + O_2$, which occurs either spontaneously or catalysed by the enzyme superoxide dismutase (EC 1.15.1.1.). Reaction of H_2O_2 with O_2^- can generate the very reactive hydroxyl radical ($OH^{\cdot}$), probably through an Fe^{2+}-catalysed Haber–Weiss reaction: $H_2O_2 + O_2^- \rightarrow OH^{\cdot} + OH^- + O_2$. This paper deals with recent investigations on the nature of the NADPH oxidase in granulocytes and macrophages and with findings related to its activation.

Nature of oxidase: the candidate components

The information now available seems to indicate that the oxidation of NADPH involves various components that form an electron transport chain in the plasma membrane. The candidate components are a flavoprotein, a b-type cytochrome, and perhaps other cofactors, including quinones. The evidence that these components are involved is indirect because so far attempts to purify NADPH oxidase have been unsuccessful.

Involvement of a flavoprotein

The evidence that a flavoprotein (with FAD as prosthetic group) forms part of the NADPH oxidase system is as follows: (1) O_2^--forming activity by membranes solubilized with Triton X-100 is enhanced by the addition of FAD to the assay system (Gabig & Babior 1979); (2) the FAD analogue 5-carbadeaza-FAD inhibits the O_2^--forming activity of the solubilized enzyme (Light et al 1981); (3) leucocytes of patients affected by chronic granulomatous disease (CGD), a condition in which there is no NADPH oxidase activity, are deficient in FAD (Cross et al 1982a, Gabig 1983); (4) membrane extracts prepared from neutrophils contain flavoproteins which are reduced by NADPH in anaerobiosis (Cross et al 1984, Gabig & Lefker 1984).

It has been suggested that the flavoprotein moiety of this oxidase is an NAD(P)H-dye reductase, that is an NAD(P)H dehydrogenase which can give electrons to an artificial electron acceptor (Green et al 1983, Wakeyama et al 1983, Sakane et al 1984, Gabig & Lefker 1984).

Involvement of cytochrome b₋₂₄₅

The involvement of a cytochrome b first discovered about 20 years ago by Hattori (1961) and Shinagawa et al (1966) has been investigated by Segal's and Jones's groups (Segal 1983). The evidence suggesting that this haemoprotein, which has an unusually low midpoint potential ($E_0 = -245\,mV$), plays a part in the NADPH oxidase activity of phagocytes is as follows: (1) patients with the X-linked form of CGD have no cytochrome b_{-245} (Segal 1983); (2) this cytochrome behaves as a typical component of a terminal oxidase, since it is reduced when the cells are activated in anaerobic conditions, is rapidly reoxidized by oxygen, and binds carbon monoxide, although with low affinity (Shinagawa et al 1966, Cross et al 1982b, Bellavite et al 1983a); (3) during cell differentiation, the cytochrome appears in parallel with the development of the ability to perform the respiratory burst (Roberts et al 1982); (4) cytochrome b_{-245} can reconstitute the oxidase activity that is lacking in cells from patients with CGD. It has been shown that the hybridization of monocytes from a cytochrome b_{-245}-negative X-linked male CGD patient with monocytes from a cytochrome b_{-245}-positive male CGD patient of unknown genetic background restores the O_2^--forming activity (Hamers et al 1984).

In spite of the above positive evidence, there are experimental findings that raise doubts about the role of cytochrome b_{-245} in NADPH oxidase activity. According to Babior (1983), the large discrepancy observed between the rate of cytochrome b_{-245} reduction needed to account for O_2^- production by stimulated neutrophils and the rate of cytochrome b_{-245} reduction by NADPH forces the conclusion that this haemoprotein cannot be an obligatory electron carrier in the O_2^--forming reactions of leucocytes. However, the rate of O_2^- production by stimulated neutrophils has been measured aerobically, while NADPH-dependent cytochrome b_{-245} reduction has been measured anaerobically. It has been suggested that the presence of oxygen might affect the affinity of cytochrome b_{-245} for its electron donor (Tauber et al 1983) or that the removal of oxygen grossly distorts the bioenergetic circumstances under which cytochrome b_{-245} must function (Segal 1983). It is worth pointing out that the oxygen requirement for the rapid reduction of cytochrome b_{-245} by NADPH in solubilized enzyme preparations has been demonstrated recently by Cross et al (1985).

An alternative explanation can be advanced for the necessity of oxygen for the reduction of cytochrome b_{-245}. Assuming that cytochrome b_{-245} is reduced by a flavin semiquinone, in the absence of oxygen this semiquinone could not be formed from the one-electron reduction of O_2 by the fully reduced flavin. A branched NADPH oxidase system which forms O_2^- through both the flavin + O_2 and the flavin + cytochrome b_{-245} + O_2 pathways, as suggested by Light et al (1981) and by Morel & Vignais (1984), would be compatible with the fact that cytochrome b_{-245} in anaerobiosis is slow.

Involvement of quinones

A role of quinones, namely of ubiquinone-50, has been proposed by Cunningham et al (1982) and by Crawford & Schneider (1982, 1983). The main evidence is the following: (1) a substantial content of ubiquinone-50 in various neutrophil fractions, including plasma membranes and phagolysosomes, has been found (Crawford & Schneider 1983); (2) ubiquinone-5 and duroquinone stimulate O_2 consumption by intact resting neutrophils and, in the presence of NADPH and NADH, by disrupted cells (Crawford & Schneider 1982). This stimulated O_2 consumption by intact neutrophils is inhibited by the ubiquinone analogues, quercetin and juglone, which also inhibit the respiratory burst induced by latex particles and the succinoxidase of rat liver mitochondria; these inhibitors act between ubiquinone and cytochrome b of the mitochondrial respiratory chain (Crawford & Schneider 1982); (3) NAD(P)H-dye reductase activities solubilized from guinea-pig polymorphonuclear leucocytes are enhanced by menadione and the enhancement is accompanied by the formation of superoxide anion (Sakane et al 1983, 1984). The enhancing effect of mendione has been explained by a mechanism in which menadione mediates the electron transfer from NAD(P)H to cytochrome c or molecular oxygen by undergoing cyclic oxidation–reduction between the quinone and semiquinone forms (Sakane et al 1983).

In our opinion these effects of quinones on neutrophil metabolism, shown about 20 years ago by our group (Rossi & Zatti 1964) and more recently by Gallin et al (1982), are independent of NADPH oxidase, and the mechanism of inhibition of the quinone analogues is not specific. Against the role of quinone is the demonstration that its very low content in neutrophils is exclusively associated with the mitochondrion (Cross et al 1983), a subcellular organelle that has nothing to do with the respiratory burst. Recently Lutter et al (1984) found no ubiquinone-50 in human neutrophils.

The electron-transport chain

From the findings so far presented, the more likely hypothesis is that NADPH oxidase is formed by a flavoprotein enzyme, which contains the substrate binding site and catalyses the transfer of electrons from NADPH to the flavin, and by cytochrome b_{-245}, which transfers the electrons from the reduced flavin

to oxygen (see Fig. 1). The flavin:cytochrome b_{-245} ratio measured in leucocyte membranes or in crude extracts varies from $2:1$ (Cross et al 1982a),
to $1:1$ (Gabig 1983) or $1:2$ (Borregaard & Tauber 1984, Lutter et al 1984).

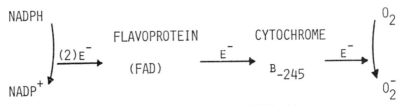

FIG. 1. Simplified hypothetical scheme for O_2^--forming NADPH oxidase.

Assuming that this is the composition of NADPH oxidase, two main problems remain to be investigated: the mechanism of the transformation of
this simple electron transport chain from the inactive to the active state, and
the mechanisms of electron transport between the various components. For
the second problem, the main points to be investigated are (a) the presence
of metal atoms (e.g. Fe, Mo, Cu) or of other groups as part of the structure
of the flavoprotein or of cytochrome b_{-245}; (b) the type of oscillation of flavin
between the oxidized and the reduced forms (e.g. $FAD \rightleftharpoons FADH_2$, $FAD \rightarrow$
$FADH_2 \rightarrow FADH \rightarrow FAD$, $FAD \rightleftharpoons FADH$, $FADH \rightleftharpoons FADH_2$), which is relevant for the mechanisms of NADPH oxidation and oxygen reduction; (c)
the actual FAD:cytochrome b_{-245} ratio; (d) the mechanism of oxidation of
the reduced flavin (e.g. by cytochrome b_{-245} and oxygen, or by cytochrome
b_{-245} only); (e) the requirement of phospholipids, suggested by Gabig &
Babior (1979).

Partial purification of NADPH oxidase

In order to clarify the nature of the oxidase, the mechanism of its activation
and the pathway of O_2^- formation, some years ago we began a series of attempts
to extract and purify the enzyme. In common with other groups we experienced
many difficulties because the enzyme has proved to be extremely unstable.
Nonetheless, in a first group of experiments on guinea-pig neutrophils we
obtained some relevant findings (Bellavite et al 1983a,b, 1984a,b, Serra et
al 1984).

Experiments on guinea-pig neutrophils

Subcellular particles were solubilized from phorbol myristate acetate (PMA)-
activated guinea-pig neutrophils with deoxycholate in the presence of glycerol

as a stabilizing agent, followed by chromatography through Ultragel AcA22 equilibrated with buffer containing glycerol but not detergents. We obtained an extract containing aggregates of high M_r formed by several proteins, including cytochrome b_{-245} and phospholipids, and endowed with high NADPH-dependent O_2^--forming activity. The extract was then further purified by centrifuging it on a glycerol density gradient and partially disaggregating it with 0.4 M-NaCl. The electrophoretic pattern of this purified preparation showed the presence of a major band of 32 000 M_r and of other protein bands. By comparing the electrophoretic analyses of preparations at different purification steps we found that only the protein of M_r 32 000 progressively increased as purification proceeded. Since the specific activities of NADPH oxidase and cytochrome b_{-245} also increased in the same preparations, we suggested that this protein belonged to NADPH oxidase and that it could be cytochrome b_{-245}.

Biochemical studies of these extracts from guinea-pig neutrophils allowed the oxidase to be characterized better and we were able to distinguish NAD(P)H-cytochrome c and NAD(P)H-dichlorophenol indophenol reductases (here called dye-reductases) from NADPH-dependent O_2^--forming activity. The main properties of leucocyte NADPH oxidase are shown in Table 1. It is worth noting that the properties of neutrophil and macrophage NADPH oxidase are similar, the only difference being that the kinetic parameters (K_m for NADPH) of macrophage oxidase can be modulated by the different activation states of these cells (Berton et al 1985).

The evidence in favour of the distinction between NADPH oxidase-forming O_2^- and dye reductase activities is as follows (Bellavite et al 1984a): (1) the dye reductase activities are similar in preparations from resting and activated

---

TABLE 1 Properties of leucocyte NADPH oxidase

(1) Catalyses the reaction
  $$NADPH + H^+ + 2O_2 \rightarrow NADP^+ + 2O_2^- + 2H^+$$

(2) Works on the plasma membrane, releasing O_2^- (and perhaps H^+) at the external side of the membrane and in the phagosome

(3) Non-active in resting cells, activated by phagocytosis and by some soluble agents. During phagocytosis the enzyme in contact with the particle is selectively activated

(4) The activated state of the enzyme in intact cells is reversible upon removal of the stimulatory agent

(5) Optimum pH: 7.0–7.5

(6) K_m for NADPH: 0.03–0.05 mM, K_m for NADH: 0.5–1.0 mM; the K_m for NADPH can change in various types of macrophages

(7) Inhibited by parachloromercuribenzoate, quinacrine, batophenanthroline sulphonate, trifluoperazine, nordihydroguaiaretic acid, cibacron blue, strong detergents, high ionic strengths, 5-carba-deaza FAD

(8) Optimum activity of solubilized enzyme requires phospholipids

cells; (2) the dye reductase activities use NADH as the preferred substrate whereas the O_2^--forming enzyme uses NADPH; (3) the dye reductase activities have a K_m for NADPH ($5\,\mu M$) that is different from the K_m for NADPH of the O_2^--forming enzyme (30–$50\,\mu M$); (4) unlike the dye reductases, the 'true' NADPH oxidase does not give electrons to artificial electron acceptors in either aerobiosis or anaerobiosis. The finding that molecular oxygen is the preferred and perhaps the obligatory acceptor suggested two considerations. The first is that, since practically all flavin dehydrogenases can be oxidized by artificial electron acceptors, the behaviour of our enzyme indicates that the role of flavin must be reinvestigated. The second is that NADPH oxidase is 'protected' from the withdrawal of electrons which are completely utilized for the formation of O_2^- and H_2O_2, the actual weapons of the bactericidal and tumoricidal oxygen-dependent system of phagocytes.

Experiments with pig neutrophils and guinea-pig macrophages

In subsequent experiments using pig neutrophils we obtained better results with purified membranes as the starting material instead of nuclei-free homogenates, with a different mixture of detergents (deoxycholate plus Lubrol PX instead of deoxycholate), and with different chromatographic procedures (Ultragel AcA34 chromatography eluted in the presence of detergents) (Bellavite et al 1984b, 1985). First, we confirmed with these procedures that a protein of M_r 31 500 progressively copurified with the NADPH oxidase activity and with cytochrome b. This protein band was present in enzyme preparations from both PMA-activated and resting neutrophils. Secondly, after gel filtration chromatography we obtained two distinct peaks (Fig. 2). The first protein peak contained practically all the NADPH oxidase activity and cytochrome b. This peak corresponded to the void volume of the column, indicating that it contained aggregate material of $M_r > 350\,000$. This material also contained phospholipids (0.27–$0.3\,mg/mg$ protein) and was totally devoid of quinones. The second protein peak was almost devoid of cytochrome b and NADPH oxidase but contained most of the FAD and NAD(P)H-dye reductase activity. Similar results have been also obtained with macrophages from guinea-pig peritoneal exudates (G. Berton et al, unpublished work 1985).

The above results clarify the following points: (1) quinones are not components of the NADPH oxidase system; (2) NAD(P)H dye reductases are different from NADPH oxidase and therefore the hypothesis that the first component of the proposed electron transport chain is an NAD(P)H dye reductase is untenable; (3) cytochrome b_{-245} is probably a true component of the NADPH oxidase system; (4) most of the flavin contained in the membrane extract does not belong to NADPH oxidase. This last finding requires

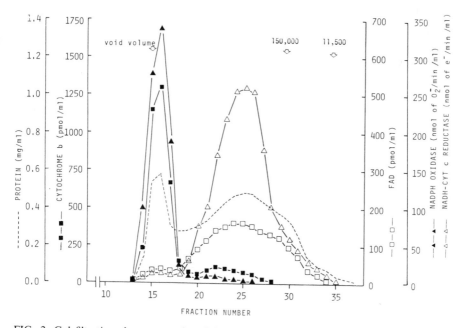

FIG. 2. Gel filtration chromatography of the solubilized extract from plasma membranes of phorbol myristate acetate (PMA)-activated pig neutrophils. Membránes were solubilized with 0.4% Lubrol PX and 0.4% deoxycholate in the presence of 20% glycerol and centrifuged at 100 000 g for 60 min; 4 ml of the supernatant (3.3 mg protein/ml; 2.31 nmol cytochrome b_{-245}/ml; 1.03 nmol FAD/ml; NADPH oxidase: 601 nmol O_2^- min^{-1} ml^{-1}; NADH cytochrome c reductase: 475 nmol cytochrome c reduced min^{-1} ml^{-1}) was chromatographed through an Ultragel AcA 34 column (LKB Produkter, Bromma, Sweden) (1.6 × 30 cm) equilibrated with phosphate buffer containing 20% glycerol, 0.15% sodium deoxycholate and 0.15% Lubrol PX. Fractions of 1.5 ml were collected at a flow rate of 18 ml/h. Assays were carried out as described by Bellavite et al (1984b). The void volume was determined with blue dextran, standards were alcohol dehydrogenase (M_r 150 000) and cytochrome c (M_r 11 500).

a revision of the cytochrome b_{-245}:FAD ratio in true NADPH oxidase, which in non-purified preparations resulted in a range between 2:1 and 1:2 (Cross et al 1982a, Gabig 1983, Borregaard & Tauber 1984, Lutter et al 1984).

Analysis of the NADPH oxidase, cytochrome b and flavin content during the various steps of purification (Table 2) points to some important observations. First, the findings confirm the previous results obtained with guinea-pig neutrophils, i.e. that cytochrome b copurifies with NADPH oxidase, since the cytochrome b_{-245}:NADPH oxidase ratio remains similar in all the preparations. Secondly, the ratio between NADPH oxidase activity and flavin content, which remains similar in the postnuclear supernatant, membranes and

TABLE 2 NADPH oxidase activity, cytochrome b_{-245} and FAD content of preparations at different stages of purification

	Postnuclear supernatant	Washed membranes	Solubilized extract	First protein peak (AcA34)
NADPH oxidase (nmol O_2^- min^{-1} mg protein^{-1})	30.8	210	182	572
Cytochrome b_{-245} (pmol/mg protein)	70.3	617.2	702	1915
Flavin (FAD) (pmol/mg protein)	35.6	290	312.5	50
NADPH oxidase: cytochrome b ratio	0.4	0.3	0.3	0.3
NADPH oxidase: FAD ratio	0.9	0.7	0.6	11.4
Cytochrome b: FAD ratio	2.0	2.1	2.2	38.3

The postnuclear supernatant from PMA-activated pig neutrophils was centrifuged on sucrose gradient and the plasma membrane fraction was collected. After being washed with 0.3 M-NaCl, membranes were treated with 0.4% Lubrol PX and 0.4% deoxycholate and centrifuged at 100 000 g for 1 h. The supernatant (solubilized extract) was chromatographed through an Ultragel AcA34 column (see Fig. 2) and the fractions were assayed as described by Bellavite et al (1984b)

first crude extract, enormously increases in the first peak of AcA34 chromatography, due either to an increase in the specific activity of the enzyme or (mostly) to a decrease in the flavin content. The decrease in the flavin content in the first peak is not due to removal of flavin from the flavoprotein of the enzyme complex because if this happened the enzymic activity would also decrease. Finally, the cytochrome b_{-245}:FAD ratio, which is about 2:1 in the postnuclear supernatant, progressively increases and becomes about 40:1 in the first peak from gel filtration chromatography. A similar ratio has been found in preparations from resting cells. All these findings strongly suggest that the content of flavin in NADPH oxidase is much lower than that previously reported in studies with crude enzyme preparations. On this basis, kinetic analysis of flavoprotein reduction and oxidation in crude membrane extracts (Gabig & Lefker 1984, Cross et al 1984) also becomes questionable, since other flavoproteins not related to the oxidase system could affect it.

As regards the small amount of flavin associated with cytochrome b_{-245} and NADPH oxidase activity, two explanations can be advanced. The first is that NADPH oxidase is an electron-transport system composed of one flavoprotein and many cytochrome b_{-245} molecules. The manner of the functional association of the flavoprotein with many cytochromes remains to be investigated. A non-equimolecular concentration of flavoprotein and cytochrome P-450 has been found in liver microsomes (Peterson et al 1976). The second explanation is that the small amount of flavin found in the first protein peak of gel filtration represents a contaminant belonging to the NAD(P)H-dye oxidoreductases or to other enzymes. If this is so, NADPH oxidase does not contain a flavoprotein. The finding that NADPH oxidase does not give electrons to artificial acceptors is compatible with either the latter explanation or with the molecular structural arrangement required by the high cytochrome b_{-245}: flavoprotein ratio.

Further purification of components of the NADPH oxidase system

Attempts to purify further the components of the NADPH oxidase system have been made by dissociating the proteolipid complex by procedures such as high concentrations of Triton X-100, deoxycholate or Lubrol PX, or extensive sonication, treatment with 1 M-NaCl and/or 1 M-KCl, or treatment with 8 M-urea. Unfortunately, all these procedures caused a complete loss of activity. In spite of this, we decided to identify some components of the oxidase.

Partially purified enzyme complexes from the first peak of AcA34 were loaded on a glycerol gradient (22–32%) and centrifuged overnight at 131 000 g. The protein peak resulting from the gradient fractionation and containing NADPH oxidase and cytochrome b_{-245} was concentrated, treated with 1% Triton X-100, 0.5% deoxycholate and 1 M-KC1, and centrifuged for 3 h at 100 000 × g. The resulting supernatant contained most of cytochrome b_{-245}, indicating that the complex had been dissociated. In fact, when the supernatant was re-chromatographed through an Ultragel AcA34 column eluted in the presence of 1% Triton X-100, 0.5% deoxycholate and 1 M-KCl, the cytochrome b_{-245} appeared in a peak in the included volume, with an apparent M_r of 170 000–230 000 (Fig. 3). During the course of this experiment, NADPH oxidase activity was progressively lost. On the other hand, cytochrome b_{-245} was more resistant to the experimental manipulations, and its overall purification compared to the starting material (postnuclear supernatant) was 147-fold. The cytochrome b_{-245} content of the most purified preparation was 10.3 nmol/mg protein.

Analytical SDS-polyacrylamide gel electrophoresis of the 147-fold purified cytochrome b_{-245} showed only one major band of 31 500 M_r with minimal contaminants (Fig. 4). This is a direct demonstration that this protein band, previously indicated as a component of the oxidase, corresponds to cytochrome b_{-245} or to a subunit of the cytochrome dissociated by SDS. The oxidized and reduced spectra of purified cytochrome b_{-245} from pig neutrophils are shown in Fig. 5. Table 3 summarizes the main properties of phagocyte cytochrome b_{-245}, as found in our laboratory and elsewhere. Harper et al

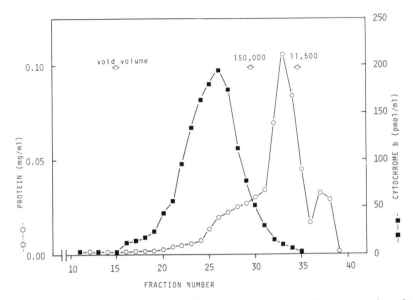

FIG. 3. Isolation of cytochrome b_{-245} by gel filtration chromatography. Enzyme complexes from AcA34 chromatography and subsequent glycerol gradient (see text) were dissociated with 1% Triton X-100, 0.5% deoxycholate and 1M-KCl. The extract (2 ml; 0.44 mg protein/ml; 1.035 nmol cytochrome b_{-245}/ml) was chromatographed through the same Ultragel AcA column as was used in the experiments illustrated in Fig. 2, but eluted with phosphate buffer containing 1% Triton X-100, 0.5% deoxycholate and 1 M-KCl. Fractions of 1.5 ml were collected.

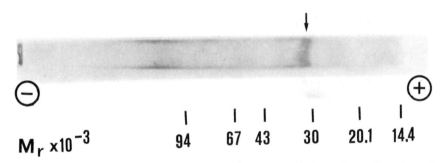

FIG. 4. SDS-polyacrylamide gel electrophoresis of 147-fold purified cytochrome b_{-245} from pig neutrophils. Cytochrome b_{-245} isolated by gel filtration chromatography (see Fig. 3) was rechromatographed through Ultragel AcA34 eluted in the absence of detergents in order to remove the excess of Triton X-100, deoxycholate and KCl. The eluted cytochrome was pelleted by centrifugation for 16 h at 131 000 g and then treated with 2% SDS and 2% 2-mercaptoethanol for 1 h at 50 °C in the presence of 2 mM phenylmethanesulphonyl fluoride (PMSF). Electrophoresis was performed with a slab gel consisting of a linear polyacrylamide gradient (4–20%), in 40 mM-Tris/HCl buffer, pH 8.0, containing 1% SDS, 1 mM-EDTA and 20 mM-sodium acetate; 7.3 µg protein were loaded on the gel. Arrow: 31 500 M_r.

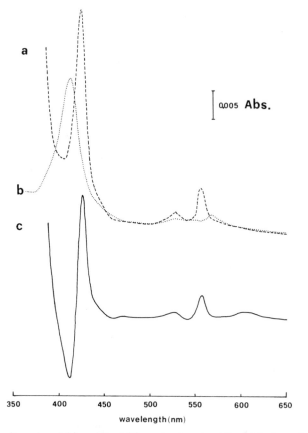

FIG. 5. Dithionite reduced (a), oxidized (b), and reduced–oxidized (c) absorption spectra of neutrophil cytochrome b_{-245}. Protein concentration, 0.017 mg/ml.

TABLE 3 Properties of leucocyte cytochrome b_{-245}

(1) Absorption peaks: oxidized 412 nm; reduced–oxidized 559 nm, 528 nm, 427 nm
(2) Difference absorption coefficient at 559–540 nm: 21.6 mM^{-1} cm^{-1}
(3) Low oxidation–reduction midpoint potential ($E_{m\,7.0}$): −245 mV
(4) Reduced by NADPH, slowly in anaerobiosis and fast in aerobiosis
(5) Reduced in intact phagocytes activated under anaerobic conditions
(6) Oxidized by oxygen with a $t^{\frac{1}{2}}$ of 4.7 ms
(7) Binds CO, although with lower affinity than O$_2$
(8) Present in neutrophils, eosinophils, monocytes, macrophages; not present in lymphocytes
(9) Copurifies with NADPH oxidase activity
(10) Relative molecular mass: 31 500 (Rossi's group); 68 000–78 000 (Segal's group); 17 000–14 000–11 000 (Pember's group)

(1984) have recently reported an M_r of 68 000–78 000 for human neutrophil cytochrome b_{-245}, whereas Pember et al (1984) indicated that three proteins of 14 000, 12 000 and 11 000 M_r were components of cytochrome purified from bovine neutrophils. The reason(s) for these discrepancies remain(s) to be investigated.

Hypotheses of the structure of NADPH oxidase

We are now working on two main hypotheses concerning the chemical composition of NADPH oxidase.

Hypothesis 1

NADPH oxidase is a two-component system made by a flavoprotein dehydrogenase (different from the NAD(P)H-dye reductase) and by many cytochrome b_{-245} molecules. The structural and functional relationship between flavoprotein and the cytochromes remains to be clarified. This clarification must take into account (a) that the ratio cytochrome b_{-245} : FAD is similar in extracts from resting and activated cells, and (b) the lack of quinones that could carry electrons between the components in the lipid milieu of the membrane.

Hypothesis 2

NADPH oxidase is made by only one molecular species, the haemoprotein with a cytochrome b-like spectrum, not containing flavin. This molecule should have a substrate binding site facing the cytoplasmic side and a haem group for the reduction of oxygen on the other side. The following points have yet to be clarified: (a) the enhancing effect of FAD on enzymic activity, and (b) how a two-electron donor (NADPH) reduces a one-electron acceptor (the haem group). This latter point could be explained if the haemoprotein contains other electron carriers such as metal atoms (e.g. Fe, Mo, Cu). The presence of non-haem iron is suggested by our finding that batophenanthroline sulphonate inhibits oxidase activity (Bellavite et al 1983b). Furthermore, the ESR spectra presented by Shinagawa et al (1966) could be indicative of some non-haem metal protein, and Pember et al (1984) mentioned the existence of an EPR spectrum atypical of haem proteins in purified cytochrome b_{-245}, suggesting the existence of another paramagnetic centre.

The above hypotheses do not consider the importance of SH-groups (Bellavite et al 1983a) and of phospholipids (Gabig & Babior 1979) for O_2^--generating activity. These properties of the oxidase are compatible with both models.

Phosphorylation of the 31 500 M_r protein

A fundamental question that remains open is the mechanism by which the NADPH oxidase system is turned on in activated cells. In the last few years the hypothesis has been advanced that the transduction mechanism responsible for many leucocyte responses to external stimuli involves the activation of a calcium- and phospholipid-dependent protein kinase (protein kinase C) and of protein phosphorylation (Sha'afi et al 1983, McPhail et al 1984). Protein kinase C may be activated either directly, for example as it is by PMA (Castagna et al 1982), or indirectly, via formation of diacylglycerol by breakdown of phosphoinositides (Grzeskowiak et al 1985). We have therefore investigated the possibility that phagocyte activation is associated with phosphorylation of some identified component of the NADPH oxidase system.

Granulocytes labelled with $^{32}P_i$ were divided in two aliquots, one of which was stimulated with PMA. The activated and resting cells were processed until partial purification of NADPH oxidase and cytochrome b_{-245} was achieved by gel filtration chromatography. Electrophoresis of these preparations, followed by autoradiography, showed that the 31 500-M_r protein was markedly phosphorylated in the enzyme obtained from activated but not from resting cells (Fig. 6). Other minor protein bands of about 26 500 and 41 000 M_r also appeared to be phosphorylated in preparations from activated cells.

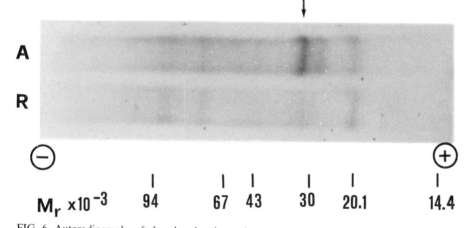

FIG. 6. Autoradiography of phosphorylated proteins present in resting (R) and PMA-activated (A) partially purified NADPH oxidase. Neutrophils were labelled with $^{32}P_i$ and divided in two parts, one of which was treated with PMA. NADPH oxidase was extracted from membranes and partially purified through Ultragel AcA34 chromatography (see Fig. 1). Fractions of the first protein peak were pooled, concentrated and subjected to SDS electrophoresis on a linear polyacrylamide gradient (4–20%) slab gel. The gel was desiccated and exposed to Kodak X OMAT R film for two days at 70 °C; 40 μg protein from each sample was subjected to electrophoresis. The arrow indicates the position of the 31 500 M_r band.

However, these proteins probably do not belong to the oxidase system because they are not enriched during the various steps of NADPH oxidase purification.

The finding that the 31 500 M_r protein which has been identified as cytochrome b_{-245} becomes phosphorylated in the extract from PMA-activated neutrophils is relevant. In fact this could be the evidence that the activation of protein kinase C is involved in the transduction mechanism for cell stimulation. If this is the case, it represents the identification of the target of protein kinase, phosphorylation of which is essential to activation of the respiratory burst. However, phosphorylation of cytochrome b by a kinase other than protein kinase C cannot be ruled out.

The mechanism by which phosphorylation of the 31 500 M_r protein changes the state of the NADPH oxidase system remains to be explained. Phosphorylation may induce a conformational modification of the haemoprotein, facilitating its functional relation with other components of the oxidase, the transfer of electrons, or—if the haemoprotein is the oxidase—the interaction with substrate NADPH. Alternatively, phosphorylation may remove or change the interaction with a regulatory factor.

It remains to be established whether phosphorylation is the only mechanism for activation of NADPH oxidase or whether other processes are involved in different conditions of stimulation. The problem will be clarified by experiments on the phosphorylation of the 31 500 M_r protein in cells stimulated by chemotactic peptides or other stimulants and on the activation of NADPH oxidase in cell-free systems.

Acknowledgements

This work was supported by grants from Ministero Pubblica Istruzione (Fondi 40%) and from the National Research Council (grant no. 84.00789.04 and Progetto Finalizzato Oncologia, sottoprogetto Immunologia).

REFERENCES

Babior BM 1978 Oxygen-dependent microbial killing by phagocytes. N Engl J Med 298:659-668
Babior BM 1983 The nature of the NADPH oxidase. Adv Host Def Mech 3:91-119
Bellavite P, Cross AR, Serra MC, Davoli A, Jones OTG, Rossi F 1983a The cytochrome b and flavin content and properties of O_2^--forming NADPH oxidase solubilized from activated neutrophils. Biochim Biophys Acta 746:40-47
Bellavite P, Serra MC, Davoli A, Bannister JV, Rossi F 1983b The NADPH oxidase of guinea pig polymorphonuclear leucocytes. Properties of the deoxycholate extracted enzyme. Mol Cell Biochem 52:17-25

Bellavite P, Della Bianca V, Serra MC, Papini E, Rossi F 1984a NADPH oxidase of neutrophils forms superoxide anion but does not reduce cytochrome c and dichlorophenol indophenol. FEBS (Fed Eur Biochem Soc) Lett 170:157-161

Bellavite P, Jones OTG, Cross AR, Papini E, Rossi F 1984b Composition of partially purified NADPH oxidase from pig neutrophils. Biochem J 223:639-648

Bellavite P, Papini E, Zeni L, Della Bianca V, Rossi F 1985 Studies on the nature and activation of O_2^--forming NADPH oxidase of leukocytes. Identification of a phosphorylated component of the active enzyme. Free Rad Res Commun 1:11-29

Berton G, Cassatella M, Cabrini G, Rossi F 1985 Activation of mouse macrophages causes no change in expression and function of phorbol diesters receptors, but is accompanied by alterations in the activity and kinetic parameters of NADPH oxidase. Immunology 54:371-379

Borregaard N, Tauber AI 1984 Subcellular localization of the human neutrophil NADPH oxidase. B-cytochrome and associated flavoprotein. J Biol Chem 259:47-52

Castagna M, Takai Y, Kaibuchi K, Sano K, Kikkawa U, Nishizuka J 1982 Direct activation of calcium-activated, phospholipid dependent protein kinase by tumor-promoting phorbol esters. J Biol Chem 257:7847-7851

Crawford DR, Schneider DL 1982 Identification of ubiquinone-50 in human neutrophils and its role in microbicidal events. J Biol Chem 257:6662-6668

Crawford DL, Schneider DL 1983 Ubiquinone content and respiratory burst activity of latex-filled phagolysosomes isolated from human neutrophils and evidence for the probable involvement of a third granule. J Biol Chem 258:5363-5367

Cross AR, Jones OTG, Garcia R, Segal AW 1982a The association of FAD with the cytochrome b_{-245} of human neutrophils. Biochem J 208:759-763

Cross AR, Higson FK, Jones OTG, Harper A, Segal AW 1982b The enzymic reduction and kinetics of oxidation of cytochrome b_{-245} of neutrophils. Biochem J 204:479-485

Cross AR, Jones OTG, Garcia R, Segal AW 1983 The subcellular localization of ubiquinone in human neutrophils. Biochem J 216:765-768

Cross AR, Parkinson JF, Jones OTG 1984 The superoxide-generating oxidase of leucocytes. NADPH-dependent reduction of flavin and cytochrome b in solubilized preparations. Biochem J 223:337-344

Cross AR, Parkinson JF, Jones OTG 1985 Mechanism of the superoxide producing oxidase of neutrophils, O_2 is necessary for the fast reduction of cytochrome b_{-245} by NADPH. Biochem J 226:881-884

Cunningham CC, DeChatelet LR, Spach PI et al 1982 Identification and quantitation of electron-transport components in human polymorphonuclear neutrophils. Biochim Biophys Acta 682:430-435

Gabig TG 1983 The NADPH-dependent O_2^--generating oxidase from human neutrophils. Identification of a flavoprotein component that is deficient in a patient with chronic granulomatous disease. J Biol Chem 258:6352-6356

Gabig TG, Babior BM 1979 The O_2^--forming oxidase responsible for the respiratory burst in human neutrophils. Properties of the solubilized enzyme. J Biol Chem 254:9070-9074

Gabig TG, Lefker BA 1984 Catalytic properties of the resolved flavoprotein and cytochrome b components of the NADPH dependent O_2^--generating oxidase from human neutrophils. Biochem Biophys Res Commun 118:430-436

Gallin JI, Seligmann BE, Cramer EB, Schiffmann E, Fletcher MP 1982 Effects of vitamin K on human neutrophil function. J Immunol 128:1399-1408

Green TR, Wirtz MK, Wu DE 1983 Delineation of the catalytic components of the NADPH-dependent O_2^--generating oxidoreductase of human neutrophils. Biochem Biophys Res Commun 110:873-879

Grzeskowiak M, Della Bianca V, De Togni P, Papini E, Rossi F 1985 Independence with respect to Ca^{2+} changes of the neutrophil respiratory burst and secretory response to exogenous phospholipase C and possible involvement of diacylglycerol and protein kinase C. Biochim Biophys Acta 844:81-90

Hamers MN, de Boer M, Meerhof LJ, Weening RS, Roos D 1984 Complementation in monocyte hybrids revealing genetic heterogeneity in chronic granulomatous disease. Nature (Lond) 307:553-555

Harper AM, Dunne MJ, Segal AW 1984 Purification of cytochrome b_{-245} from human neutrophils. Biochem J 219:519-527

Hattori H 1961 Studies on the labile, stable NADi oxidase and peroxidase staining reactions in the isolated particles of horse granulocyte. Nagoya J Med Sci 23:362-378

Light DR, Walsh C, O'Callaghan AM, Goetzl EJ, Tauber AI 1981 Characteristics of the cofactor requirements for the superoxide-generating NADPH oxidase of human polymorphonuclear leukocytes. Biochemistry 20:1468-1476

Lutter R, van Zwieten R, Weening RS, Hamers MN, Roos D 1984 Cytochrome b, flavins, and ubiquinone-50 in enucleated human neutrophils (polymorphonuclear leukocyte cytoplasts). J Biol Chem 259:9603-9606

McPhail LC, Wolfson M, Clayton C, Snyderman R 1984 Protein kinase C and neutrophil (PMN) activation. Differential effects of chemoattractants and phorbol myristate acetate (PMA). Fed Proc 43:1661 (abstr 1430)

Morel F, Vignais PV 1984 Examination of the oxidase function of the b-type cytochrome in human polymorphonuclear leucocytes. Biochim Biophys Acta 764:213-225

Pember SO, Heyl BL Kinkade JM Jr, Lambeth JD 1984 Cytochrome b_{558} from (bovine) granulocytes. Partial purification from Triton X-114 extracts and properties of the isolated cytochrome. J Biol Chem 259:10590-10595

Peterson JA, Ebel RE, O'Keeffe DH, Matsubara T, Estabrook RW 1976 Temperature dependence of cytochrome P-450 reduction. A model for NADPH-cytochrome P-450 reductase: cytochrome P-450 interaction. J Biol Chem 251:4010-4016

Roberts PJ, Cross AR, Jones OTG, Segal AW 1982 Development of cytochrome b and an active oxidase system in association with maturation of a human promyelocytic (HL-60) cell line. J Cell Biol 95:720-726

Rossi F, Zatti M 1964 Changes in the metabolic pattern of polymorphonuclear leucocytes during phagocytosis. Br J Exp Pathol 15:548-559

Rossi F, Berton G, Bellavite P, Della Bianca V 1982 The inflammatory cells and their respiratory burst. Inflammation Res 3:329-340

Sakane F, Takahashi K, Koyama J 1983 Separation of three menadione-dependent, O_2^--generating, pyridine nucleotide-oxidizing enzymes in guinea pig polymorphonuclear leukocytes. J Biochem (Tokyo) 94:931-936

Sakane F, Takahashi K, Koyama J 1984 Purification and characterization of a membrane-bound NADPH-cytochrome c reductase capable of catalyzing menadione-dependent O_2^--formation in guinea pig polymorphonuclear leukocytes. J Biochem (Tokyo) 96:671-678

Segal AW 1983 Chronic granulomatous disease: A model for studying the role of cytochrome b_{-245} in health and disease. Host Def Mech 3:121-143

Serra MC, Bellavite P, Davoli A, Bannister JV, Rossi F 1984 Isolation from neutrophil membranes of a complex containing active NADPH oxidase and cytochrome b_{-245}. Biochim Biophys Acta 788:138-146

Sha'afi RI, White JR, Molski TFP et al 1983 Phorbol 12-myristate 13-acetate activates rabbit neutrophils without an apparent rise in the level of intracellular free calcium. Biochem Biophys Res Commun 114:638-645

Shinagawa Y, Tanaka C, Teraoka A, Shinagawa Y 1966 A new cytochrome in neutrophilic granules of rabbit leucocyte. J Biochem (Tokyo) 59:622-624

Tauber AI, Borregaard N, Simons E, Wright J 1983 Chronic granulomatous disease: a syndrome of phagocyte oxidase deficiencies. Medicine (Baltimore) 62:286-309

Wakeyama H, Takeshige K, Minakami S 1983 NADPH-dependent reduction of 2,6-dichlorophe-nol-indophenol by the phagocytic vesicles of pig polymorphonuclear leucocytes. Biochen J 210:577-581

DISCUSSION

Roos: There are now four reports from groups who have purified cytochrome b from phagocytic cells, and there are four different M_r values. This may be due to species differences, but it is hard to believe that species differences alone would account for the difference between the M_r we find (127 000) and Dr Bellavite's protein of 31 500 M_r. It might be argued that yours is a subunit of our protein from human neutrophils, but we cannot obtain a lower M_r by SDS treatment, in either reducing or non-reducing conditions.

Another possibility is that proteins of lower M_r have been partly degraded, because neutrophils are loaded with proteinases. So I would be very careful about calling your preparation intact cytochrome b. If purified cytochrome b can be incorporated into the chronic granulomatous disease cell, and if it restores the function, that would show that it is a protein that is still working. It would also prove that the cytochrome is part of the oxidase system.

Bellavite: Pember et al (1984) reported that cytochrome b from bovine neutrophils showed three protein bands with M_r of 14 000, 12 000 and 11 000. Harper et al (1984) and you (D. Roos, personal communication), using human neutrophils, get 68 000 and 127 000 respectively. It is tempting to suggest that the three M_r bands that Dr Pember gives come to a value not far from the M_r we indicated, 31 500, which is close to half of 68 000, which in turn is about half of 127 000 ... As you suggest, this may be a problem of the aggregation of different subunits. Segal indicates that there is a strong tendency for cytochrome b to aggregate, even in the presence of SDS. We took many precautions against proteolysis. We pretreated the cells with diisopropylphosphorofluori-date and we always included phenylmethanesulphonyl fluoride in the buffer. So in our case it is not a problem of proteolysis but perhaps one of aggregation in different conditions. Finally, the existence of marked species differences seems to be excluded because we found the same M_r of cytochrome b in pig guinea-pig neutrophils (Serra et al 1984).

Roos: An important point is that we find one haem per protein molecule of 127 000, which indicates that our preparation is an intact protein.

Bellavite: Your preparation seems less dissociated than ours but we cannot estimate the haem: protein ratio in our preparation because it is not 100% pure. We indicated the M_r of cytochrome b by looking at the relative increase in the 31 500 band during purification. With very sensitive methods we can find other bands but these cannot be cytochrome b because their intensity decreases during purification. Our procedure takes three to four days and some loss of haem would be expected in that time. Taking these limitations into consideration I think that in our cytochrome b preparation the haem:protein ratio approaches 1:1.

Whaley: What are the specific functional activities of these two proteins? Dr Roos, have you tried limited proteolytic digestion of your protein and examined the relative molecular mass of the digests?

Roos: Once we have purified cytochrome b we don't find any activity. We have given up trying to purify the oxidase activity. When we solubilize the oxidase we lose most of the activity, and we didn't want to draw conclusions from the 2–3% of the activity we can really purify. Therefore, we purified one of the components that we believe is part of the oxidase system and concentrated our efforts on that. From there, we want to go back to the oxidase system with chemical cross-linkers and try to identify the other possible components.

Whaley: What happens after proteolytic digestion?

Roos: We did that but for completely other reasons. We had a very pure protein so we wanted to make digests, do amino acid sequence analyses and try to make a DNA probe to go to the gene level. It turned out that trypsin treatment generated an enormous amount of small peptides. Using cyanogen bromide, we found two peptides of about equal M_r.

Springer: Dr Bellavite, you are isolating oxidase from plasma membranes of PMA-activated cells. What are the normal storage sites of the oxidase and the cytochrome b? Is there a translocation process during activation?

Bellavite: Fractionation studies indicate that a significant proportion of cytochrome b is in specific granules in the resting cells but is translocated to the membrane after the activation process. However, nobody demonstrated that this is the actual mechanism by which the oxidase is activated. The translocation is not necessary for the activation of neutrophil cytoplasts, which are practically devoid of specific granules and contains cytochrome b on the membrane only (Roos et al 1983).

Another piece of evidence against the role of translocation is that the release of the granules can be blocked by suitable inhibitors without affecting activation of the respiratory burst (Korchak et al 1980).

Finally, we have some data indicating that a lot of cytochrome b is present on the membrane in resting cells. If we treat macrophages with a small amount of a reducing agent, sodium dithionite, practically all the cytochrome b is reduced without reduction of intracellular chromophores such as mitochondrial and mitosomal cytochromes and peroxidase. The membrane of the cell therefore seems to be impermeable to the reducing agent. This indicates that cytochrome b is available on the surface of the cells.

Roos: We found that cytochrome b in the plasma membrane is a transmembrane antigen, because we can iodinate it from the outside and monoclonal antibodies against cytochrome b bind to the inside of the plasma membrane. For this last reaction, we have to spin the cells on a coverslip, so they become permeable to antibodies. This indicates that cytochrome b sticks out of the membrane on both sides.

Singer: But does that require the active site to be externalized?

Roos: I don't know whether the cytochrome needs a flavoprotein to form an active oxidase complex, but I think the active site is inside the cells because it somehow has to receive its electrons from NADPH, either directly or via a flavoprotein. On the other hand, cytochrome b also has to react with oxygen, and it does that on the outside of the cells or maybe in the membrane.

Singer: What about ubiquinone?

Roos: If you purify the neutrophils very carefully hardly any ubiquinone is present. We suspect that most of the ubiquinone that has been reported as part of the oxidase system has been derived from platelet-contaminated neutrophils.

Cohn: What about the localization of NADPH oxidase?

Bellavite: The active oxidase works on the membrane. In particular conditions, for example in the presence of cytochalasin B, practically all the superoxide produced is released outside the cell. The production of free radicals takes place on the membrane but obviously during phagocytosis free radicals and hydrogen peroxide are also released inside the cell.

Nathan: In your review of the evidence for the involvement of flavin, the only strong point is the genetic evidence that in some patients with chronic granulomatous disease the membrane proteins lack flavin fluorescent spectral signals. Have you confirmed that, in CGD neutrophils, membrane flavins are absent in the cytochrome b-containing population?

Bellavite: CGD is a very complex disease and many other defects have been described besides cytochrome b deficiency. For example there are also defects of the red cell antigens. The demonstration of the lack of flavin is not a direct demonstration that flavin is involved in the oxidase. Secondly, I wonder how a cell can be completely free of flavin, as described by one of these reports (Gabig 1983). The activity of cytochrome c reductase, diaphorase enzymes and so on suggests that other flavoprotein dehydrogenases are present in these cells. It is a bit contradictory.

Roos: We have looked at cells from eight CGD patients: X-linked, autosomal and a third group. Using cytoplasts for simplicity, we found completely normal amounts of non-covalently bound flavin in the membrane fraction and in the soluble fraction of the cytoplasm. That does not completely invalidate the published results but I have been wondering why such large deficiencies have been found in whole membranes and even in whole cells.

Nathan: It is difficult to prove, by either time or quantity, that phosphorylation of cytochrome *b* represents an activation step. Couldn't it either be unrelated to activation or represent deactivation? We know that the oxidase begins to be suppressed shortly after it starts to be activated.

Bellavite: The phosphorylation of cytochrome *b* is not due to deactivation, as the preparations where we observed phosphorylation were fully active. Certainly we cannot be sure that this is the only mechanism of NADPH oxidase activation. For example activation may consist of phosphorylation of cytochrome *b*, which could allow interaction with other factors necesary for the activity. This does not mean that activation affects only cytochrome *b* molecules *per se*.

Nathan: Have you looked for any other covalent modifications after stimulating the cell, such as acylation, for example?

Bellavite: No.

Dean: Is the system a self-inactivating one? In other words, if electron transport occurs, do enzymes in the system have to be progressively inactivated? It looks as if that is what happens with electron transport in chloroplasts, in relation to the 32K protein, and perhaps also in mitochondria (Dean & Pollak 1985).

Bellavite: The system is not self-inactivating. Oxidase activity can be turned on and off but this is due to the activation mechanism of the cell. For example, we can turn off the function of the oxidase by destroying the activator factor. If we activate the cells with arachidonic acid and then add albumin, this binds to the arachidonic acid and stops activation immediately. This is due to the removal of the stimulant that should be continuously present if activation is to be maintained. Addition of new stimulants can reactivate the oxidase.

Dean: So after a burst of activity you would expect the system to activate equally well again?

Bellavite: Yes.

Nathan: That is not what happens in macrophages. Once they are triggered they are refractory for at least three days, which is as long as anyone has looked, although they are viable (Murray 1982).

Dean: Is there any evidence that during the refractory period there are still components which are active and reconstitutable?

Nathan: No one has tried that.

Bellavite: The refractory period depends on the function of the receptor, because if you add a different stimulus the cells are responsive in terms of the respiratory burst.

Gordon: With large doses of PMA there is total deactivation to all stimuli.

Singer: Wouldn't this have to be a very unusual cytochrome to be in the plasma membrane? Most electron transport chains are in the endoplasmic reticulum. Does this suggest that the same cytochrome might be present in other cells but is for some reason stuck in the endoplasmic reticulum and never gets to the cell surface, so never expresses this kind of activity? Or is it a unique cytochrome that is characteristic of neutrophils and is not present in any other cells? Dr Roos, have you shown that your monoclonal antibody that reacts with this cytochrome is on the cytoplasmic face of the plasma membrane by *in situ* labelling?

Roos: Those experiments are being done now.

Singer: Is it present in homogenates of other cells?

Roos: Segal has shown that it is present in monocytes, some macrophages, eosinophils and neutrophils, that is in all the real phagocytes that are able to produce superoxide and hydrogen peroxide (Segal et al 1981).

The term cytochrome is perhaps a bit misleading. It was given the name because of the light absorbance spectrum, which is reminiscent of *b* type cytochromes. However, we think that it is a protein of high M_r and we prefer to call it a haem-containing protein. Indeed, as Dr Bellavite said, there may be other active centres in the same protein.

*Bellavite:*It should be stressed that this 'cytochrome *b*' has a very low mid-point potential, which is completely different from the potential of other *b* cytochromes present in other systems. This is necessary so that the reaction with oxygen can generate superoxide.

Unkeless: Does the monoclonal antibody that binds to the macrophages correlate with the capacity to evoke superoxide in, say, cells stimulated with IFN-γ, or is that a different component?

Roos: Those experiments are also on the programme.

Stanley: Is the protein of M_r 127000 phosphorylated in response to PMA?

Roos: Yes, and also in response to serum-opsonized zymosan. We have not tried other stimuli yet.

Stanley: Do you use solubilized membranes, or what?

Roos: Several groups have already shown that when the neutrophils are stimulated dozens of proteins are phosphorylated, giving different patterns with different stimuli. We took the simplest system that we could think of, the phagosomes from neutrophil cytoplasts. We used Oil Red 0 to form phagosomes and then floated them up in a gradient. We looked at the protein bands in the homogenate from the phagosomes. The 127000 M_r protein was phosphorylated.

Stanley: Were other proteins phosphorylated as well?

Roos: Yes, a couple of others.

Gordon: With G. Berton, H. Rosen and other collaborators we used the almost final stage of purified guinea-pig 'oxidase' to raise monoclonal antibodies. We produced rat hybridomas which were screened for the ability to trigger a respiratory burst on intact guinea-pig neutrophils. Most of the antibodies do not trigger a respiratory burst but we have isolated two which dramatically stimulate a burst. This requires the presence of cytochalasin B. If we treat the cells with intact antibody there is an efficient respiratory burst after a very short lag period. We can shorten the lag period slightly by preincubation with antibody. We can also trigger a burst by taking $F(ab')_2$ fragments of the antibody and cross-linking it with a second $F(ab')_2$ antibody. The $F(ab')_2$ fragment by itself does not trigger the burst any more, although the cells are still responsive to PMA. The second antibody, OX-12, is a mouse anti-rat hybridoma which also does not trigger the burst by itself.

Both monoclonal anti-'oxidase' antibodies see the same antigen, which is a novel proteolipid molecule found in macrophages and neutrophils only. It is present in the preparation originally used for immunization and is found in lysates and on the cell surface. It is very hydrophobic. We can extract with chloroform–ethanol and get rid of most of the other cellular proteins. In addition to the respiratory burst it also triggers degranulation. Although it is physically associated with the respiratory burst oxidase preparation, it may be more generally involved in signal transduction. Although we can trigger the burst in intact neutrophils, we cannot trigger it in macrophages even with cross-linking.

Cohn: Does its relative molecular mass fit in with the others we have heard about?

Gordon: It is smaller than $10\,000\ M_r$ but it has very distinctive properties. It is very hydrophobic, and extremely resistant to proteolysis even if we boil it in SDS.

Roos: Why didn't you get enough cross-linking with the Fab_2 fragments? Would you get better cross-linking with the intact antibody?

Gordon: We don't understand the role of Fc on the first antibody. The two antibodies we have used have different effects. With one antibody the intact antibody will trigger but $F(ab')_2$ fragment will not until we cross-link. In the other case neither the intact antibody nor the $F(ab')_2$ will trigger unless we cross-link with the second antibody. We have done controls to exclude that the Fc fragment of the intact immunoglobulin could be involved directly in stimulation. We assume that aggregation of the antibody and antigen within the membrane is facilitated by the intact molecule and not the $F(ab')_2$. That is a bit of a puzzle.

Springer: There are antibodies to a human neutrophil component, *N*-acetyl lactosamine (X-hapten). This carbohydrate moiety is present in both glycolipids and glycoproteins. Antibodies to the moiety can trigger a respiratory burst on human neutrophils. The density of this antigen on the cell surface is much greater than that of any other antigen that we looked at during the Second

International Leukocyte Workshop. Cross-linking of this high density antigen may non-specifically trigger the respiratory burst. What is the density of your antigen? Could you be looking at a glycolipid?

Gordon: We have purified the antigen by HPLC and find protein. We don't know if there is sugar as part of the proteolipid as well.

Singer: Was that measured by immunoprecipitation?

Gordon: When we blot we pick up a single band which is very characteristic. We looked at several other antibodies and they don't do this.

Cohn: There is no evidence that the antigen is part of the oxidase synthesis, is there?

Gordon: The antigen is physically associated with the oxidase preparation. It cofractionates with it in detergent-solubilized membranes until activity is lost.

REFERENCES

Dean RT, Pollak JK 1985 Endogenous free radical generation may influence proteolysis in mitochondria. Biochem Biophys Res Commun 126:1082-1089

Gabig TG 1983 The NADPH-dependent O_2^--generating oxidase from human neutrophils. Identification of a flavoprotein component that is deficient in a patient with chronic granulomatous disease. J Biol Chem 258:6352-6356

Harper AM, Dunne MJ, Segal AW 1984 Purification of cytochrome b_{-245} from human neutrophils. Biochem J 219:519-527

Korchak HM, Eisenstat BA, Hoffstein ST, Dunham PB, Weissmann G 1980 Anion channel blockers inhibit lysosomal enzyme secretion from human neutrophils without affecting generation of superoxide anion. Proc Natl Acad Sci USA 77:2721-2725

Murray HW 1982 Pretreatment with phorbol myristate acetate inhibits macrophage activity against intracellular protozoa. J Reticuloendothel Soc 31:479

Pember SO, Heyl BL, Kinkade JM Jr, Lambeth JD 1984 Cytochrome b_{558} from (bovine) granulocytes. Partial purification from triton X-114 extracts and properties of the isolated cytochrome. J Biol Chem 259:10590-10595

Roos D, Voetman AA, Meerhof LJ 1983 Functional activity of enucleated human polymorphonuclear leukocytes. J Cell Biol 97:368-377

Segal AW, Garcia R, Goldstone AH, Cross AR, Jones OTG 1981 Cytochrome b_{-245} of neutrophils is also present in human monocytes, macrophages and eosinophils. Biochem J 196:363-367

Serra MC, Bellavite P, Davoli A, Bannister JV, Rossi F 1984 Isolation from neutrophil membranes of a complex containing active NADPH oxidase and cytochrome b_{-245}. Biochim Biophys Acta 788:138-146

Bacterial lipopolysaccharides modify signal transduction in the arachidonic acid cascade in macrophages

ALAN A. ADEREM and ZANVIL A. COHN

Laboratory of Cellular Physiology & Immunology, The Rockefeller University, 1230 York Avenue, New York, NY 10021, USA

Abstract. Macrophages are a potent source of arachidonic acid (20:4) metabolites. When macrophages interact with an appropriate stimulus, phospholipase activity is induced, resulting in the liberation of 20:4 from the membrane phospholipid and its quantitative oxygenation via either the lipoxygenase or cyclooxygenase pathways. We have attempted to dissect the molecular events coupling the initial membrane-perturbing signal to the phospholipase activity. Using a variety of stimuli and uncoupling agents we have found that receptor-mediated 20:4 release is triggered by a series of sequential signals, including ligand–receptor binding, receptor clustering, Na^+-dependent events, the synthesis of a rapidly turning over protein and finally an influx of Ca^{2+} into the cell. Bacterial lipopolysaccharides (LPS) are poor triggers of the 20:4 cascade. However, pretreatment of cells with LPS leads to the establishment of a 'primed' or 'intermediate' state which can act synergistically with subsequent signals. Hence, the amount of 20:4 metabolites secreted in response to a variety of triggers is increased 3–10-fold in LPS-primed cells, and the lag phase usually observed in 20:4 secretion disappears. The observations presented suggest a two-stage mode of signalling in the receptor-mediated induction of the 20:4 cascade.

1986 Biochemistry of macrophages. Pitman, London (Ciba Foundation Symposium 118) p 196-210

Macrophages are a potent source of arachidonic acid (20:4) metabolites. When macrophages interact with an appropriate stimulus, phospholipases are activated, resulting in the liberation of 20:4 from membrane phospholipids. Quantitative oxygenation via either the cyclooxygenase or lipoxygenase (EC 1.13.11.12) pathways then ensues (Bonney et al 1978, Scott et al 1980). The specific profile of the 20:4 metabolites secreted varies with the tissue localization and activation state of the macrophage and has been the object of detailed studies in murine resident peritoneal macrophages (Scott et al 1982a). In these cells the major cyclooxygenase products synthesized are prostacyclin

(PGI_2) and prostaglandin E_2 (PGE_2) (Bonney et al 1978) while leukotriene C_4 (LTC) and 5-hydroxyeicosatetranoic acid (5-HETE) are the chief lipoxygenase metabolites (Rouzer et al 1980a).

A number of triggers which initiate the 20:4 cascade in macrophages have been described. They include particulate stimuli such as zymosan, immune complexes and some bacteria which exert their effects via specific receptors on the cell surface, as well as soluble agents such as phorbol myristate acetate (PMA), the Ca^{2+} ionophore A23187 and bacterial lipopolysaccharides (LPS) (for review see Bonney & Humes 1984). Very little is known about the nature or cellular localization of the enzymes involved in the 20:4 cascade. The enzymes associated with the cyclooxygenase pathway have in some cells been associated with the endoplasmic reticulum while the 5-lipoxygenase appears to be a soluble enzyme. A number of acylhydrolases have been described in macrophage lysates, including two phospholipase A_2 enzymes, a phospholipase C and a diacylglycerol lipase (Wightman et al 1981). It is not known which, if any, of these lipases are involved in the 20:4 cascade.

The triggers discussed above stimulate the mobilization and metabolism of endogenous membrane 20:4. Cells also metabolize exogenously supplied 20:4 via both the cyclooxygenase and lipoxygenase pathways (Scott et al 1982b). In all the investigations described here we studied the endogenous pathway using radiolabelled 20:4, the metabolites of which were identified by high-pressure liquid chromatography (HPLC).

The nature of the signal between the ligand–receptor complex and the phospholipase is the focus of our discussion. Here we report studies of the events which follow the binding of a particle to its receptor and lead to phospholipase activity and 20:4 release. Second, we describe the profound influence which LPS has on the facilitation of the signal sequence.

Triggers of the 20:4 cascade

The 20:4 cascade is triggered by both particulate and soluble stimuli. In general, particle–receptor complexes result in the release of both cyclooxygenase and lipoxygenase products while soluble stimuli (with the exception of the Ca^{2+} ionophore, A23187) often trigger only the secretion of cyclooxygenase metabolites (Bonney & Humes 1984). This suggests that the lipoxygenase and cyclooxygenase pathways might be independently regulated. Receptors which are known to trigger the 20:4 cascade include (a) Fc receptors for IgG and IgE immune complexes (Rouzer et al 1982), (b) the mannose–fucose receptor (MFR), as evidenced by stimulation with zymosan particles, and (c) a third, as yet unidentified, receptor. Evidence for this putative receptor (c) includes our recent observations that (1) zymosan-mediated 20:4 release

is only inhibited 50% by an excess of mannans (which block the MFR) and
(2) interferon-γ down-regulates zymosan-induced 20:4 release by 50%, an
event paralleled by the complete down-regulation of the MFR. Zymosan is
also known to bind the complement receptor (Ezekowitz et al 1984) but neither
the ligated C3b nor C3bi receptors are capable of causing 20:4 secretion
(Aderem et al 1985). Finally, a variety of lectins have also been shown to
trigger the 20:4 cascade.

Monovalent ligands (mannans and Fab fragments of antibodies directed
against the Fc receptor) do not trigger the 20:4 cascade, suggesting that events
in addition to receptor binding must be required (C. A. Rouzer & A. A.
Aderem, unpublished). Such events may include receptor clustering or cross-
linking, or both. Neither internalization of the receptor–ligand complexes
nor phagosome–lysosome fusion are required for 20:4 release (Rouzer et al
1980b).

An Na⁺ flux is an early signal in receptor–ligand-mediated 20:4 release

The Fc receptor for IgG2b functions as a monovalent cation channel when
it interacts with immune complexes or the divalent monoclonal antibody directed against its active sites (Young et al 1983). We have addressed the question of whether this potential influx of Na^+ is involved in the signalling of
phospholipase activity. When the Na^+ in the external medium is replaced
with either K^+ or choline, receptor-mediated 20:4 release is markedly inhibited, while 20:4 release triggered by soluble stimuli is unimpaired (Aderem
et al 1984). Furthermore, the Na^+-channel blocker amiloride inhibits both
zymosan and immune complex-induced 20:4 release, while PMA- and A23187-
triggered secretion is not affected. Raising the intracellular Na^+ concentration
with the Na^+–H^+ exchanger monensin or by inhibiting Na^+ efflux with ouabain
does not cause 20:4 release from cells. None of these agents inhibit the release
or metabolism of 20:4 triggered by either PMA or A23187, suggesting that
they do not interefere with phospholipase activity or any step distal to it
in the 20:4 cascade. These observations are compatible with a model in which
receptor-associated Na^+ influx is sufficient as a signal, although a generalized
increase of intracellular Na^+ is not. If the Na^+-independent soluble stimuli
trigger the same pathway as that mediated by the receptor–ligand complex,
the Na^+-requiring step must be proximal to the signals generated by either
PMA or A23187 and would therefore be an early signal in the cascade.

The influx of Na^+ has been shown to be an early event after stimulation
of neutrophils with the chemotactic peptide f-Met-Leu-Phe (Naccache et al
1977). Furthermore, removal of Na^+ from the medium decreases chemotactic
responsiveness in neutrophils as well as f-Met-Leu-Phe-stimulated lysosomal

enzyme secretion and O_2^- generation (Simchowitz & Spilberg 1979). Immune complex and concanavalin A (con A)-stimulated O_2^- production and lysosomal enzyme secretion in human neutrophils also have a requirement for external Na^+ (Korchak & Weissman 1980).

The role of Ca^{2+} ions in 20:4 secretion

The observation that the Ca^{2+} ionophore A23187 triggers the 20:4 cascade led us to examine the role of Ca^{2+} in 20:4 secretion. Fc receptor-mediated 20:4 release is abolished by the removal of Ca^{2+} from the external medium (EGTA medium). If the cells are then exposed to Ca^{2+} a rapid release of 20:4 is observed. The usual lag phase associated with immune complex-induced 20:4 release is eliminated, suggesting that some necessary intermediate signals have already been established and that an influx of external Ca^{2+} is a late signal in the induction of phospholipase activity. This is also supported by the observations that 20:4 secretion mediated by particulate as well as soluble triggers is dependent on Ca^{2+} (A. A. Aderem, unpublished data) and that the phospholipases described in macrophages have a Ca^{2+} requirement (Wightman et al 1981).

Protein synthesis is required for signal–response coupling in the 20:4 cascade

Bonney et al (1980) have shown that treatment of macrophages with protein synthesis inhibitors results in the rapid inhibition of PGE_2 secretion in response to zymosan and PMA. We have found that zymosan-, immune complex- and PMA-induced 20:4 release is inhibited 80–90% by protein and RNA synthesis inhibitors, while A23187-induced and basal secretion of 20:4 are relatively unaffected.

Kinetic analysis shows that the effect of protein synthesis inhibitors is very rapid, with 80% inhibition occuring within 15 min (Bonney et al 1980). Inhibition with actinomycin D occurs within 40 min, suggesting a precursor product relationship. These findings suggest that a rapidly turning over protein is synthesized which regulates the release of 20:4 from macrophage membranes in response to PMA, zymosan and IgG immune complexes. As the A23187-induced and basal secretion of 20:4 are unimpaired we conclude that either (1) basal and ionophore-stimulated 20:4 release are mediated via a different phospholipase to that induced by PMA and the receptor–ligand complexes or (2) a rapidly turning over protein modulates the 20:4 cascade at a step proximal to the phospholipase.

Sequential signals trigger the activation of phospholipase(s) in macrophages

Receptor-mediated phospholipase activation in macrophages clearly involves a number of complicated steps. The findings presented thus far can most simply be described by a pathway which is linear with respect to early and late intermediates (Fig. 1). As monovalent ligands do not trigger the 20:4 cascade, further events in addition to receptor binding must be required. Such events may include receptor clustering or cross-linking, or both. An early signal in the 20:4 cascade has an Na^+-dependent component, probably reflecting the influx of Na^+ into the cell. For further transduction of the signal there is a requirement for the synthesis of a rapidly turning over protein. If the soluble stimuli trigger the same pathway as that mediated by the receptor–ligand complex, PMA would stimulate the pathway at a point proximal to the protein synthetic step while A23187 would bypass this step. This implies that an increase in intracellular Ca^{2+} is the terminal event in the release of 20:4 from membrane phospholipids.

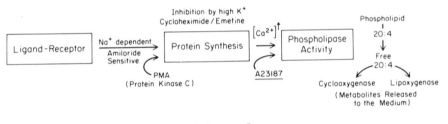

Scheme I

FIG. 1. Possible sequence of signals in the 20:4 cascade in macrophages. Receptor–ligand complexes first generate an Na^+-dependent, amiloride-sensitive signal. This is followed by the synthesis of a rapidly turning over protein. Finally, an increase in intracellular Ca^{2+} results in the activation of the phospholipase(s). If the soluble triggers activate the same pathway, phorbol myristate acetate (PMA) would stimulate the pathway at a point proximal to the protein synthetic step, while A23187 would bypass this step

LPS primes macrophages for enhanced 20:4 release in response to subsequent stimulation

Lipopolysaccharides (LPS) are a major component of the cell wall of Gram-negative bacteria. In its native state LPS consists of four subunits which are covalently attached: lipid A; 2-keto, 3-deoxyoctonate (KDO); a core polysaccharide moiety; and O-specific antigenic polysaccharide side-chains. Under certain growth conditions the O-antigen side-chain is not synthesized and rough LPS is formed. The lipid A moiety, a D-glucosamine disaccharide backbone substituted with four fatty acid side-chains, is considered responsible for the biological effects of LPS (for review see Morrison & Ulevitch 1978).

LPS induces a variety of biological effects. Some of the effects are deleterious, such as endotoxic shock, while others may be beneficial to the host, such as increased resistance to infection. In addition, LPS exerts multiple effects on cells *in vitro*, including B-cell mitogenicity (Morrison & Ulevitch 1978) and the secretion from macrophages of neutral proteases (Gordon et al 1974) and prostaglandins (Kurland & Bockman 1978). LPS is known to prime macrophages (Pabst & Johnston 1980) and neutrophils (Guthrie et al 1984) for enhanced release of reactive oxygen intermediates in response to subsequent stimulation with a variety of triggers.

LPSs are by themselves poor triggers of the 20:4 cascade. However, preincubation of cells for 30–60 min in LPS enhances both the amount and the rate of 20:4 secretion in response to a second stimulus. For example, PMA-induced 20:4 secretion is increased 3–15-fold in cells pretreated with LPS. Similarly, LPS also synergizes with zymosan, immune complexes and A23187 (Table 1). Secretion of 20:4 commences only after a lag phase when unprimed cells are stimulated. This lag phase is abolished in LPS-treated cells. This suggests that the lag phase seen in the absence of LPS priming might reflect the accumulation of intermediates which are necessary for signal transduction and that LPS might induce such intermediates in the cell.

Further support for this hypothesis is provided by the ability of LPS to render macrophages responsive to latex particles. Latex particles are ingested by macrophages without the release and metabolism of 20:4 (Bonney & Hume 1984) (Table 1). Interestingly, when LPS-primed cells ingest latex beads, up to 30% of the cellular 20:4 is released as PGI_2 and PGE_2 (Table 2).

TABLE 1 LPS priming potentiates 20:4 release in macrophages

Stimulus	Control cells		LPS-treated cells	
	20min	120 min	20 min	120min
No stimulus	1.0	1.8	1.6	5.1
PMA	3.1	11.2	20.9	37.8
Zymosan	6.1	20.8	24.5	41.6
Immune complexes	5.4	15.1	22.8	31.2
A23187[a]	8.5*	18.8+	24.2*	41.3+

Murine resident peritoneal macrophages were isolated and labelled overnight with [³H]20:4. The cells were then preincubated for 60 min in minimal essential medium (MEM) plus or minus LPS (0.5 µg/ml). The indicated trigger was added and the secreted 20:4 metabolites were determined 20 min and 120 min after addition of the stimulus. The results are expressed as percentage of radiolabel released.

[a] Time points for A23187 were 5 min (*) and 30 min (+).

TABLE 2 Macrophages primed with LPS secrete 20:4 metabolites in response to latex beads

Stimulus	Control cells 20 min	120 min	LPS-treated cells 20 min	120 min
No stimulus	0.9	2.1	1.3	6.1
Latex beads	1.2	3.0	18.2	30.5
C3b/C3bi-coated beads	1.0	2.0	1.5	7.3

Murine resident peritoneal macrophages were isolated and labelled with [^{3}H]20:4. The cells were then preincubated for 60 min in MEM plus or minus LPS (0.5 μg/ml). The particles were then added and the secreted 20:4 metabolites were determined 20 min and 120 min after addition of the stimulus. The results are expressed as percentage of radiolabel released.

While some particles which do not usually induce 20:4 release can do so when cells are primed with LPS (e.g. latex beads), this is not a general phenomenon. For example, particles phagocytosed via the C3b or C3bi receptors are incapable of triggering the 20:4 cascade even after LPS priming of the cells (Table 2).

We have tested different rough and smooth LPSs and lipid A for various strains of *Salmonella minnesota*, *Salmonella typhosa*, *Salmonella typhimurium* and *Escherichia coli*. All were capable of triggering the 20:4 cascade and priming the cells for enhanced 20:4 release in response to PMA, zymosan, immune complexes and A23187, suggesting that lipid A is the active moiety.

Since lipid A activates the protein kinase C (Wightman & Raetz 1984) we investigated whether the activation of this enzyme was responsible for inducing macrophages to secrete 20:4 in response to latex beads. Pretreatment of the cells with PMA, a known activator of protein kinase C (Nishizuka 1984), could not substitute for LPS in this system. This suggests that the activation of protein kinase C by LPS is not the mechanism by which LPS-primed cells are rendered capable of secreting 20:4 metabolites in response to latex particles.

LPS priming might modify a rate-limiting step in the activation sequence

The mechanism of LPS priming was further investigated by manipulating the ion content of the medium. LPS-induced 20:4 release is unaffected when extracellular Na$^+$ is replaced with choline, as is observed with other soluble stimuli. Zymosan-induced 20:4 release is dependent on Na$^+$ in the medium and therefore the baseline of secretion in response to this stimulus can be modified by varying the extracellular Na$^+$. Under these conditions we found that LPS priming always potentiated 20:4 release in proportion to baseline secretion (Table 3). These findings suggest that an intermediate on the linear pathway

TABLE 3 Effect of media of differing ionic composition on zymosan-induced 20:4 release from cells primed with LPS

Medium	Control cells	LPS-treated cells	Ratio
High Na$^+$	15.4	32.3	2.1
High K$^+$	2.8	6.4	2.3
High choline	5.8	13.9	2.4

Murine resident peritoneal macrophages were isolated and labelled with [^{3}H]20:4. The cells were preincubated for 60 min in MEM plus or minus LPS (0.5 μg/ml). The cells were then overlaid with either an Na$^+$-based medium, a K$^+$-based medium or a choline medium. Secretion was triggered with zymosan and the 20:4 metabolites were determined after 2 h. The results are expressed as percentage of radiolabel released.

(Fig. 1) is the rate-limiting step and that LPS priming modifies the equilibrium, thereby potentiating 20:4 release.

LPS and the 20:4 cascade in LPS-unresponsive mice

Macrophages from C3H/Hej mice, which are unresponsive to LPS by other criteria (Sultzer 1968), also do not release 20:4 in response to smooth LPS. The 20:4 cascade in these macrophages is intact, as the cells secrete about 20–25% of their cellular 20:4 in response to zymosan and A23187 (Table 4). Cyclooxygenase and lipoxygenase products are secreted and the amount and profile of the metabolites are comparable to those secreted by macrophages from other strains of mice.

Interestingly, PMA does not cause the secretion of 20:4 by macrophages from C3H/Hej mice. However, PMA causes the characteristic spreading response in these cells. This suggests that the 20:4 cascade is selectively unresponsive to PMA while other physiological responses to PMA are unimpaired.

TABLE 4 Effect of LPS on 20:4 secretion by C3H/Hej mice

Stimulus	Control	Smooth LPS	Rough LPS	Lipid A
None	2.1	2.4	1.9	2.0
Zymosan	20.4	21.1	27.4	30.6
A23187[a]	17.1	18.3	23.5	24.0
PMA	1.9	2.2	12.8	10.5

Macrophages were isolated from C3H/Hej mice and labelled with [^{3}H]20:4. The cells were then preincubated for 60 min in MEM containing either no addition, smooth LPS (1.0 μg/ml), rough LPS (1.0 μg/ml) or lipid A (1.0 μg/ml). The indicated trigger was then added and the secreted 20:4 metabolites were determined 120 min after addition of the stimulus. The results are expressed as percentage of radiolabel released.
[a] Time point for A23187 was at 30 min.

Next we investigated whether macrophages from C3H/Hej mice could be primed by LPS for enhanced 20:4 secretion in response to other stimuli. Smooth LPS does not cause potentiation of 20:4 secretion in response to zymosan or A23187 (Table 4). In contrast, while rough LPS and lipid A were unable to trigger 20:4 release, they were capable of potentiating secretion induced by zymosan (twofold) and A23187 (1.5-fold). Furthermore, priming C3H/Hej macrophages with either rough LPS or lipid A (but not with smooth LPS) results in the cells secreting 10% of their 20:4 content in response to PMA (Table 4).

Concluding remarks

We have explored the sequence of events leading to the activation of phospho-lipases in the macrophage. We have identified a number of steps in the activation sequence and have been able to situate them temporally (Fig. 1). While this simplified pathway is by no means complete, it provides us with a framework for further experimentation.

LPS induces a primed state in macrophages in which signal–response coupling in the 20:4 cascade is markedly modified. Priming cells with LPS results in enhanced 20:4 secretion in response to a second stimulus, possibly due to a shift in the equilibrium of certain rate-limiting steps. Other mechanisms by which LPS potentiates 20:4 secretion may include the activation of additional phospholipases. Another alternative is that LPS may induce an altered association of enzymes with the plasma membrane or with each other, resulting in more efficient coupling. Finally, the time course of priming may be attributed to a requirement for the metabolism of LPS. These questions are being investigated in our laboratory.

Acknowledgements

We thank Dan Cohen for excellent technical assistance and Drs Ellen Pure and Gilla Kaplan for reading the manuscript. This work was partially supported by National Institutes of Health Grant AI 07012.

REFERENCES

Aderem AA, Scott WA, Cohn ZA 1984 A selective defect in arachidonic acid release from macrophage membranes in high potassium media. J Cell Biol 99:1235-1241
Aderem AA, Wright SD, Silverstein SC, Cohn ZA 1985 Ligated complement receptors do not

activate the arachidonic acid cascade in resident peritoneal macrophages. J Exp Med 161:617-622

Bonney RJ, Humes JL 1984 Physiological and pharmacological regulation of prostaglandin and leukotriene production by macrophages. J Leuk Biol 35:1-10

Bonney RJ, Wightman PD, Davies P, Dadowski SJ, Kuehl FA, Humes JL 1978 Regulation of prostaglandin synthesis and the select release of lysosomal hydrolases by mouse peritoneal macrophages. Biochem J 175:433-442

Bonney RJ, Wightman PD, Dahlgren ME, Davies P, Kuehl FA, Humes JL 1980 Effect of RNA and protein synthesis inhibitors on the release of inflammatory mediators by macrophages responding to phorbol myristate acetate. Biochim Biophys Acta 633:410-421

Ezekowitz RAB, Sim RB, Hill M, Gordon S 1984 Local opsonization by secreted macrophage complement components. J Exp Med 159:244-260

Gordon S, Unkeless JC, Cohn ZA 1974 Induction of macrophage plasminogen activator by endotoxin stimulation and phagocytosis. J Exp Med 140:995-1010

Guthrie LA, McPhail LC, Henson PM, Johnston RB 1984 Priming of neutrophils for enhanced release of oxygen metabolites by bacterial lipopolysaccharide. J Exp Med 160:1656-1671

Korchak HM, Weissman G 1980 Stimulus-response coupling in the human neutrophil–transmembrane potential and the role of extracellular Na^+. Biochim Biophys Acta 601:180-194

Kurland JL, Bockman RJ 1978 Prostaglandin E production by human blood monocytes and mouse peritoneal macrophages. J Exp Med 147:952-957

Morrison DC, Ulevitch RJ 1978 The effects of bacterial endotoxins on host mediation systems. Am J Pathol 93:527-617

Naccache PH, Showell HJ, Becker EL, Sha'afi RI 1977 Transport of sodium, potassium, and calcium across rabbit polymorphonuclear leukocyte membranes. Effect of chemotactic factor. J Cell Biol 73:428-444

Nishizuka Y 1984 The role of protein kinase C in cell surface signal transduction and tumour promotion. Nature (Lond) 308:693-698

Pabst MJ, Johnston RB 1980 Increased production of superoxide anion by macrophages exposed in vitro to muramyl dipeptide or lipopolysaccharide. J Exp Med 151:101-114

Rouzer CA, Scott WA, Cohn ZA, Blackburn P, Manning JM 1980a Mouse peritoneal macrophages release leukotriene C in response to a phagocytic stimulus. Proc Natl Acad Sci USA 77:4928-4932

Rouzer CA, Scott WA, Kempe J, Cohn ZA 1980b Prostaglandin synthesis by macrophages requires a specific receptor–ligand interaction. Proc Natl Acad Sci USA 77:4279-4282

Rouzer CA, Scott WA, Hamill AL, Liu FT, Katz DH, Cohn ZA 1982 IgE immune complexes stimulate arachidonic acid release by mouse peritoneal macrophages. Proc Natl Acad Sci USA 79:5656-5660

Scott WA, Zrike JM, Hamill AL, Kempe J, Cohn ZA 1980 Regulation of arachidonic acid metabolites in macrophages. J Exp Med 152:324-335

Scott WA, Pawlowski NA, Murray HW, Andreach M, Zrike J, Cohn ZA 1982a Regulation of arachidonic acid metabolism by macrophage activation. J Exp Med 155:1148-1160

Scott WA, Pawlowski NA, Andreach M, Cohn ZA 1982b Resting macrophages produce distinct metabolites from exogenous arachidonic acid. J Exp Med 155:535-547

Simchowitz L, Spilberg I 1979 Chemotactic factor induced generation of superoxide radicals by human neutrophils: evidence for the role of Na^+. J Immunol 123:2428-2435

Sultzer BM 1968 Genetic control of leukocyte responses to endotoxin. Nature (Lond) 219:1253-1255

Wightman PD, Humes JL, Davies P, Bonney RJ 1981 Identification and characterization of two phospholipase A_2 activities in resident mouse peritoneal macrophages. Biochem J 195:427-433

Wightman PD, Raetz CRH 1984 The activation of protein kinase C by biologically active moieties of lipopolysaccharide. J Biol Chem 259:10048-10052
Young JD-E, Unkeless JC, Kaback HR, Cohn ZA 1983 Mouse macrophage Fc receptor for IgG$_{2b/a1}$ in artificial and plasma membrane vesicles functions as a ligand-dependent ionophore. Proc Natl Acad Sci USA 80:1636-1640

DISCUSSION

Gordon: Is the LPS effect for the neutrophil the same as for the macrophage, or is the neutrophil already primed? Would some of the results you describe for the complement receptor hold for the neutrophil as well?

Aderem: I have not done any of these experiments on neutrophils. However, a great deal of work has been done on neutrophils with respect to the generation of reactive oxygen intermediates (ROI). For example, McPhail and Snyderman (McPhail et al 1984) have shown that pre-exposing neutrophils to suboptimal doses of one type of stimulus results in potentiated ROI production when the cells are subsequently challenged with a second, heterologous, trigger. Also, Dick Johnston and co-workers have recently reported that neutrophils can be primed with LPS for enhanced ROI production (Guthrie et al 1984).

I do not know whether the complement receptors trigger the arachidonic acid (20:4) cascade in neutrophils.

Humphrey: LPS binds to these and other cells. Is it internalized after that?

Aderem: This is a very controversial area. Cell surface LPS receptors have been reported by some workers but none has been rigorously defined. It is probable that LPS binds to the cell surface, is internalized and then metabolized. Hall & Munford (1983) have recently reported that the granule fraction of neutrophils contains one or more enzymes that partially deacylate lipid A. We are currently investigating whether this metabolic process has anything to do with priming.

Cole: When you incubate cells in the presence of the smaller LPS derivatives, is there any way to check what physical state they are in? Do they form micelles or are they single molecules in the fluid phase? We have had some trouble trying to determine that ourselves.

Aderem: As I reported, we found that the monoacyl derivative and the dephospho compound were as capable as lipid X in priming macrophages for enhanced 20:4 release. We were worried that we had the wrong compounds but then we repeated Wightman & Raetz's (1984) observation that lipid X was capable of triggering the secretion of 20:4 metabolites while the deacylated derivative was not. So I guess that the structural requirements defined by Raetz and co-workers holds for some but not all biological effects. On the other hand, it is possible that the monoacyl derivative gets reacylated in the cell, although there is no evidence for that yet.

We have had trouble with the solubility too. The dephospho compound is extremely insoluble. The phosphate group seems to keep it in solution. The monoacyl derivative appears to be rather soluble. We have had less trouble when delivering these compounds in DMSO. Micelles appear to be formed at high concentrations, making it very difficult to know exactly how much LPS or derivative you are actually delivering to the cells.

Cole: Have you used butanol-extracted LPS rather than phenol-extracted LPS?

Aderem: No.

Cole: A protein (endotoxin-associated protein) is co-isolated with butanol extraction to which the C3H/H3j mouse macrophage responds. Butanol-extracted LPS also causes an increase in C3 synthesis in the same way as Westphal LPS.

Aderem: Pabst & Johnston (1980) compared the capacity of butanol-extracted LPS and phenol-extracted LPS to prime macrophages for enhanced ROI secretion. They found no difference in the priming capacity of these two LPS preparations in macrophages from Swiss mice or from C3Heb/FeJ mice. However, butanol-extracted LPS primed macrophages isolated from C3H/Hej mice to secrete more ROI than did phenol-extracted LPS.

Werb: How much LPS is needed to get this effect?

Aderem: We need at least 10–100 ng LPS/ml.

Werb: Is that also true for the derivatives?

Aderem: We sometimes need higher concentrations of the derivatives. All the experiments described here were done at 500 ng LPS derivative/ml.

Cole: The derivatives are so much smaller than the LPS that you don't know whether to control for weight or for molarity.

Schreiber: Have you compared LPS priming on either interferon-treated macrophages or macrophages in different states of activation?

Aderem: Immune activated macrophages (those elicited with *C. parvum* or BCG) are down-regulated with respect to the secretion of 20:4 metabolites. We are currently investigating whether LPS is capable of priming these cells for enhanced 20:4 release.

We have examined the effect of IFN-γ on 20:4 metabolism in macrophages. In general, treatment of macrophages with IFN-γ for 24–48 hours does not result in any modulation of the 20:4 cascade, even though the cells now secrete much larger quantities of ROI. The only effect we have found is a 50% down-regulation in 20:4 secretion in response to zymosan, which can be directly ascribed to the down-regulation of the mannose–fucose receptor. LPS appears to prime IFN-γ-treated cells to the same extent as control cells.

Schreiber: The high dose of LPS that you require in these assays may go to much lower concentrations if you use IFN-treated cells.

Humphrey: Polymyxin binds to lipid A and prevents the biological effects in whole animals. If you added it at various times after the triggering so as to block the LPS at that stage, it might block the effect.

Aderem: I have not tried using polymyxin.

Cole: We have treated LPS with polymyxin and then exposed it to cells. That did not seem to abolish the effect on C3 synthesis, while polymyxin treatment usually abolishes most of the other biological effects of LPS.

Ezekowitz: The calcium-dependent sodium exchange seems to be a distal event. Is it involved in any way?

Aderem: I don't know.

Ezekowitz: If you prime cells, challenge them and some time later challenge them again, can you get a similar response?

Aderem: We are currently investigating this question.

Ezekowitz: Why doesn't PMA give a maximal response? Is that because you need some early surface event? PMA seems to give two-thirds of the response you see with zymosan.

Aderem: PMA is a very poor trigger of the 20:4 cascade. It appears that, in addition to the phosphorylations mediated by the protein kinase C, other signal(s) are required for effective triggering of the 20:4 cascade. For example, we have evidence that suboptimal doses of the Ca^{2+} ionophore A23187 and PMA synergize and result in much-enhanced 20:4 release. This enhancement is most pronounced with respect to leukotriene C production. This suggests a synergy between increased intracellular Ca^{2+} and the protein kinase C, as has been described in other systems (Nishizuka 1984).

Certain triggers of the 20:4 cascade (such as zymosan, which triggers the secretion of both cyclooxygenase and lipoxygenase metabolites) might be capable of generating a specific sequence of signals: for example, a priming signal followed by a second signal which triggers the secretion of 20:4 metabolites. PMA might not be capable of priming the cell. This could result in poor stimulation of the 20:4 cascade. LPS, on the other hand, is probably capable of generating the primed state in the macrophage. The primed state thus established might synergize with the PMA-induced phosphorylation, resulting in much-enhanced 20:4 release.

Gordon: Does the PMA effect normally depend on endotoxin?

Aderem: We control quite rigorously for the endotoxin levels in our media, but it is possible.

Nathan: Does the C3H/HeN counterpart respond normally to PMA?

Aderem: I don't know. Experiments with C3H/HeN mice are in progress.

Springer: Do you know what receptor mediates the response to zymosan?

Aderem: The mannose–fucose receptor appears to mediate approximately half of the zymosan-induced 20:4 secretion from macrophages. This is inferred from our observation that one can inhibit zymosan-induced 20:4 release by 50% with high concentrations of mannan. Furthermore, treatment of the cells with IFN-γ results in a 50% down-regulation of 20:4 secretion, which correlates nicely with an almost complete down-regulation of the mannose–fucose receptor.

We have to explain the release of the remaining 50% of 20:4 metabolites. Zymosan is also known to bind the C3b and C3bi receptors but we have recently shown that neither of these two receptors is capable of triggering the 20:4 cascade (Aderem et al 1985). So that leaves us with at least one further, as yet undefined, receptor which must bind zymosan and which will mediate the release of 20:4 metabolites. Certain lectins are capable of triggering the 20:4 cascade in macrophages and it is possible that a lectin receptor might mediate some of the zymosan-induced 20:4 release, but we have no direct evidence for that yet.

Gordon: If you opsonize the zymosan particles do you deposit an excess of C3bi on it?

Aderem: Opsonized zymosan triggers the cascade.

Springer: Is it any more effective than unopsonized zymosan?

Aderem: Opsonization of the particles does not affect the levels of zymosan-mediated 20:4 secretion from murine resident peritoneal macrophages.

However, the situation with human monocytes is quite different. Nick Pawlowski (personal communication) has found that unopsonized zymosan is poorly bound by the cell and also does not trigger the release of 20:4 metabolites. In this regard it is worth noting that freshly explanted human monocytes have very low levels of mannose–fucose receptor. On the other hand, opsonized zymosan which is both bound and phagocytosed is a very good stimulus of 20:4 secretion from human monocytes.

Dean: We have published much complementary information on the role of the mannose receptor in triggering lysosomal enzyme secretion, rather in agreement with what you and Alan Ezekowitz have described (Bodmer & Dean 1983a,b,c, Leoni & Dean 1984, Jessup et al 1985). Have you compared the membrane potential changes in cells which have and have not been primed with LPS?

Aderem: No, we have not. We have looked at the effect of membrane potential on 20:4 release triggered by other stimuli such as zymosan. We concluded that depolarization *per se* is not very important in the triggering event.

Humphrey: Does your work suggest that the effect of endotoxaemia *in vivo* is due to the arachidonic acid metabolites?

Aderem: Endotoxin has so many effects *in vivo* that I wouldn't want to comment on that.

Cohn: Is there any evidence that endotoxin primes macrophages for enhanced release of vasoactive components *in vivo.*

Aderem: We have not done any *in vivo* experiments so I cannot answer the question.

Gordon: There is ATPase on the surface of macrophages but what is its function?

Aderem: The presence of an ecto-ATPase on the surface of macrophages has been inferred from the observation that free ^{32}Pi is detected in the medium when the cells are incubated with γ-^{32}Pi-labelled ATP. This is not watertight evidence for an ecto-ATPase as there are multiple mechanisms by which the ^{32}Pi could be liberated. For example one could get a phosphorylation reaction followed by phosphatase activity.

There is no evidence that cell surface ATPase activity has anything to do with the 20:4 cascade.

REFERENCES

Aderem AA, Wright SD, Silverstein SC, Cohn ZA 1985 Ligated complement receptors do not activate the arachidonic acid cascade in resident peritoneal macrophages. J Exp Med 161:617-622

Bodmer JL, Dean RT 1983a Does the induction of macrophage lysosomal enzyme secretion involve the mannose receptor? Biochem Biophys Res Commun 113:192-198

Bodmer JL, Dean RT 1983b A comparison of iodinated and technetium labelled zymosan for measurement of particle binding and internalisation by macrophages. Biochem J 214:277-278

Bodmer JL, Dean RT 1983c Receptor-mediated phagocytosis of zymosan is unaffected by some conditions which reduce lysosomal enzyme secretion. Biosci Rep 3:1053-1061

Guthrie LA, McPhail LC, Henson PM, Johnston RB 1984 Priming of neutrophils for enhanced release of oxygen metabolites by bacterial lipopolysaccharide. J Exp Med 160:1656-1671

Hall CL, Munford RS 1983 Enzymatic deacylation of the lipid A moiety of Salmonella typhimurium lipopolysaccharides by human neutrophils. Proc Natl Acad Sci USA 80:6671-6675

Jessup W, Leoni P, Dean RT 1985 Constitutive and triggered lysosomal enzyme secretion. In: Dean RT, Stahl PD (eds) Developments in cell biology. Butterworths, Sevenoaks, UK, vol. 1, p 38-57

Leoni P, Dean RT 1984 Cell surface events which may initiate lysosomal enzyme secretion by human monocytes. Eur J Immunol 14:997-1002

McPhail LC, Clayton CC, Snyderman R 1984 The NADPH oxidase of human polymorphonuclear leukocytes; evidence for regulation by multiple signals. J Biol Chem 259:5768-5775

Nishizuka Y 1984 The role of protein kinase C in cell surface signal transduction and tumour promotion. Nature (Lond) 308:693-698

Pabst MJ, Johnston RB 1980 Increased production of superoxide anion by macrophages exposed in vitro to muramyl dipeptide or lipopolysaccharide. J Exp Med 151:101-114

Wightman PD, Raetz CRH 1984 The activation of protein kinase C by biologically active lipid moieties of lipopolysaccharide. J Biol Chem 259:10048-10052

Secretion of toxic oxygen products by macrophages: regulatory cytokines and their effects on the oxidase

CARL F. NATHAN and SHOHKO TSUNAWAKI

The Rockefeller University, 1230 York Avenue, New York, NY 10021, USA

Abstract. We are attempting to identify cytokines that regulate macrophage secretion of reactive oxygen intermediates (ROI) and to analyse the biochemical basis of their effects. In both humans and mice, interferon-γ (IFN-γ) appears to be the chief factor secreted by clonally unselected lymphocytes that enhances macrophage oxidative metabolism and antiprotozoal activity. *In vivo* administration of recombinant IFN-γ enhances the ROI secretory capacity of monocytes in humans, and the secretion of ROI and killing of protozoa by peritoneal macrophages in mice. A protein secreted by murine tumours and certain non-malignant cells exerts opposing effects. This macrophage deactivation factor (MDF) both blocks the induction of activation by IFN-γ and reverses pre-existent activation. MDF action is non-toxic and selective, suppressing the secretion of ROI, killing of intracellular protozoa, and expression of Ia antigen, without inhibiting secretion of several other products, or synthesis of protein, ingestion of particles or adherence to culture vessels. The suppressive effect of MDF is reversed over several days after its removal. This reversal is hastened by IFN-γ. Profound suppression of oxidative metabolism accompanies the differentiation of murine monocytes into Kupffer cells. The capacity of Kupffer cells to secrete ROI and kill intracellular protozoa remains deficient even after exposure to IFN-γ. Thus, four states of macrophage activation can provisionally be discerned: the transition of mouse peritoneal macrophages from the (a) non-activated to the (b) activated state is accompanied by a ninefold increase in affinity of the superoxide-producing enzyme for NADPH, without a marked increase in cellular V_{max} or content of cytochrome b_{559}. The MDF-induced transition of mouse peritoneal macrophages from the activated to the (c) deactivated state is accompanied by both an increase in K_m and a decrease in apparent V_{max} of the oxidase. There are no changes in the phorbol myristate acetate receptor number or affinity, glucose transport, NADPH levels, cytochrome b_{559} content, catalase (EC 1.11.1.6) GSH, GSH peroxidase (EC 1.11.1.9), GSH reductase (EC 1.6.4.2) or myeloperoxidase, consistent with the suppressed ROI secretory capacity and antiprotozoal activity of these cells. The Kupffer cell, whose non-responsiveness to IFN-γ may mark it as (d) inactivated, appears to lack detectable NADPH oxidase activity, despite the probable presence of cytochrome b_{559}, and in this regard differs from both non-activated and deactivated macrophages. Further biochemical analysis of macrophages in these four states of differentiation may illuminate the workings of the oxidase and its regulatory apparatus.

1986 Biochemistry of macrophages. Pitman, London (Ciba Foundation Symposium 118) p 211-230

211

Defence of the host by secretion of reactive oxygen intermediates (ROI) is a strategy used by organisms of surprising phylogenetic diversity. Certain marine algae equipped with haloperoxidase secrete alkyl halides that may deter feeding by predators and suppress the growth of epiphytic microflora (Gschwend et al 1985). The bombardier beetle (*Brachinus crepitans*) maintains an enormous concentration of H_2O_2 in a specialized reservoir (Schildknecht 1970). When attacked, the beetle injects the H_2O_2 into an adjoining chamber rich in catalase, whose exergonic action pressurizes peroxide, peroxidase products and oxygen in a jet of steam spewed at the foe (Aneshansley et al 1969). The defence of the sea urchin egg against polyspermy includes responding to fertilization by secreting H_2O_2 that reacts with a peroxidase in the heads of approaching sperm (Boldt et al 1981). Finally, the vertebrate phagocyte, triggered by microbes, immune complexes or other stimuli, including phorbol esters, secretes O_2^-, H_2O_2, OH^-, and in some cases hypohalous acids, which not only kill microorganisms and tumour cells (Badwey & Karnovsky 1980, Nathan 1983) but can also exert wide-ranging effects on normal host cells and their products (Table 1). Such effects extend beyond cytotoxic and mutagenic actions to include non-cytotoxic regulation of secretion and other functions of leucocytes, as well as activation or inactivation of inflammatory mediators. Thus, many interests converge in seeking to understand how the secretion of ROI by phagocytes is regulated. Study of the oxidase itself is more advanced with the abundant polymorphonuclear leucocyte (Babior 1984) than with the sparingly generated mononuclear phagocyte. However,

TABLE 1 Effects of reactive oxygen intermediates

On cells	*On factors involved in inflammation*
Killing of viruses, bacteria, fungi, protozoa, nematodes, trematodes	Activation of chemotactic lipids
	Inactivation of leukotrienes B, C, D
Injury of tumour cells	Inactivation of α_1-antiprotease
Injury of erythrocytes, lymphocytes, leucocytes, platelets, endothelial cells, fibroblasts, lung cells, spermatozoa	Inactivation of chemotactic peptides
	Inactivation of Met-enkephalin
	Inactivation of leucocyte hydrolases
Inhibition of leucocyte lysosomal enzyme release	Inactivation of bacterial toxins
Stimulation of secretion by platelets, mast cells, endothelial cells, glomerular cells	*On subcellular components*
	Oxidation of glycolytic intermediates
	Hydrolysis of NAD
Suppression of lymphocytes directly (NK cells) or through SIRS	Oxidation of proteins
	Peroxidation of lipids
Mutagenesis of bacterial and eukaryotic cells	Depolymerization of mucopolysaccharides
Tumour promotion and carcinogenesis	
	Syndromes with evidence for a major role
	Acute respiratory distress syndrome
	Post-ischaemic reperfusion injury

SIRS, soluble immune response suppressor

the latter lives long enough in the tissues to come under external controls, both by those cells that coordinate the immune response (T cells) and those that confound it (tumour cells). Below are reviewed our preliminary attempts to identify such regulatory factors and their mechanisms of action.

Results and discussion

Macrophage activation: role of interferon-γ

Five lines of evidence support the identification of interferon-γ (IFN-γ) as the predominant lymphocyte-derived factor that activates macrophages for enhanced secretion of ROI and oxygen-dependent antimicrobial function. Three of these are summarized in Table 2. (a) Human peripheral blood lymphocytes stimulated with any of three different polyclonal or oligoclonal activators (lentil lectin plus mezerein, concanavalin A or toxoplasma lysate using cells from toxoplasma-immune donors) secreted IFN-γ. The IFN-γ containing, lymphocyte-conditioned media quadrupled the ability of human macrophages, derived by culture of blood monocytes, to secreted H_2O_2 when challenged with phorbol myristate acetate (PMA). The enhancing effect was abolished by incubating the lymphokines with a monoclonal antibody that neutralizes

TABLE 2 Identification of the lymphokine enhancing human macrophage oxidative metabolism as interferon-γ[a]

Lymphokine preparation and means of induction	Concentration before dilution, or specific activity	Macrophage H_2O_2 release [mean ± SEM (number of expts.)]	
		Ratio, experimental[b]: control	% inhibition by anti-IFN-γ MAb
Crude lymphokines (U/ml)			
Lentil lectin, mez	$0.1–1 \times 10^3$	3.8 ± 1.5 (6)	207[c] ± 43 (3)
Concanavalin A	$1.0–3 \times 10^3$	3.6 ± 0.5 (5)	86 ± 9 (5)
Toxoplasma antigen	$2–6 \times 10^3$	4.1 ± 0.5 (4)	108 ± 12 (4)
Purified native IFN-γ (U/mg)			
Lentil lectin, mez	10^6	7.2 ± 1.9 (4)	113 ± 8 (2)
Staphylococcal enterotoxin A	10^7	9.7 ± 2.4 (8)	91 ± 13 (5)
Recombinant IFN-γ (U/mg)	3×10^6	17.7 ± 4.8 (14)	

[a] From Nathan et al 1983.
[b] Mean ± SEM for 41 experimental sets = 643 ± 57 nmol H_2O_2/mg cell protein/h.
[c] Inhibition in excess of 100% probably represents unmasking of suppressive activity in the same preparation.
MAb, monoclonal antibody; mez, mezerein.

IFN-γ. This suggests that IFN-γ is necessary for macrophage activation by these supernatants but does not rule out the possibility that another molecule is also required or even that the antibody neutralized an activating factor other than IFN-γ. (b) IFN-γ was partially or highly purified from these lymphokines by either of two independent protocols, as monitored by bioassay for antiviral activity. The active fractions were enriched in the ability to activate macrophage oxidative metabolism. (c) Pure, recombinant IFN-γ (rIFN-γ) was a potent macrophage-activating factor, with effective concentrations in the picomolar range (Nathan et al 1983). The results in Table 2 were duplicated with regard to the ability of macrophages to kill *Toxoplasma gondii* (Nathan et al 1983), and were confirmed for macrophage antileishmanial function (Murray et al 1983). Together, these observations support the interpretation that IFN-γ is both necessary and sufficient for macrophage activation by the lymphokine preparations studied, keeping in mind our definition of 'activation': enhanced oxidative metabolism and antiprotozoal function.

However, these observations do not exclude the possibility that other cytokines may also activate macrophages—cytokines that may not have been present in sufficient concentration in the lymphocyte supernatants studied. Several investigators have approached this question by screening media conditioned by lymphocyte clones or hybridomas. A contribution by IFN-γ to the activity of such media can be difficult to exclude, given that cloned lymphocytes secrete multiple cytokines, IFN-γ is a frequent product of such clones, IFN-γ can activate macrophages at concentrations far below the limits of sensitivity of antiviral assays, and antibodies that neutralize IFN-γ's antiviral activity may not neutralize its macrophage-activating capacity (Schreiber et al 1985). Several laboratories are attempting to establish firmly the existence of non-IFN-γ macrophage-activating factors through their purification and physico-chemical characterization.

In the meantime, we have taken an alternative approach, the individual testing of all cytokines already known to have an effect on mononuclear phagocytes and available to us as natural products in highly purified form or as pure, recombinant molecules (Nathan et al 1984). The results are summarized in Fig. 1. With rIFN-γ as a positive control in each experiment, the combination of markedly enhanced oxidative metabolism and antitoxoplasma activity was not observed after incubation of human macrophages with native IFN-α, rIFN-αA, rIFN-αD, rIFN-β, colony-stimulating factor type 1, colony-stimulating factor for granulocytes and macrophages, pluripotent colony-stimulating factor (an interleukin-3-like molecule), or migration inhibitory factor. (With the last of these, some enhancement of H_2O_2 secretion was induced without antitoxoplasmal activity.) In addition, we tested native and recombinant interleukin-2, and native tumour necrosis factor. These findings indicate that macrophage activation is a highly restricted property among cytokines with effects

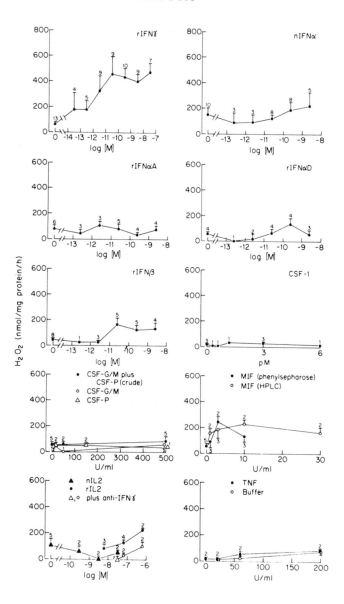

FIG. 1. Hydrogen peroxide release by phorbol myristate acetate-challenged human macrophages after incubation for three days in the indicated cytokines. Means ± SEM for the number of experiments noted above each point, each with cells from a different donor. (From Nathan et al 1984.) CSF-1, colony-stimulating factor type 1; CSF-G/M, CSF for granulocytes and macrophages; CSF-P, pluripotent CSF; MIF, migration inhibitory factor; nIL2, native interleukin-2; rIL2, recombinant interleukin 2; TNF, tumour necrosis factor.

on macrophages, and provide the fourth line of evidence for the predominant role of IFN-γ in this regard.

A fifth test of the role of IFN-γ as a macrophage-activating factor is whether it functions *in vivo*. Until this is demonstrated, the possibility remains that the effects observed above may be an artifact of *in vitro* cell culture. An opportunity to approach this question has arisen with the initiation of phase 1 trials of rIFN-γ in patients with cancer. In order to conduct serial studies on monocytes isolated from the blood of such patients, we have adapted a quantitative assay for cellular H_2O_2 production to a semi-automated microscale (de la Harpe & Nathan 1985). Using this technique, we conducted 170 assays on cells from 13 patients with advanced malignancy who underwent 20 cycles of intravenous administration of rIFN-γ in dosages ranging from 0.1 to 1.0 mg/m^2 of body surface per infusion. Eighty-five per cent of these subjects responded, by the criterion that their post-treatment monocytes released more H_2O_2/mg cell protein than their pretreatment monocytes, in $\geq 67\%$ of tests conducted > 1 h after the start of infusion of rIFN-γ (Nathan et al 1985). Since monocytes normally can secrete abundant H_2O_2, they may be a suboptimal population in which to look for an increase. Nonetheless, combined data for all 13 patients revealed statistically significant increases averaging from 1.4-fold to 2.8-fold above the pretreatment controls (Nathan et al 1985). These findings may be the first to suggest that mononuclear phagocytes can be activated in humans by a lymphocyte product.

It remains to be shown whether human tissue macrophages can also be activated *in vivo* by IFN-γ, and whether the manifestations of activation extend to antimicrobial or cytotoxic functions. Studies addressing these questions are under way. Meanwhile, work in the mouse has already provided affirmative answers for that species.

The murine studies first recapitulated key points of the *in vitro* work described above with human cells and reagents. Thus, concanavalin A-stimulated supernates of mouse spleen cells augmented the H_2O_2-releasing capacity of resident mouse peritoneal macrophages, and this was abolished by a monoclonal antibody against murine IFN-γ. The results shown in Table 3 for oxidative metabolism were affirmed when we studied the ability of macrophages to kill *Toxoplasma gondii* and *Leishmania donovani* (Murray et al 1985). Similar results with other monoclonal anti-murine IFN-γ antibodies have been reported for macrophage antitumour activity by Schreiber et al (1985). The concentrations of rIFN-γ required *in vitro* for enhancement of H_2O_2-releasing capacity are illustrated for a representative experiment in Fig. 2, which compares polyclonally derived lymphocyte supernates, the supernate of a cloned T-T hybridoma, and pure recombinant material as sources of IFN-γ. All three were potent activators of resident peritoneal macrophages, in contrast to IFN-α, IFN-β, and human rIFN-γ. Fig. 3 illustrates the time

TABLE 3 Monoclonal antibody to murine interferon-γ inhibits the enhancement of macrophage oxidative metabolism induced by lymphokines and murine rIFN-γ[a]

Cytokine	No. of expts.	H_2O_2, nmol/mg protein per 60 min (mean ± SEM)[b] Control	Cytokine	Inhibition by antibody (%)[c]
Con A supernate	3	83 ± 7	313 ± 92	109 ± 16
Hybridoma supernate	4	94 ± 11	788 ± 118	88 ± 6
rIFNγ-mu (CHO)	3	97 ± 14	419 ± 59	93 ± 19
rIFNγ-mu (E. coli)	2	91 ± 4	495 ± 134	114 ± 23

[a] Resident macrophages were incubated with the indicated materials for 2 d with or without 3–18 μg/ml monoclonal anti-IFN-γ antibody. At the dilutions used, the cytokines contained the following concentrations of IFN-γ, in U/ml: concanavalin A lymphokine, 10–65; hybridoma (from R. Schreiber, Scripps Research Institute), 2–69; murine rIFN-γ produced in Chinese hamster ovary (CHO) cells (a glycosylated form), 4; and murine rIFN-γ purified from E. coli, 0.1–1. The recombinant materials were from Genentech, Inc.
[b] Means ± SEM for three to four experiments or ± range for two experiments.
[c] Percentage inhibition = $100[1 - (A - C)/(E - C)]$, where A = results with cytokine plus antibody, E = results with cytokine alone, and C = results for the control (no cytokine) From Murray et al 1985.

course of activation by rIFN-γ, in this case using inflammatory macrophages. Summarizing a number of experiments, we can say that enhancement of oxidative metabolism, antitoxoplasma function and antileishmania activity were half-maximally induced by rIFN-γ in concentrations ranging from 0.03 to 0.14 antiviral unit/ml (subpicomolar range) (Murray et al 1985).

A single intraperitoneal injection of rIFN-γ was administered to mice, and peritoneal cells were collected 18 h later. The injection had no effect on either the number or the differential count of peritoneal cells. However, as illustrated in Fig. 4, the macrophages displayed dose-dependent increases in H_2O_2-releasing capacity and antiprotozoal activity, with half-maximal enhancement after the injection of 85–250 units (Murray et al 1985). The rIFN-γ was diluted in protein-free buffer and over 90% was lost by adherence to the tubes and syringes used for its administration. Thus, the amounts actually injected were probably far less than stated above. Peritoneal macrophages were also activated by intravenous or intramuscular administration of rIFN-γ. These results complement those showing reduction of Listeria monocytogenes counts (Kiderlen et al 1984) and decreased mortality from Toxoplasma gondii in rIFN-γ-treated mice (McCabe et al 1984).

From these studies, we conclude that IFN-γ is the predominant macrophage-activating factor secreted by clonally unselected lymphocytes in at least two species, that this pertains both to splenic lymphocytes (in the mouse) and to peripheral blood lymphocytes (in humans), that IFN-γ acts not only on

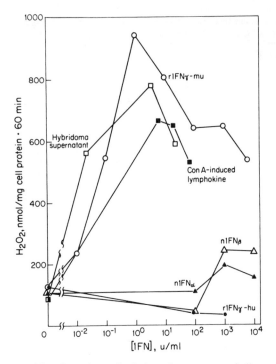

FIG. 2. Hydrogen peroxide release from phorbol myristate acetate-challenged resident mouse peritoneal macrophages after incubation for two days in the indicated cytokines, whose IFN-γ concentrations are expressed in terms of their antiviral activity (units/ml). IFN-γ-rich supernate of a T-T hybridoma was a gift of R. Schreiber, Scripps Research Institute. Pure murine rIFN-γ (rIFNγ-mu) was from Genentech, Inc. Concanavalin A (ConA)-induced lymphokine was prepared from splenocytes of *Listeria*-infected mice. Native IFN-α and nIFN-β were partially purified preparations from Lee Biomolecular. Pure human rIFN-γ (rIFNγ-hu) was from Genentech, Inc.

macrophages derived *in vitro* from monocytes but also on tissue macrophages, that it is effective both *in vitro* and *in vivo*, and that its potency in both milieus is remarkable.

Macrophage deactivation: pathological and physiological

In 1980, we observed that activated mouse peritoneal macrophages incubated with murine tumour cells lost their capacity to secrete H_2O_2 after 1-2 days (A. Szuro-Sudol & C. F. Nathan, unpublished). This proved to be the result of a trypsin- and heat-sensitive factor found in the medium of each of 13

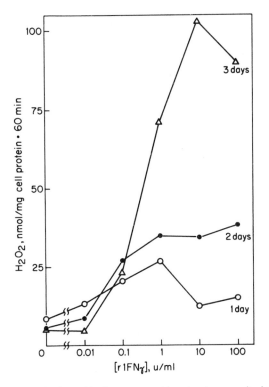

FIG. 3. Time course of induction of hydrogen peroxide-releasing capacity in protease peptone-elicited mouse peritoneal macrophages by pure murine rIFN-γ (from Genentech, Inc.). Concentrations of rIFN-γ are expressed in terms of antiviral activity.

murine tumour cell lines so far examined (Szuro-Sudol & Nathan 1982, and unpublished). A similar activity was found in lower titre in medium conditioned by some but not all non-malignant cells. Biochemical characterization of the macrophage-deactivating factor (MDF) is at an early stage. MDF appears to be distinct from IFN-β and p15E retroviral protein (Snyderman & Cianciolo 1984). The chief effects on macrophages exposed to MDF *in vitro* or *in vivo* (by injection of MDF into the peritoneal cavity) are three: suppression of ability to release ROI, to kill intracellular protozoal pathogens (Szuro-Sudol et al 1983), and to express Ia antigens (A. Szuro-Sudol & C. F. Nathan, unpublished). In contrast, there is little or no effect on macrophage morphology, adherence, phagocytic rate, DNA or protein synthesis, or secretion of lysozyme and plasminogen activator (Szuro-Sudol & Nathan 1982).

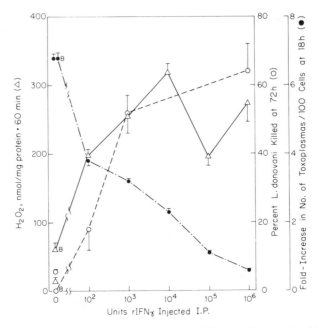

FIG. 4. Enhancement of mouse peritoneal macrophage H_2O_2-releasing capacity ($\triangle$), inhibition of toxoplasma replication ($\bullet$), and killing of leishmania amastigotes ($\circ$) when macrophages were collected 18 h after intraperitoneal injection of murine rIFN-γ. The doses indicated were calculated on the basis of dilution in protein-free buffer, assuming no loss of rIFN-γ by adsorption. In fact, adsorption under these conditions is extensive. The symbol B denotes results for mice injected with buffer alone. The other data points at 0 dose are for untreated mice. (From Murray et al 1985.)

When MDF is added to macrophages which have already been activated, their enhanced ability to secrete ROI is lost ($t^{1/2} \sim 18\,\mathrm{h}$). When MDF and lymphokines (Szuro-Sudol & C. F. Nathan 1982, Szuro-Sudol et al 1983) or rIFN-γ (A. Szuro-Sudol & C. F. Nathan, unpublished) are added simultaneously to resident peritoneal macrophages, the onset of activation is forestalled (Table 4). However, when MDF is removed from macrophages and replaced with rIFN-γ, the ability to secrete H_2O_2 can be restored much faster than occurs spontaneously (S. Tsunawaki & C. F. Nathan, unpublished). By this criterion, the deactivated macrophage, defined as one which was previously activated but now displays deficient secretion of ROI and impaired killing of intracellular protozoal pathogens, appears to retain responsiveness to IFN-γ.

Because some non-malignant cells, notably fibroblasts, produce low levels of MDF-like activity, whose suppressive effect is much more rapidly reversed than that of tumour-derived MDF (Szuro-Sudol & Nathan 1982), we speculate

TABLE 4 Macrophage deactivation factor (MDF) blocks induction of activation by murine rIFN-γ

Treatment of resident p.c. (48 h)		H_2O_2 release
MDF, % v/v	rIFN-γ, U/ml	nmol/(mg h)[a]
0	0	73 ± 13
100	0	9 ± 3
0	1	247 ± 1
100	1	63 ± 2

[a] Means ± SEM for triplicates.
p.c., peritoneal cells.

that the ability to suppress the macrophage respiratory burst at least transiently may be a physiological mechanism for limiting tissue damage during the late phases of the inflammatory response, for example when macrophages ingest debris during wound healing. Another possible role for physiological suppression of the macrophage respiratory burst might be in sinusoidal lining cells, such as those in the liver, spleen and marrow, whose clearance of large numbers of senescent erythrocytes, other particulates and complexes from the circulation might thereby be accomplished with less damage to blood cells and endothelium. The potent MDF released from tumour cells may represent an exaggeration of such a physiological regulatory mechanism, one that may favour tumour growth.

The foregoing hypothesis may receive some support from recent findings with the resident macrophage of the mouse liver. Lepay et al (1985a) have developed a procedure for the isolation of murine Kupffer cells in yields which are up to 10-fold higher than with conventional techniques and which approach 100% of the number of Kupffer cells estimated to be present. These peroxidase-negative resident hepatic phagocytes undergo an almost negligible respiratory burst in response to PMA, zymosan or protozoal pathogens. The absence of an increment in O_2 consumption in response to such agents (Fig. 5) indicates

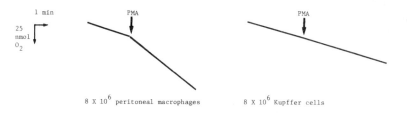

FIG. 5. Lack of a respiratory burst by mouse Kupffer cells in comparison to caseinate-elicited peritoneal macrophages. Freshly collected cells in suspension were added to a water-jacketed chamber at 37 °C and O_2 consumption was measured polarigraphically before and after addition of 100 ng/ml phorbol myristate acetate (PMA). From an experiment by D. A. Lepay and C. F. Nathan.

that ROI are not being formed and directs attention away from accelerated catabolism of ROI or interference with their detection as explanations for their apparent absence. Although the Kupffer cells respond to lymphokines and rIFN-γ with an increased display of Ia antigens, a capacity to undergo the respiratory burst is not induced. As predicted from this metabolic picture, murine Kupffer cells are markedly deficient in the ability to inhibit the growth of *T. gondii* and *L. donovani* (Lepay et al 1985a).

Among the particulates cleared from the blood by sinusoidal lining cells are pathogenic microorganisms. If Kupffer cells have deficient microbicidal capacity, at least in terms of O_2-dependent mechanisms, how does the liver cope with infection by facultative or obligate intracellular pathogens? Lepay et al have addressed this question by studying experimental murine listeriosis. Earlier studies established that *L. monocytogenes* replicates within macrophages and that its elimination depends on macrophage activation. Lepay showed that as listeria multiplied in the liver, the number of hepatic macrophages and the capacity of the macrophage population as a whole to secrete ROI increased, peaking just before the onset of clearance of bacteria. However, when the macrophage population was separated into morphologically and functionally distinct subpopulations of sinusoidal lining cells and immigrant inflammatory macrophages, only the latter were able to secrete ROI (Lepay et al 1985b). Thus, Kupffer cells remained oxidatively inactive and microbicidally deficient even during a brisk cell-mediated immune response in their surroundings. It is not known how monocytes taking up residence in hepatic sinusoids and possibly other sinusoids are induced into this state of suppressed oxidative metabolism. It has not been excluded that a cytokine akin to MDF may be involved.

Although in some regards the Kupffer cell thus resembles the peritoneal macrophage deactivated by MDF, the differences may prove informative. The Kupffer cell's oxidative metabolism is more severely suppressed, without inhibition of Ia antigen expression, and its ROI secretory capacity is not re-induced by IFN-γ. In all three respects, it differs from the 'deactivated' macrophage described earlier. In addition, the kinetic features of the Kupffer cell NADPH oxidase seem to differ, as discussed below. For these reasons, we have provisionally designated the Kupffer cell as 'inactivated' rather than 'deactivated.'

NADPH oxidase in macrophages in four different states of activation

Above we have described four states of macrophage activation with regard to the capacity to secrete ROI and associated antimicrobial activity, together with identification of cytokines controlling at least some of the transitions of macrophages from one state to the next. Such cells may represent a valuable panel for comparative studies of the NADPH oxidase and its regulation. This elusive and unusual plasma membrane electron transport chain has been extremely difficult to analyse by conventional approaches. Its lability on subcellular fractionation and partial purification may result from at least three features. The enzymic activity used to monitor its purification may depend on association of physicochemically distinct components with a propensity to sort separately during fractionation based on size, charge or hydrophobicity. The functional association of these components may require a lipid milieu which is destroyed by detergent extraction. Finally, there is evidence that the respiratory burst is normally terminated by oxidative autoinactivation of the oxidase, a process that in the intact macrophage may be under control by antioxidant defences, including the glutathione redox cycle. Such regulation may be ablated when the cells are disrupted, allowing the oxidase to self-destruct. New approaches, such as use of monoclonal antibodies, are needed for purification and characterization of the oxidase complex. A panel of otherwise highly similar phagocytes whose oxidase complexes differ in defined respects could be invaluable for strategies involving screening, complementation or subtraction. We are now characterizing the oxidase complex in non-activated, activated, deactivated and inactivated macrophages in pursuit of this goal.

Our first two steps have been to estimate the cells' content of the cytochrome b_{559} identified as an integral component of the oxidase complex by Segal, Jones and their colleagues (Segal et al 1983), and to measure the apparent K_m and V_{max} of the oxidase as a whole in lysed cells.

As shown in Table 5, no differences in cytochrome b_{559} have been identified in resident, activated or deactivated peritoneal macrophages that could account for the differences in the ROI secretory capacity of the intact macrophages (Tsunawaki & Nathan 1984, and S. Tsunawaki & C. Nathan, in preparation). Preliminary observations with Kupffer cells suggest that they, too, have a substantial complement of cytochrome b_{559}. Characterization of its CO binding, anaerobic reduction, and midpoint potential is under way (A. Ding & C. Nathan, unpublished).

To measure the kinetics of the oxidase, we have paid particular attention to developing assay conditions in which the activity of the enzyme in cell lysates is no less than in the intact cell. This excludes the techniques commonly used in work on the oxidase of polymorphonuclear leucocytes that depend on sonication or homogenization followed by differential centrifugation, as these often result in loss of 90% or more of activity in macrophage preparations. Instead, we have adapted the method of Bellavite et al (1981) to mouse peritoneal macrophages, taking care to use acetylated cytochrome c, the optimal type and concentration of detergents, suitable buffer and appropriate timing of additions. In addition, where necessary, endogenous superoxide dismutase (EC 1.15.1.1) was inhibited before cell lysis (Tsunawaki & Nathan 1984).

The results are summarized in Table 5. They suggest that each of the four states of macrophage activation (as functionally and operationally defined) is associated with a different set of kinetic parameters of the oxidase. The transition from a non-activated to an activated macrophage is accompanied by a ninefold reduction in K_m for NADPH, without a change in V_{max}. As calculated by Sasada et al (1982), based on their measurements of intracellular NADPH concentrations in macrophages, such a change in K_m is adequate to account for the observed differences in ROI secretion by the intact cells. The transition from an activated to a deactivated macrophage involves marked increases in K_m, together with variable decreases in V_{max}. In contrast, MDF induces no changes in the affinity or number of macrophage receptors for phorbol diesters, in affinity or capacity of the transport mechanism for glucose, in NADPH levels, or in the rate of degradation of exogenously supplied H_2O_2. Thus, the changes detected in the oxidase probably account for the impaired capacity of deactivated macrophages to secrete ROI and kill protozoa (S. Tsunawaki & C. Nathan, in preparation). Finally, in preliminary experiments, the Kupffer cell displays no oxidase activity under the assay conditions used for the other macrophages (A. Ding & C. Nathan, unpublished). We are now exploring whether this may be due to disappearance of a component of the oxidase or to the appearance of a suppressive factor.

TABLE 5 Oxidative metabolism of murine macrophages: four contrasting states

Distinguishing features	*Functional state*			
	Non-activated	*Activated*	*Deactivated*	*Inactivated*
Site (examples)	Peritoneum	Peritoneum	Peritoneum	Liver
Elicitation	None	IFN-γ	MDF	None
H_2O_2, nmol/(mg h)	50–100	350–650	0–100	0–20
Antiprotozoal activity	Modest	Marked	Minimal	Minimal
Activation by IFN-γ	Occurs	Sustained	Reversed or blocked but restorable	Absent
NADPH oxidase complex				
K_m (mM)	0.4	0.05	0.3–0.6	—
V_{max} (nmol/[min 10^6])	0.8	0.8	0.4–1.0	0
Cytochrome b_{559} (pmol/mg)	~100	~100	~100	present?

Non-distinguishing features:
- PMA receptors
- Glucose transport
- NADPH levels
- Myeloperoxidase
- Catalase
- GSH
- GSH peroxidase
- GSSG reductase

Acknowledgements

We thank A. Szuro-Sudol and A. Ding for contributing unpublished results. The work reported here was supported by NIH grant CA22090 and by scholarships to C.N. from the Irma T. Hirschl Trust and the Rita Allen Foundation.

REFERENCES

Aneshansley DJ, Eisner T, Widom JM, Widom B 1969 Biochemistry at 100 °C: explosive secretory discharge of bombardier beetles (Brachinus). Science (Wash DC) 165:61-63

Babior BM 1984 The respiratory burst of phagocytes. J Clin Invest 73:599-601

Badwey JA, Karnovsky ML 1980 Active oxygen species and the functions of phagocytic leukocytes. Annu Rev Biochem 49:695-726

Bellavite P, Berton G, Dri P, Soranzo MR 1981 Enzymatic basis of the respiratory burst of guinea pig resident peritoneal macrophages. J Reticuloendothel Soc 29:47-60

Boldt J, Schuel H, Schuel R, Dandekar PV, Troll W 1981 Reaction of sperm with egg-derived hydrogen peroxide helps prevent polyspermy during fertilization in the sea urchin. Gamete Res 4:365-377

de la Harpe J, Nathan CF 1985 A semi-automated microassay for hydrogen peroxide release by human blood monocytes and mouse peritoneal macrophages. J Immunol Methods 78:323-336

Gschwend PM, MacFarlane JK, Newman KA 1985 Volatile halogenated organic compounds released to seawater from temperate marine macroalgae. Science (Wash DC) 227:1033-1035

Kiderlen AF, Kaufmann SHE, Lohman-Matthes ML 1984 Protection of mice against the intracellular bacterium *Listeria monocytogenes* by recombinant immune interferon. Eur J Immunol 14:964-967

Lepay DA, Nathan CF, Steinman RM, Murray HW, Cohn ZA 1985a Murine Kupffer cells: mononuclear phagocytes deficient in the generation of reactive oxygen intermediates. J Exp Med 161:1079-1096

Lepay DA, Steinman RM, Nathan CF, Murray HW, Cohn ZA 1985b Liver macrophages in murine listeriosis: cell-mediated immunity is correlated with an influx of macrophages capable of generating reactive oxygen intermediates. J Exp Med 161:1503-1512

McCabe RE, Luft BJ, Remington JS 1984 Effect of murine interferon gamma on murine toxoplasmosis. J Infect Dis 150:961-962

Murray HW, Rubin BY, Rothermel CD 1983 Killing of intracellular *Leishmania donovani* by lymphokine-stimulated human mononuclear phagocytes. Evidence that interferon-γ is the activating lymphokine. J Clin Invest 72:1506-1510

Murray HW, Spitalny GL, Nathan CF 1985 Activation of mouse peritoneal macrophages in vitro and in vivo by interferon-γ. J Immunol 134:1619-1622

Nathan CF 1983 Mechanisms of macrophage antimicrobial activity. Trans R Soc Trop Med Hyg 77:620-630

Nathan CF, Murray HW, Wiebe ME, Rubin BY 1983 Identification of interferon-γ as the lymphokine that activates human macrophage oxidative metabolism and antimicrobial activity. J Exp Med 158:670-689

Nathan CF, Prendergast TJ, Wiebe ME et al 1984 Activation of human macrophages. Comparison of other cytokines with interferon-γ. J Exp Med 160:600-605

Nathan CF, Horowitz KCR, de la Harpe J, Vadhan-Raj S, Sherwin SA, Oettgen HC, Krown SE 1985 Administration of recombinant interferon-γ to cancer patients enhances monocyte secretion of hydrogen peroxide. Proc Natl Acad Sci USA, in press

Sasada M, Pabst MJ, Johnston RB Jr 1983 Activation of mouse peritoneal macrophages by lipopolysaccharide alters the kinetic parameters of the superoxide-producing NADPH oxidase. J Biol Chem 258:9631-9635

Schildknecht H 1970 The defensive chemistry of land and water beetles. Angew Chem Int Ed Engl 9:1-9

Schreiber RD, Hicks LJ, Celada A, Buchmeier NA, Gray PW 1985 Monoclonal antibodies to murine γ-interferon which differentially modulate macrophage activation and antiviral activity. J Immunol 134:1609-1618

Segal AW, Cross AR, Garcia RC et al 1983. Absence of cytochrome b_{-245} in chronic granulomatous disease: A multicenter European evaluation of its incidence and relevance. N Engl J Med 305:245-251

Snyderman R, Cianciolo GJ 1984 Immunosuppressive activity of the retroviral envelope protein P15E and its possible relationship to neoplasia. Immunol Today 5:240-244

Szuro-Sudol A, Nathan CF 1982 Suppression of macrophage oxidative metabolism by products of malignant and nonmalignant cells. J Exp Med 156:945-961

Szuro-Sudol A, Murray HW, Nathan CF 1983 Suppression of macrophage antimicrobial activity by a tumor cell product. J Immunol 131:384-387

Tsunawaki S, Nathan CF 1984 Enzymatic basis of macrophage activation. Kinetic analysis of superoxide production in lysates of resident and activated mouse peritoneal macrophages and granulocytes. J Biol Chem 259:4305-4312

DISCUSSION

van Furth: How many molecules of IFN-γ are needed to stimulate the cell?

Nathan: We didn't want to inject the mouse with foreign protein, so the diluent was protein-free and most of the interferon was adsorbed to the tubes. Thus I can't comment on the number of molecules *in vivo*. *In vitro*, an EC_{50} of 0.3 U/ml would correspond to about 100 molecules per cell (Murray et al 1985).

van Furth: Is IFN-γ taken up by the cells?

Schreiber: IFN-γ binds to the cell surface, is internalized and is degraded somewhat at 37°C.

Bellavite: Dr Giorgio Berton, of our laboratory, has data that confirm Dr Nathan's findings. In mouse peritoneal macrophages treated with *Corynebacterium parvum*, superoxide production was much higher than in resident peritoneal macrophages. The main difference was in the K_m for NADPH. The cytochrome b potential was almost identical in the two kinds of cells. An interesting difference was found in the ability of the two kinds of macrophages to reduce cytochrome b in anaerobiosis: *C.parvum*-activated macrophages reduced 30–40% of their cytochrome b_{-245} when stimulated by PMA in anaerobiosis, whereas resident macrophages did not reduce an appreciable amount of cytochrome b_{-245}.

Roos: I would be very hesitant to conclude from the spectrum you showed that there were comparable amounts of cytochrome *b* in the cells, Carl. Peaks in the spectrum were very close to other peaks, and both the position and the height of a peak may be influenced by other peaks in the vicinity.

Nathan: I agree. The next step will become possible with the availability of antibodies to the cytochrome as reagents.

Roos: The reagents test for the presence of the protein and not for the activity, of course. When you treat Kupffer cells with PMA they don't generate superoxide but do they react by activation of the arachidonic acid metabolism?

Nathan: Yes. Superoxide is not detected, but Ai-hao Ding and Alan Aderem found that arachidonic acid is released. We haven't yet characterized what the products are but there may be as much release as one sees from an activated peritoneal cell. Thus, there isn't a complete defect in these cells in response to triggering agents. On the other hand, the defect in the respiratory burst is not just seen in response to PMA. As the parasite data show, it is also seen in response to *Toxoplasma* or *Leishmania*, as well as PMA and zymosan.

Roos: Can these cells provide the oxidase system with enough reducing equivalents, or might that be rate-limiting? Did you test the monophosphate shunt capacity?

Nathan: We are testing that now. We have done some tests on the capacity to reduce the cytochrome anaerobically.

Roos: That is a very difficult test. When you test the cytochrome under anaerobic conditions and add NADPH, reduction is very slow.

Nathan: This work was done with intact cells that were made anaerobic and then challenged with PMA. We are asking endogenous reductive reactions to proceed, which may be even more relevant than measuring the shunt. We are doing both, but the results aren't ready.

Gordon: Alan Ezekowitz showed that there was a time-dependent deactivation by IFN-β of IFN-γ-mediated effects. This is quite similar to the Kupffer cell deactivation. How stable or how long-lasting is the deactivation in the Kupffer cell? If you explant in culture and wait a day or two, does it reverse?

Nathan: Not just after a few days. We are now testing much later periods.

Gordon: Control cells plated under the same conditions of adherence might also lose their responsiveness because of adhesion.

Nathan: The response tends to run down with human and mouse cells but it is readily detectable. Even after culture for several weeks one can still see something.

Humphrey: Dr V. Sundaram in my laboratory is interested in whether mice which have been lethally irradiated and then given bone marrow can be protected against *Listeria monocytogenes* infection, in the early stages before the bone marrow function is recovered, by T cells from syngeneic mice primed against *Listeria*. With suitable controls for the susceptibility of the mice, it proved to be impossible to protect them until circulating monocytes became detectable. This implied that the Kupffer cells and other macrophages which survived irradiation could not protect even with T cell help. Dr Sundaram tested whether Kupffer cells supplied with the supernatant from primed T cells incubated with killed *Listeria* could kill *Listeria in vitro*. It was difficult to show convincingly that they could, although peritoneal and spleen macrophages were quite effective. She was unable to explain this but it seems to fit in with what you are saying.

Nathan: If Kupffer cells are so deficient in antimicrobial defence, how does the liver cope when it is infected? David Lepay injected the mice with *Listeria* (Lepay et al 1985). He showed a logarithmic increase by colony counts in the organs, followed by a plateau phase and then resolution. He harvested livers at these times and found that just before the clearance phase there was a dramatic increase in the peroxide-releasing capacity of the total population, which went back to an undetectable level after clearance was complete. He found there were two morphologically different adherent cell populations that could be separately isolated. All of the peroxide-releasing capacity was in a population that looks different from the Kupffer cell and does not take up colloidal carbon after intravenous injection. This appears to be an emigrant monocyte and it is responsive to IFN-γ *in vitro*. The carbon-labelled, circumferentially spread cells I described did not change in number, oxidative metabolism or antiprotozoal activity.

Schreiber: Have you characterized the factor released by tumour cells?

Nathan: It appears to be a protein of between 30 000 and 60 000 M_r, but that's all I can say at present.

Schreiber: If you isolate macrophages from tumour-bearing mice or from cancer patients, what is their constitutive level of hydrogen peroxide production? It is low normally but is it further depressed?

Nathan: We haven't done that. The extraction of unaltered macrophages from solid tumours is a tricky business. George Spitalny (1980) has reported that the capacity of macrophages taken from malignant sites to kill *Listeria* is completely eliminated. That may be the counterpart of what we have seen. Certainly we can reproduce this effect simply by co-culturing macrophages and tumour cells.

Ezekowitz: When you added anti-γ monoclonal antibody you got an effect which was below normal. Does that effect disappear if you add anti-IFN-α antiserum?

Nathan: That was only seen with supernatant prepared with mezerein and lentil lectin which had little IFN-γ and had to be used at high concentrations. It doesn't reverse to anti IFN-α or β. When we assayed for IFN-α or IFN-β we could not find any.

Ezekowitz: Is there something in the local environment of the liver which affects the Kupffer cell activity or the monocyte as it seeds out of the blood-stream to become a Kupffer cell? Have you co-cultivated monocytes and hepatocytes to see whether monocytes can be made like Kupffer cells?

Nathan: Hepatocytes consume the fluorescent indicator or alter it in some way that is independent of hydrogen peroxide or exogenous peroxidase. The experiments therefore have to be done either with a different assay or by separating the macrophages from the hepatocytes before the assay. We will be trying to test this.

Ezekowitz: Have you taken the supernatant from hepatocyte cultures and tried to transfer that?

Nathan: Yes, it was toxic, so again the answer isn't clear. We need better methods, including hepatocyte cultures of good functional state, to do this.

Gordon: The cells after IFN-γ administration *in vivo* looked very similar to cells seen during intravascular activation of macrophages in mouse malaria.

Nathan: That change was seen in only about a third of the patients. It did not correlate with the change in peroxide secretory capacity so I don't know what it means.

Moore: You said that a 1-h infusion in the phase 1 trial on alternate days suppressed peroxide release whereas the 6-h infusion enhanced it. How do you explain the difference?

Nathan: Suppression was seen with cells taken immediately after the end of the 1-h infusion but if they were taken any time after that, they were markedly enhanced. Suppression was restricted to that sampling time. At that time the number of mononuclear cells recoverable from Ficoll-Hypaque gradients was markedly less and the percentage of those which were adherent monocytes was markedly less. As a result the total adherent mononuclear cell protein/ml blood was about 75% less, and the adherent cells looked different. Typical monocytes may have marginated or somehow redistributed themselves so that we are not sampling from peripheral blood in a normal way at that time. In other words the adherent cells we were measuring at the 1-h time point were probably a different subpopulation.

Stanley: Are spleen cells inactivated like the Kupffer cells?

Nathan: Work on the spleen cells is being done by Ali Nusrat. It is too soon to comment on it but the picture is beginning to emerge that if you put peritoneal, pleural, alveolar and breast milk cells in, they are all oxidatively quite active.

Cohn: The spleen is a little harder to deal with. The studies done so far have not shown any activity.

Gordon: We have isolated spleen cells and obtained some well-spread adherent cells. They have quite a high basal plasminogen-activator secretory and respiratory burst activity. That may reflect the fact that the spleen is haemo-poietically active and that there are immature stages.

van Furth: Do you take the cells after perfusion of the spleen or does your suspension contain monocytes as well?

Gordon: We took them after perfusion.

Cohn: Its secretory profile shows that the Kupffer cell has all the normal constituents seen in the peritoneal cell. If it is labelled with [^{35}S]methionine and the products are then secreted in the environment, all the same bands are present on SDS gels. It seems to be a rather selective defect.

Gordon: Mac-1 and other antigens are missing as well.

Cohn: Mac-1 is present on the Kupffer cell.

REFERENCES

Lepay DA, Steinman RM, Nathan CF, Murray HW, Cohn ZA 1985 Liver macrophages in murine listeriosis: cell-mediated immunity is correlated with an influx of macrophages capable of generating reactive oxygen intermediates. J Exp Med 161:1503-1512

Murray HW, Spitalny GL, Nathan CF 1985 Activation of mouse peritoneal macrophages in vitro and in vivo by interferon-gamma. J Immunol 134:1619-1622

Spitalny GL 1980 Suppression of bactericidal activity of macrophages in ascites tumors. J Reticu-loendothel Soc 28:223-235

Final general discussion

Effects of free radicals

Dean: Some of our observations on the effects of free radicals on proteins, including proteins within complex structures, may relate to the mechanisms applicable in cytolysis and so on during the oxidative burst. We have been using a variety of radical-generating systems but have concentrated on radicals produced by steady-state radiolysis. In this system we irradiate aqueous solutions and can generate defined radicals such as superoxide radicals, hydroxyl radicals or hydroperoxy radicals (Dean et al 1984). We can also define quantities. We usually use a system in which there is a characteristic rate of radical generation and in the experiments I'll describe not more than a micromole of radicals has been generated in the system. We can also convert these radicals into peroxy radicals of biochemical interest, including lipid radicals, and we have begun to study those effects as well.

This work arose from some studies on the degradation of proteoglycans within cartilage disks by macrophages. We then moved to studying the breakdown of those proteoglycans directly by radicals, using the generating systems I have just outlined. Degradation is measured in terms of labelled sulphate released from pre-labelled cartilage disks which are killed before the experiment. We measured the degradation effected by hydroxyl radicals in relation to the amount of irradiation and therefore to the radical dose: it was substantial. We looked at a mixture of hydroxyl and superoxide radicals and at the degradation product when the system is initially generating superoxide radicals and these conditions also lead to degradation. Within the cartilage disks a whole variety of other radicals will apply but the implication is that these radical-generating systems can produce something which can degrade. An interesting control, which rules out a role for direct radiation damage, is that the generating system for hydroperoxy radicals achieves extremely little degradation of these disks (Dean et al 1984).

The degradation products were similar in size to intact chondroitin sulphate side-chains. Various pieces of evidence led us to the idea that the main site of the radical damage was on the polypeptide core of the proteoglycan, with rather little damage (unless we irradiated it with much higher radical doses) on the glycosaminoglycan itself.

This led us to studies on protein *per se* and we have studied the degradation of bovine serum albumin in great detail (Dean & Wolff 1985, and unpublished work). These kinds of observations are general in the sense that they can be made with mixtures of radiolabelled proteins and with a variety of other purified proteins. When there is hydroxyl radical attack in the absence of oxygen, the native monomer of BSA can be converted into cross-linked SDS and mercaptoethanol-resistant cross-linked aggregates of high M_r. In the presence of oxygen the major band of 65 kDa is lost and there is much fragmentation. There is rather little attack by the superoxide and some of the other peroxy radical generating systems.

When one does silver-staining or looks at the products in more sensitive ways, the hydroxyl radical attacking in the presence of oxygen can be shown to convert the initial somewhat impure commercial preparations into a variety of quite specific fragments which are produced in a dose-dependent manner. Eventually there is virtual obliteration of these fragments and a whole range of small products results. These characteristic fragments probably result from attack selectively on proline residues within the molecule. There is a kind of synergy between the attack of the hydroxyl radical and the superoxide radical in the presence of oxygen. We fail to protect against fragmentation with glycine in the system but we have achieved protection with certain other amino acids.

So site-specific fragmentation and cross-linking occur. And from earlier published reports (see Pryor 1976–1982) we knew that modification of amino acid residues within the protein, which is a salient feature of radical attack, may be inactivating, as happens with α_1 proteinase inhibitor. We have now found that all these modifications tend to produce a form of a protein which is very susceptible to proteolysis (S.P. Wolff & R.T. Dean, unpublished).

This enhancement of proteolytic susceptibility of the products might result in an increased overall degradation in the system because of synergy between the radical attack and the proteinase attack. With John Pollak we have shown that the sort of results implied by that synergy are obtained in mitochondria, which have their own protein-degrading system. In other words when mitochondria are generating more radical fluxes they show higher rates of protein breakdown (Dean & Pollak 1985).

We also have evidence that in some circumstances lipid radicals can be fragmenting. One can have an indirect effect, therefore, of the primary oxygen radical, via a lipid radical, on protein fragmentation. Overall we would suggest that within cells inevitable rates of radical fluxes may set a basal level of proteolysis, and changes in radical flux may change that rate. Similarly, extracellular radicals may have a role in connective tissue metabolism and perhaps in the cytolytic mechanisms we heard about earlier.

Nathan: There is some evidence that low density lipoprotein (LDL) modified by oxidation becomes a ligand for the macrophage's so-called scavenger LDL receptor. Has anyone looked at other oxidized proteins in a general way? Have you found whether proteins modified in this way are more rapidly taken up by macrophages?

Dean: Some are, but not all. We have confirmed the LDL work and we have evidence that 4-hydroxynonenal, which is a product of lipid peroxidation, is able to modify LDL such that it is no longer recognized by the fibroblast LDL receptor (W. Jessup et al., unpublished). One can convert albumin into a much more rapidly recognized form. We haven't enough data to talk about competition between the different molecules and therefore to identify whether it is really the same receptor.

Cohn: Is there much unfolding of proteins with the exposure of hydrophobic residues?

Dean: Yes, there are fluorescence changes and other indications of unfolding.

Roos: Not long ago we showed that lysosomal enzymes are inactivated during activation of neutrophils (Voetman et al 1981). This was an oxygen-dependent reaction: it did not occur under anaerobic conditions or in CGD cells. Subsequently Bob Clark has shown that this reaction is completely myeloperoxidase-dependent (Clark & Borregard 1985). At least in that system it seems that hypochlorous acid is needed for this kind of damage to these enzymes. Other enzymes or other nearby proteins might be directly degraded by the oxygen radicals generated by these cells.

Dean: That mechanism is not a necessary general feature. Robin Willson (Kittridge & Willson 1984, Gee et al 1985) has shown that some of the peroxy radicals, such as uric acid peroxy radicals, can sensitize damage, for instance by hydroxyl radicals on an enzyme such as alcohol dehydrogenase. One can have a whole range of these effects, both damaging and protective.

Cohn: If you generate these radicals extracellularly, what do you think the targets are in cytolysis?

Dean: Damage to a protein is a very sensible thing to consider. If it was an ion-transporting protein, for instance, this could be a catastrophic magnifying effect, whereas damage to something like peptidoglycan or maybe the lipid of a membrane might be less immediately damaging and easier to repair.

Springer: Are halides present in your system?

Dean: No.

Springer: Have you tested whether they would have any additional effect?

Dean: Not yet.

Effects of interferon-γ on macrophages

Schreiber: We have heard throughout this meeting about the potent effects interferon-γ has on macrophages. We have looked specifically at the first contact interferon makes with the macrophage. Last year we showed that murine macrophages have a specific IFN-γ receptor (Celada et al 1984).

Recently, we have studied the interferon receptor on human mononuclear phagocytes (A. Celada et al, unpublished observations). This receptor was defined first on the basis of ligand-binding experiments, using radiolabelled, recombinant human IFN-γ. Both monocytes and U937 bound rIFN-γ in a saturable and reversible manner. Specific binding represented about 95% of the total binding. Scatchard plot analysis of the binding data indicated that the binding was to a single class of receptors in a non-cooperative manner and that mononuclear phagocytes carried between 4000 and 8000 receptors per cell.

We have observed the receptor on a number of different mononuclear phagocytes. Peripheral blood monocytes express about 7000 receptors per cell while U937 or HL60 carry about half that number. When the cells were differentiated, either by culture of the monocytes in Teflon beakers for six to eight days, or by induction of U937 and HL60 to monocyte-like cells with phorbol myristate acetate, or even by induction of HL60 with DMSO to a granulocyte-like cell, there was no change in the receptor number. The affinity of the receptors for ligand on all cells was about $5 \times 10^{-8}M$.

Binding of radiolabelled rIFN-γ was inhibitable by natural IFN-γ but not by IFN-β or IFN-α. Natural IFN-γ was quantitatively equivalent to unlabelled rIFN-γ as a competitor. In the presence of a threefold excess of natural IFN-γ, binding of ^{125}I-labelled IFN-γ was reduced by about two-thirds. IFN-α had no inhibitory effect while IFN-γ, in a 50-fold excess, had a very minor effect.

We have raised two monoclonal antibodies against human IFN-γ. Both monoclonals inhibit the binding of human interferon to human monocyte surfaces while an anti-murine interferon and two monoclonal antibodies to the various complement receptors on monocytes had no effect. These findings indicated that the binding was saturable and specific. The binding is also reversible. The dissociation half-time of the interferon bound to human monocytes was about 67 minutes and the dissociation kinetics were linear throughout two half-lives. These results thus indicated that the binding of IFN γ to mononuclear phagocytes was a classic receptor-mediated event.

The receptor appears to be a protein since trypsin or Pronase treatment of the cell abrogated binding of the radiolabelled interferon to the cell surface. Evidence was also obtained that the interferon–receptor complex was internalized at 37°C and the interferon was degraded.

Our first attempts to extrinsically label the receptor on the cell surface with lactoperoxidase and iodide have failed, probably because of the limited expression of surface receptors. Our alternative approach was to utilize homogeneous radiolabelled rIFN-γ, bind it to the cell surface, and cross-link the ligand–receptor complex with a bifunctional cross-linking agent. After dissolving the membrane in detergent, we analysed the cross-linked complexes by SDS polyacrylamide gel electrophoresis and autoradiography. IFN-γ bound to U937 plasma membranes produced a wide, rather diffuse band of about 100000 M_r. This band was not observed when (1) the membranes were pre-treated with unlabelled interferon in a 100-fold excess, (2) the cross-linking agent was omitted, or (3) the IFN-γ was treated with the monoclonal antibody that inhibited IFN-γ binding. Because of the specificity of the reaction we assume that this band represents the receptor–ligand complex. Based on the molecular weight of the ligand we estimate that the receptor may be composed, at least in part, of a 70000-M_r polypeptide chain. This result will need to be confirmed by isolating the receptor in the absence of ligand and demonstrating its ligand-binding capacity. Nevertheless I think that is the first approximation of the receptor on human monocytes.

Cohn: Is the receptor also degraded for its entire life during the lifespan of the cell, or does it cycle?

Schreiber: We have observed an intracellular or cryptic pool of receptor. It is of approximately equal size to the receptor pool that is expressed at the cell surface. In the presence of protein synthesis inhibitors, there is constant expression of unbound surface receptor at 37°C. Based on these data we presume that the receptor recycles and that it is not degraded during the recycling process. In fact if we use lysosomal trophic agents, we can block the enhanced uptake of ligand at 37°C.

Werb: Since there are so few receptors, how few have to be triggered to get a biological effect?

Schreiber: That is highly dependent on the biological effect being measured. A single round of receptor occupancy may be all that is required to induce increased production of hydrogen peroxide. In terms of tumour cell killing or in terms of Ia antigen induction, a single, saturating amount of ligand is not sufficient. In fact a preincubation period of 4 h is required, which we calculate represents at least three cycles of receptor–ligand complex internalization. This difference may reflect a simple signal transduction mechanism for one biologic-al effect and a more complicated mechanism involving an intracellular effect of degraded ligand for other biological activities.

Werb: Can you trigger any effect by treating cells in the cold with IFN-γ then washing it away?

Schreiber: In our assay systems, that is antigen expression on cell surfaces and tumour cell killing, we have not been able to do that.

Nathan: We held an adherent monocyte-containing coverslip with a pair of forceps in a well, added interferon to the well, removed the coverslip and immersed it in three successive beakers of saline. When we replaced the coverslip in a new well with medium lacking interferon, two days later the peroxide-releasing capacity was as high as if we had added interferon and left it.

Cohn: Does the ligand induce the expression of more receptors with time?

Schreiber: We haven't been able to show that. It neither down-regulates nor up-regulates receptor number, nor does it change the affinity of the receptor for ligand.

Cohn: How does the number of receptors on the human monocytes compare with the number on mouse macrophages?

Schreiber: The human monocyte has a higher affinity for ligand, by about a factor of 2, and it has about half the number of receptors on the surface.

Ezekowitz: Does priming the macrophages affect the receptor numbers?

Schreiber: No; LPS, IFN-α and IFN-β are all ineffective in regulating receptor expression.

Cohn: Do all cells that respond to IFN-γ have the same high affinity receptors as endothelial cells and fibroblasts?

Schreiber: We have begun to compare receptors on a number of different cells. In the mouse, the fibroblast, the macrophage, the T cell and even the T cell hybridoma that is making interferon all have IFN-γ receptors. All cell types show receptors with similar affinity. When we directly compare the receptors on macrophages and fibroblasts in the same experiment, we have seen a threefold difference in binding affinity. That may not be representative of different receptor classes but there is a reproducible difference in binding affinity. It may be a reflection of the cell surface itself.

Stanley: When you do the chemical cross-linking experiments and then reduce, do you still observe an M_r of 100000 for the chemically cross-linked species?

Schreiber: Yes.

Stanley: In uptake experiments at 37°C do you see accumulation of ligand beyond the levels at which you observe maximal binding at 0°C?

Schreiber: Yes, at 37°C we see higher levels of cell-associated ligand although not twofold higher than at 4°C. This is probably because the ligand is rapidly degraded once it gets inside the cell.

Stanley: So the level would be less than twice the number of receptors that you can demonstrate on the cell surface at 0°C?

Schreiber: Correct.

Springer: Some time ago we reported that thioglycollate-elicited macrophages were of course positive for Mac-1 and negative for the LFA-1 antigen (Kürzinger et al 1982). We were careful not to generalize the absence of LFA-1 to other types of macrophages. Recently, with Drs Strassmann and Adams (Strassman et al 1985), we screened a number of types of peritoneal macrophage populations for expression of a panel of antigens in order to look for markers of macrophage activation. We found that pyran-induced macrophages and BCG macrophages express the LFA-1 antigen, and we confirmed the previous observation that resident macrophages and thioglycollate-elicited macrophages are LFA-1 negative. With thioglycollate-elicited macrophages stimulated with LPS, we see a very dramatic expression of LFA-1. One also sees very dramatic LFA-1 expression on induction with IFN-γ. On lymphoid cells LFA-1 is involved in natural killing and antigen-specific killing responses, so it is possible that LFA-1 plays a role in the tumoricidal responses by activated macrophages. We have no evidence yet that anti-LFA-1 inhibits tumour cell responses but so far we have only tested this in one system.

Gordon: Is that true if you treat human monocytes with γ-interferon?

Springer: The blood monocyte is LFA-1-positive and Mac-1-negative in the mouse. So after migration into the peritoneal cavity and differentiation towards a resident macrophage, LFA-1 expression is lost. Human monocytes start out being LFA-1 positive so one would have to look at tissue macrophages. We have not done that.

Gordon: Dr T. Mokoena has looked at monocytes treated with IFN-γ and found no effect on LFA-1 expression.

Cohn: Does anti-LFA-1 trigger some of these cascades or oxygen production?

Springer: That would be an interesting thing to look at.

Werb: Human monocytes and macrophages seem to express a whole host of proteinase inhibitors that mice do not express at all. In human cells, the α-proteinase inhibitor and $α_2$-macroglobulin are made, as well as several inhibitors of metalloproteinases, particularly the one that inhibits collagenase, gelatinase and elastase made by the human monocyte-derived-macrophages.

It has been notoriously difficult to find any activity of metalloproteinases such as elastase or collagenase in the human. The mouse is different and all these proteinases are found in the mouse. However, the mouse makes a rather modest amount of these proteinases compared to the human, but because mice make no inhibitors it is very easy to demonstrate the proteinases by classic enzyme assays. These observations will affect how we think about regulation of macromolecules in the extracellular matrix and extracellular milieu. When cells are polarized cells, for example cells placed on immune complexes, we don't know whether the proteinases are secreted in one direction and inhibitors in another. There certainly can be polarized secretion in the macrophage into sites of ligand–receptor interaction, but whether there is a divergence in secretory routes we don't yet know.

Work on angiogenesis factors has been done by several groups. It is clear that the macrophage can be an important producer of factors that promote the directed migration of capillary endothelial cells and blood vessels into sites of inflammation (Knighton et al 1983). These factors are clearly not the same as those that promote proliferation of endothelial cells, although both angiogenesis factor and nitrogen are produced coordinately (Banda et al 1982). Oxygen tension seems to regulate the production of these factors in rabbit macrophages. Probably some lymphocyte interaction is also involved but that hasn't been well worked out.

Polverini & Leibovich (1984) have separated tumour cells and macrophages from buccal tumours in hamsters. Virtually all the angiogenic activity that comes out of a tumour separates with the macrophages. Much of the old work on tumour angiogenesis factors was done using the Walker 256 tumour grown in ascites. There are probably a few macrophages there as well.

Cohn: I thought the tumour factor had been purified now?

Werb: The reports are very confusing. People talk about angiogenesis factor, but measure mitogenesis. The mitogens definitely bind to heparin (Shing et al 1984). The macrophage-derived angiogenesis factor does not bind to heparin. It is still possible that it is one big molecule which during purification gets chopped into two domains. However it is clear that vascular sprouting can occur in the absence of proliferation (Sholley et al 1984).

Unkeless: Mike Klagsbrun did most of the work on angiogenesis binding factor, which is a heparin-binding protein. They have a tumour angiogenesis factor purified to homogeneity, giving a single band on a silver-stained gel.

Cohn: Does this have specific mitogenicity on endothelial cells and not on other cells?

Unkeless: I don't know. Apparently there is a whole family of fibroblast growth factors/angiogenesis factors that bind to heparin–Sepharose with varying affinities, as measured by the concentration of salt that is required to elute them.

Cohn: Wouldn't you expect some of the other growth regulatory factors that macrophages make to be influential in angiogenesis as well?

Werb: Yes. None of these things are made in isolation. The findings suggest that angiogenesis is accompanied by a remodelling of extracellular matrix, by proliferation of fibroblasts and by proliferation of endothelial cells as well. Macrophages can make at least two or three distinct growth factors. The reported ones for endothelial cells are probably distinct from those for fibro-blasts. I don't know whether the reported ones for cells like chondrocytes (Rifas et al 1984) are similar or different. Russell Ross's group has shown that at least a small portion of the growth factor made by macrophages is related to platelet-derived growth factor and can be precipitated by antibodies (unpub-lished work). That doesn't account for most of it, though, and I think that macrophages under appropriate conditions will express c-*sis*, which is the appropriate oncogene. But that work is not well developed.

Cohn: In delayed-type reactions such as the tuberculin reaction one sees many more blood vessels. Is there any evidence that T cell factors, whether IFN-γ or others, influence the production of these products by macrophages?

Werb: Experiments by Auerbach and others (Auerbach 1981) suggest that a lot of these factors are made under those conditions. Exactly who is doing what to whom has not been established. It is not clear whether things can be made separately by lymphoid cells, whether it is the result of macrophage–lymphocyte interaction, or whether IFN-γ is the mediator.

Humphrey: We have heard almost nothing about interleukin 1 at this meeting. This seems to have a large number of biological activities, ranging from the thymocyte activation assay by which it is usually measured to endogeneous pyrogen and the muscle necrosis factor. My colleagues Dr Diane Scott and L. Borysiewicz have found that early cytomegalovirus-infected cells release a very potent inhibitor of IL-1. A culture supernatant diluted 1000-fold prevents IL-1 from stimulating ConA-activated thymocytes. I have heard that when humans have a fever an inhibitor of IL-1 is found in the urine which is stoichiometrically combined with IL-1 (Rosenstreich). Does anyone know any more about these products which are biologically rendered?

Cohn: IL-1 has been cloned now and is available in pure form. I am sure there will be a lot more information on it. Has anybody used the products?

Werb: We have. It is not angiogenic. It is a very potent inducer of a whole family of proteinases and proteinase inhibitors in humans and in rabbit endothelial cells and fibroblasts (Murphy et al 1985).

Cohn: Gimbrone's group has shown that it induces tissue factor production by endothelial cells.

Springer: Gimbrone and coworkers (Bevilacqua et al 1985) have also shown that after four hours of treatment with IL-1, endothelial cells express a receptor for granulocyte adherence. Adherence goes up 20-fold so it is probably important in diapedesis.

Hogg: What is the state of information on natural macrophage-activating factors other than IFN-γ?

Cohn: A fair amount of information has been obtained from the supernatants of cloned T cells. That is somewhat suspect though. Most of the results can probably be explained by IFN-γ.

Nathan: Those supernatants often also contain IFN-γ. The argument relies heavily on neutralizing antibodies, some of which in fact neutralize rather poorly. One has to begin to worry about the affinity of the antibody versus that of the receptor on the macrophage. Host defence systems always seem complex and redundant, and the existence of non-IFN activating factors seems highly likely, but to prove it conclusively will require purification of other factors and their physicochemical characterization.

Hogg: Anne Rees and her colleagues (Andrew et al 1984) have looked at factors from cloned T cell lines specific to mycobacterial antigens. They have done column purifications for all their clones and one of the supernatants apparently does not contain any IFN-γ, or at least the active fraction has a different M_r to that of IFN-γ. They feel this is evidence of something different.

Nathan: The next question in studies like that is whether the factor induces interferon in the responding population, which usually is not totally devoid of lymphoid cells.

Hogg: They tested the fractions directly on U937, looking at the respiratory burst activity.

Schreiber: We have just completed some experiments to study the physiological role of IFN-γ in which we took the opposite approach to Carl Nathan's of injecting exogenous interferon into experimental animals. We have generated a very potent neutralizing monoclonal antibody to murine IFN-γ. We have attempted to study the effects of this antibody in an *in vivo Listeria* infection model, since this model has been reported to involve macrophage activation and interferon production. We quantitated interferon production and examined whether the neutralizing monoclonal anti-IFN-γ could prevent resolution of the bacterial infection (N. Buchmeier & R.D. Schreiber, unpublished observations). We were unable to detect interferon in the circulation of infected mice but observed a 20-fold increase in the ability of T cells from infected mice to produce interferon *in vitro*. In addition, we isolated activated tumoricidal macrophages from the peritoneal cavity of infected mice. After a single dose of monoclonal antibody administered one day after infection, no activated macrophages were found, and, more importantly, the clearance of the bacteria from both the spleen and the peritoneal cavity of the mice was prevented. This indicated to us that interferon was an integral part of the immune response of the mouse against *Listeria*. We are not certain at present whether we are blocking the development of the immune response or blocking the effector cell-inducing function of interferon. Nevertheless this is one of the first pieces of evidence that endogenous interferon production is required for the resolution of *Listeria* infection.

Springer: What happened to the mice?

Schreiber: We stopped the experiment after seven days. A third of the mice had died by then, and the rest were not very healthy.

Aderem: An activated macrophage is generally regarded as a cell with enhanced reactive oxygen production. However, an activated macrophage may also be defined as one in which 20:4 metabolite production is down-regulated. While IFN-γ up-regulates the oxygen burst in macrophages, it does not affect the down-regulation of arachidonic acid metabolite secretion. This suggests that factors in addition to IFN-γ are involved in immune activation of macrophages.

Cohn: Agents such as *C. parvum* complicate what is happening in the peritoneal cavity. Huge numbers of granulocytes accumulate in these lesions. The products of granulocytes on macrophages could be an important factor, as well as all the humoral factors that are generated.

Gordon: We have also noticed antigenic differences between *in vivo* and *in vitro* activated cells. Clearly the maturity of the target population is very important, as well as the response to cytokines.

REFERENCES

Andrew PW, Rees ADM, Scoging A et al 1984 Secretion of a macrophage-activating factor distinct from interferon-γ by human T cell clones. Eur J Immunol 14:962-964

Auerbach R 1981 Angiogenesis-inducing factors: a review. In: Pick E (ed) Lymphokines. Academic Press, New York, vol 4, p 69

Banda MJ, Knighton DR, Hunt TK, Werb Z 1982 Isolation of a nonmitogenic angiogenesis factor from wound fluid. Proc Natl Acad Sci USA 79:7773-7777

Bevilacqua MP, Pober JS, Wheeler ME, Mendrick D, Cotran RS, Gimbrone MAJ 1985 Interleukin-1 (IL-1) acts on vascular endothelial cells to increase their adhesivity for blood leukocytes. Fed Proc 44:1494(abstr)

Celada A, Gray PW, Rinderknecht E, Schreiber RD 1984 Evidence for a gamma-interferon receptor that regulates macrophage tumoricidal activity. J Exp Med 160:55-74

Clark RA, Borregaard N 1985 Neutrophils autoinactivate secretory products by myeloperoxidase-catalyzed oxidation. Blood 65:375-381

Dean RT, Pollak JK 1985 Endogenous free radical generation may influence proteolysis in mitochondria. Biochem Biophys Res Commun 126:1082-1089

Dean RT, Wolff SP 1985 Free radicals and connective tissue catabolism. In: Venge P (ed) The inflammatory process. Uppsala University Press, in press

Dean RT, Roberts CR, Forni L 1984 Oxygen derived free radicals can efficiently degrade the polypeptide of proteoglycans in whole cartilage. Biosci Rep 4:1017-1026

Gee CA, Kittridge KJ, Willson RL 1985 Peroxy free radicals, enzymes and radiation damage: sensitisation by oxygen and protection by superoxide dismutase and antioxidants. Br J Radiol 58:251-256

Kittridge KJ, Willson RL 1984 Uric acid substantially enhances the free radical-induced inactivation of alcohol dehydrogenase. FEBS (Fed Eur Biochem Soc) Lett 170:162-164

Knighton DR, Hunt TK, Scheuenstuhl H, Halliday BJ, Werb Z, Banda MJ 1983 Oxygen tension regulates the expression of angiogenesis factor by macrophages. Science (Wash DC) 221:1283-1285

Kürzinger K, Ho MK, Springer TA 1982 Structural homology of a macrophage differentiation antigen and an antigen involved in T-cell mediated killing. Nature (Lond) 296:668-670

Murphy G, Reynolds JJ, Werb Z 1985 Biosynthesis of tissue inhibitor of metalloproteinases by human fibroblasts in culture. Stimulation by 12-O-tetradecanoylphorbol-13-acetate and interleukin 1 in parallel with collagenase. J Biol Chem 260:3079-3083

Polverini PJ, Leibovich SJ 1984 Induction of neovascularization in vivo and endothelial cell proliferation in vitro by tumor-associated macrophages. Lab Invest 51:635-642

Pryor WA 1976-1982 Free radicals in biology. Academic Press, Orlando, Florida, vols. 1-5

Rifas L, Shen V, Mitchell K, Peck WA 1984 Macrophage-derived growth factor for osteoblast-like cells and chondrocytes. Proc Natl Acad Sci USA 81:4558-4562

Shing Y, Folkman J, Sullivan R, Butterfield C, Murry J, Klagsbrun M 1984 Heparin affinity: purification of a tumor-derived capillary endothelial cell growth factor. Science (Wash DC) 233:1298-1300

Sholley MM, Ferguson GP, Seibel HR, Montour JL, Wilson JD 1984 Mechanisms of neovascularization. Vascular sprouting can occur without proliferation of endothelial cells. Lab Invest 51:624-634

Strassmann G, Springer TA, Adams DO 1985 Studies on antigens associated with the activation of murine mononuclear phagocytes: kinetics of and requirements for induction of lymphocyte function associated (LFA)-1 antigen in vitro. J Immunol 135:147-151

Voetman AA, Weening RS, Hamers MN, Meerhof LJ, Bot AAM, Roos D 1981 Phagocytosing human neutrophils inactivate their own granular enzymes. J Clin Invest 67:1541-1549

Chairman's closing remarks

ZANVIL A. COHN

Laboratory of Cellular Physiology & Immunology, The Rockefeller University, 1230 York Avenue, New York NY 10021-6399, USA

1986 Biochemistry of macrophages. Pitman, London (Ciba Foundation Symposium 118) p 242-243

Rather than review the excellent discussions we have had during this meeting I want to point out a few areas we haven't touched on that might be productive in the future. One of these areas concerns problems in cell biology. First there is the efficacy of macrophage populations for studying the secretory pathway, as Zena Werb mentioned in her paper. In some ways it seems perhaps easier to modulate the system *in vitro* than it is with hepatocytes. Secondly, there are the problems of intracellular parasitism and the question of membrane–membrane fusion. Microorganisms and their products presumably have a number of significant effects, both in lysing the endocytic vacuole and allowing the microbe to escape into the cytosol and in blocking fusion of membranes. This again gives us an opportunity for study in the future. None of these problems are easy and I imagine that equally good, or better, systems exist with some of the enveloped viruses.

We have not talked much about the mechanisms of endocytosis, though the role of contractile elements was mentioned by Dr Hartwig, nor about membrane dynamics, recycling, the differential effects of ligand valency on the fate of receptors, or the mechanism by which receptor–ligand interactions dissociate and where they dissociate in the vacuolar system.

The second area has to do with the overall study and evaluation of discrete immunological lesions in the animal. With some of the reagents that are being generated we will have the possibility, if we can dissociate these lesions and isolate individual components, of converting what has always been a black box based on sections to something in which we can evaluate temporally the emigration of cells, the presence of different phenotypes and their possible interactions. As someone who has been interested in the general problems of inflammation I think this is of considerable interest. In addition one can look at the cells accumulating in tumour beds.

Perhaps we will even be able to approach problems such as the Shwartzman reaction in the future. Lipopolysaccharides are still with us and their interaction with membranes can be of considerable interest. Some of the problems are really tough ones. Studying the oxidases is one such problem. We should be heartened by the fact that until a year or so ago the study of lymphokines was a great problem, then overnight, with cloning, the whole situation changed.

The role of macrophages in the overall initiation of the immune response has not been discussed either and should perhaps be left to a future meeting.

Index of contributors

*Non-participating co-author
Indexes compiled by John Rivers

Subject index